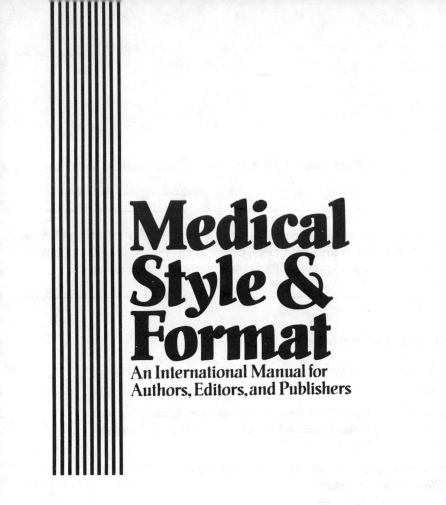

Medical Style & Format

An International Manual for
Authors, Editors, and Publishers

The Professional Editing and Publishing Series

This volume is one of a series published by ISI Press®. The Professional Editing and Publishing Series provides timely, practical information to help publishers and editors of professional, scholarly, and scientific publications.

---

90 91 92 93 94   10 9 8 7 6 5 4 3 2

Medical Style & Format

An International Manual for Authors, Editors, and Publishers

Edward J. Huth, M.D.

Foreword by Stephen Lock

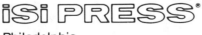

iSi PRESS®

Philadelphia

Published by

iSi PRESS® A Subsidiary of the
Institute for Scientific Information®
3501 Market St., Philadelphia, PA 19104 U.S.A.

Library of Congress Cataloging-in-Publication Data

Huth, Edward J.
   Medical style and format.

   (The Professional editing and publishing series)
   Bibliography: p.
   Includes index.
   1. Medical writing—Handbooks, manuals, etc.
2. Authorship—Style manuals.   I. Title.   II. Series.
[DNLM: 1. Publishing.   2. Writing.   WZ 345 H979m]
R119.H875   1987   808′.06661021   86-27609
ISBN 0-89495-063-0

Printed in the United States of America.

Contents

Foreword

What of 1986, I wonder, will surprise a scientist most a hundred years hence? Anybody can play this game, of course — and nobody can win — but the answer is likely to depend on one's discipline. To a physician-editor two things might stand out: firstly, our society's tolerance, if not blatant encouragement, of proven disabling and lethal habits — certainly cigarette smoking and probably also drinking alcohol and driving automobiles in the way that we do — and, secondly, the quixoticness of our scientific communication. If this prediction has any truth, then fortunately our retrospector might also be able to see that the late 20th century was the time when something began to be done about both problems. Remembering Wilfred Trotter's aphorism "the most powerful antigen known to man is a new idea," he or she would understand why it had taken so long to achieve sanity. And, finally in 2086, would come the recognition that the author of this book, Ed Huth, had had a major role in the reforms of both types of abuses, with *Medical Style and Format* a milestone to high standards in medical communication.

The time is past when editors could adopt a passive role, claiming with Virchow that anybody is free to make a fool of himself in the papers of their journals. To be sure, much published work will be shown to be false and superseded by new hypotheses, but our society's investment in science, in terms of money, manpower, and prestige — not to mention the direction of the research thrust — now depends so highly on the communication of new research findings that it is unethical for anybody concerned not to achieve the maximum possible. This can be achieved at four main stages. Firstly, authors can be taught how to write clearly and succinctly, using words with the same sort of accuracy that they expect from their laboratory apparatus; at this stage the advice of colleagues on the draft manuscript can have a major role. Secondly, through peer review, both in house and using external referees, editors can achieve the three objectives cited by Waksman: to prevent publication of bad work; improve scholarship; and improve the language and presentation of data. The third stage, deft copy editing of the accepted manuscript, will continue this last objective, and, finally, by allowing free debate in his correspondence columns, an editor will see that the published article is weighed in the balance by knowledgeable experts — resulting in the findings being discarded by the scientific community, superseded by further work, or incorporated into the knowledge base of the discipline.

Activities have been going on in three of these four stages for some time. Several universities, journals, and editors' organisations now hold regular courses in medical writing. Editors, realizing that they have paid scant attention to auditing their own activities, particularly peer review, have started research into both the process and the outcome, which with luck should materialise in a world congress in Chicago in 1989. And the whole discipline of citation analysis, effectively pioneered by Gene Garfield over 20 years ago, has given us one gold standard of considerable help in judging our editorial efforts.

Nevertheless, in one part of the third stage, copy editing, progress has been difficult and slow; for this reason a small group of medical editors came together in Vancouver 8 years ago to try to sort out the chaos. Despite their recommendations some of the scientific community still ignores, or debates with the passion once accorded to counting angels on pinheads, these international agreements on publication style, particularly standardized abbreviations and the method of quoting references. Yet the decision taken by the International Committee of Medical Journal Editors to recommend the sequential numbering system of references in the text reduced the number of possible reference styles from 2632 to one at a stroke. As Ed Huth points out in this book, the decision had been anticipated by several American clinical and biochemical journals; the style was based on that used by the *Index Medicus*; and, anyway, surveys had shown that on grounds of speed and ease of comprehension readers preferred a numbering system to the Harvard style (names of authors and dates in text and reference list in alphabetical order). But I am in no doubt that had the majority of medical journals been found to be using the Harvard style, and readers to have preferred this, the Vancouver group of editors would have recommended it. Their decision was largely pragmatic, reflecting the view that conventions are like traffic laws, necessary, sensible, and helpful, but in the background and unobtrusive — and there can be no more *logic* in whether you drive on the right or the left of the road than in the way you style references.

Fortunately, medical journals all over the world have recognised the good sense of these proposals and well over 300 have taken the trouble to write to say that they are using the Vancouver style. Some editors and their boards still carry on a tedious debate — claiming that the style is less informative than another (theirs) or that it and other conventions threaten the authors' freedom to express themselves in their own way. We even have the spectacle, which would have delighted Dean Swift, of one journal published in two parts, each using a different reference system (neither of them the Vancouver style). The truth is, however, much more mundane. Conventions actually free an author to devote his main energies to expanding his scientific findings. By extending these conventions from their humble beginnings in metric units and reference systems further to definitions of duplicate publications, the criteria for authorship, and the statistical presentation of results, editors' organisations will improve the accuracy and readability of the articles printed in their journals; that is the essence of scientific communication, and there are still more problems to be tackled. We need many more such international conventions.

As I have intimated before, Ed Huth has played a major part in putting the whole editorial process on a much more professional basis, in which explicitness has the fundamental role. I congratulate him on a superb book, which, as the reader will find out, ranges much further than mere conventions in medical papers. As he listens for the thousandth time to a debate by the unknowledgeable on Vancouver versus Harvard, or metric versus SI, may I advise him to do as I do, hearing the same fatuities only for the 500th time—to take heart from the way the conductor Sir Thomas Beecham dealt with another unseeing pedant many years ago:

I was hardly surprised when the [leading Strauss devotee and watchdog] got in touch with me over *Elektra*.

Sir,

What is coming over you? Last night from my coign of vantage in the gallery I counted your orchestra and could discover no more than ninety-eight players. As you well know, Strauss has stipulated for no less than one hundred and eleven. What have you done with the rest? Please reply at once.

Yours anxiously
SYLVESTER SPARROW

Surely it was impossible for a company of them to have trouped out while I was conducting without my observing it. To satisfy myself I ascended to Mr Sparrow's exalted spot and discovered the explanation of the mystery. From there it was impossible to see the full orchestra, some having been concealed in and under certain boxes, and greatly relieved I was able to send a reply that all was well and the temple had not been profaned. (Beecham T. *A Mingled Chime*. London: Hutchison, 1943.)

STEPHEN LOCK

Preface

If scientific information is to be transmitted accurately in print and understood readily by its readers, journals carrying that information must use conventions in style and format widely recognized and readily understood. This manual describes and recommends formats and publication style for journals in the medical sciences, clinical medicine, and closely associated fields. The term *publication style* includes all the conventions in word choice, spelling, capitalization, choice of typefaces, symbols and abbreviations, and presentation of numeric data characteristic of a publication. In this manual, *style* means *publication style* unless another meaning is specified; this meaning is distinguished from that of *style* in general (the characteristics of a work in the arts or letters; the characteristics of a person's behavior) and of *literary style* (characteristics of literary works).

The logic and clarity of a journal's format, notably the format of its articles and their pages, determine in part whether its readers see the journal as a reliable source of important information. Similarly the logic and consistency of the details of its publication style and the degree to which they represent standard practice affect readers' judgments of the journal's legitimacy within its scientific community. So editors should consider adherence to standards in format and style not to be slavish conformity but one means of gaining respect for their journals.

The recommendations in this manual are based as far as possible on published international and American national standards and on well-established practice. Authoritative manuals of style were consulted and the information-for-authors pages of many journals were reviewed with particular regard to style in special fields, but the recommendations in this manual differ with those in some of these sources; in some instances the differences are rationalized. I have also drawn on my experience as an editor of a major journal for more than 20 years and my work for the Council of Biology Editors and the International Committee of Medical Journal Editors.

A leading aim in writing this manual has been to bring into convergence, if not identity, conventions presently differing among disciplines and among the medical journals of the various regions in the English-language world. At some points this aim has led to recommendations based on British style, at other points to recommendations based on American style. A strong effort has been made to promote international standards and conventions, especially for nomenclature, symbolization, and units of measurement. I have long had a strong belief that such convergences in publication style will benefit all authors, editors, publishers, and readers around the world. Further, I believe that some of the recommendations will lessen the work of typists and the cost to journals of composition. Some recommendations may be rejected by some users of this manual. I am fully aware that habit and taste do not always succumb to logic, but I hope that the logic leading to some recommendations likely to seem unorthodox to some users of the manual may convince them of their value.

Efforts have been made to further the work and accomplishments of the International Committee of Medical Journal Editors embodied in the Vancouver agreement (see section 15.4). But the Committee has not taken part in the writing and review of this manual, and I do not mean to imply any endorsement of its content by the Committee.

Editors and publishers may be the main users of this manual, but many authors should find help in it with aspects of style not specified by the journals for which they are writing. When authors find differences in style between that expected by a journal and what this manual recommends, they may be acting in their best interests if they use the journal's style.

Some users of this manual will see some duplication of statement at a number of points. This duplication is deliberate; this manual will be mainly a reference work, and such duplication cuts down the extent to which its readers will have to turn to other pages.

I will welcome both criticisms of this manual and recommendations on what to add to it; they should be addressed to me at ISI Press, 3501 Market Street, Philadelphia, PA 19104, USA.

Acknowledgments

I am grateful to many persons who have helped me in various ways while I was writing this book: directions to source materials, recommendations on style, copies of their house-style manuals: Pamela T Allen (*Journal of the National Cancer Institute*), Roberta Arnold (*Radiology*), Sharon G Boots (*Journal of Pharmaceutical Sciences*), Lois Ann Colaianni (National Library of Medicine), Kenneth A Foon (University of Michigan Medical Center), Margaret Foti (*Cancer Research*), Stephen R Geiger (The American Physiological Society), Christopher T George (*American Journal of Epidemiology*), Dolores E Henning (*Journal of the American Dietetic Association*), Jane L Holland (American National Metric Council), Debbie Hull (BRS/Saunders), Betsy L Humphreys (National Library of Medicine), Robert W Keith (*Ear and Hearing*), J Stanton King (*Clinical Chemistry*), Sidney D Leverett, Jr (*Aviation, Space, and Environmental Medicine*), R E F Matthews (The University of Auckland), Braxton D Mitchell (Urban & Schwarzenberg), Sandra J Ott (*Journal of the National Cancer Institute*), Raymond A Palmer (Medical Library Association), Margaret H Seward (*British Dental Journal*), Alfred Soffer (*Chest*), Dale R Spriggs (*The Journal of Infectious Diseases*), Annette Terzian (University of California, Los Angeles), Frances R Zwanzig (*Proceedings of the National Academy of Sciences*).

Two experts in matters editorial closely and carefully read this manual in manuscript and gave me their unsparing, and thus invaluable, criticisms: Bernard K Forscher (Mayo Clinic) and Peter Morgan (*Canadian Medical Association Journal*). I wish to make clear that though I have named them here to make public my deep gratitude to them, they are not responsible in any way for any errors or poor judgments this book may carry.

My greatest gratitude is to Robert A Day (University of Delaware; formerly director of ISI Press), who challenged me to write this book. He thought I could do it decently well; I hope I have not disappointed him.

I promised my wife, Carol M Huth, that I would not give her the stereotypic public thanks for her patience, support, and other virtues; I am not doing so!

19 October 1986   EDWARD J HUTH

Chapter 1

Journal Format

The characteristics of a journal—title, arrangement, content and location of sections, cover design—determine in large part how readily it is located by librarians and bibliographers and how easily it is used by its readers. Decisions on its characteristics should be careful and deliberate. The clarity of information conveyed by title and other content, and by format, ought to take priority over any aesthetic considerations not defined by functional needs; as in architecture, function should define form.

The recommendations in this chapter are based in large part on the *American National Standard for Periodicals: Format and Arrangement* (ANSI Z39.1-1977) (1) and recommendations from the Institute for Scientific Information (2,3).

JOURNAL TITLE

TITLE FUNCTION AND LENGTH

1.1 The title should define clearly but concisely the scope and content of the journal. The title should be as short as possible but specific:

> *Clinic*
> A clinic is a place for care of patients. Is the journal about the practice of medicine, nursing care, veterinary practice, dental hygiene?
>
> *The American Journal and Archives of the History of Medicine and Closely Related Fields*
> Excessively long; "journal" and "archives" carry similar meaning. What "fields" are closely related?

A long title may be needed to describe a journal adequately; in view of the growing use of microcomputers with displays of 80-character width, titles could be reasonably limited to a maximum length of 65 characters, including the spaces between the words of the title.

Titles that are abbreviations (such as initial letters of a parallel title or an acronym formed from the name of the publishing organization) should be avoided. Such titles rarely convey a sense of the journal's scope and content; if they appear on the cover with a full formal title, they may confuse authors as to the correct title for references and librarians for catalogs.

TITLE UNIQUENESS

1.2 The title should be unique. A newly devised title may already identify another journal; adoption of that title by the new journal could, at the least, confuse librarians and bibliographers but could also lead to legal defense of right to the title by the publisher with the prior claim. Titles already in use can be identified through catalogs of serials, such as the SERLINE of the National Library of Medicine and the *Bowker International Serials Database* searchable through the BRS and DIALOG database online systems [fn1]. The National Serials Data Program (see section 1.4) will search these and other sources in response to requests for information on the uniqueness of a proposed title.

TITLE LOCATIONS AND FORM

1.3 The title will appear at many locations in the journal: cover, spine, table of contents, masthead, text, running heads or footlines. The identical complete form of the title should be used at each location; where an abbreviated title must be used to save space, it should be a standard abbreviation, based on *Documentation — Rules for the abbreviation of title words and titles of publications* (ISO 4-1984 [E]) (4); see *List of Journals Indexed in Index Medicus* (5) for examples of abbreviated title words based on this standard.

The title should be unambiguously identifiable by its character and typography from any other text near it; the acronymic name for an organization should not be placed close to a title lest it be confused with being a title.

INTERNATIONAL STANDARD SERIAL NUMBER

1.4 After a unique title with satisfactory characteristics has been selected (see section 1.2), a request should be made to the National Serials Data

---

fn1: For further information contact: R. R. Bowker Company, 245 West Seventeenth Street, New York, NY 10011, telephone (212) 916-1600; Bibliographic Retrieval Services, Inc., 1200 Route 7, Latham, NY 12110, telephone (800) 833-4707; Dialog Information Services Inc., 3460 Hillview Avenue, Palo Alto, CA 94304; or a library subscribing to the BRS or DIALOG services.

Program [Library of Congress, National Serials Data Program, Washington, DC 20540; telephone (202) 287-6452] for prepublication assignment of an International Standard Serial Number (ISSN) for the journal so that the number can be shown on the first issue. The ISSN will uniquely identify the journal. The international authority for ISSNs is International Serials Data System (ISDS), CIEPS, 20, rue Bachaumont, 75002 Paris, France.

TITLE CHANGE

1.5   An established title should not be changed without a compelling reason. If the title must be changed, additional proper steps will reduce the risk of confusing readers, authors, librarians, indexers, bibliographers, and dealers (see section 1.35).

THE UNITS OF A JOURNAL: VOLUME AND ISSUE

For efficiency in organizing the content of a journal and sending it to its subscribers in readily handled units easily mailed, and for ease of bibliographic identification of the contents, journals are organized into smallest units called issues, with issues organized into groups called volumes.

1.6   Issues ought to be published and sent to subscribers at a constant frequency and at fixed dates. The most widely used frequencies are weekly, semimonthly (twice per month), monthly, bimonthly (every other month), and quarterly; journals published less frequently than at these intervals should be organized simply into volumes, without individual issues. The choice of frequency is usually determined after weighing the relative merits of getting the journal's content to readers rapidly and in easily handled units against the lower costs of less frequent publication, with lower costs in printing, binding, and distribution of a given number of pages.

- Weekly journals should be issued on the same day of each week.
- Semimonthly journals should be issued on dates representing equal intervals; the most convenient dates are the first and fifteenth days of the month (for example, 1 January 1999 and 15 January 1999) even if the actual mailing date cannot be the issue date.
- Monthly journals are identified simply with the month of issue; the date of mailing need not be identified but it should be as constant as possible from month to month.
- Bimonthly journals should be identified with the pair of months in which issued, for example, January–February, even if the mailing date

is not in the first month of the pair. As with monthlies, the mailing date should be as constant as possible from issue to issue.

- Quarterly journals are most unequivocally identified, as for bimonthly journals, with the span of months represented by each issue: January–March, April–June, July–September, and October–December. Designation of issues by season may be ambiguous with regard to the year in which a "Winter" issue has been issued.

See sections 1.8 and 1.12 for identification of dates of issues.

VOLUMES

1.7   Volumes (a grouping of 2 or more issues) are best organized by year or even divisions of a year, for simplicity in bibliographic identification, convenience in ordering by, and billing to, subscribers, and convenience in bookkeeping by the publisher. The decision to use 1 volume per year or a greater number, such as 2, 3, or 4, should be determined mainly by the frequency and size of issues; unnecessarily thin volumes raise binding costs and produce excessive shelving needs for libraries, but very thick volumes are hard to handle and their bindings may not last long. Volumes representing issues of smaller units than a year should contain equal numbers of issues per volume. For identification of volumes see sections 1.27 and 1.28.

ISSUES

ISSUE COVER

1.8   The front cover of each issue should carry at least 6 elements.

Complete title and subtitle (if one is used)
    See section 1.1.
Volume number and issue number, both in arabic numerals
    If issues are usually monthly and 2 or more must be combined, 2 issue numbers may be used together (for example, Volume 33, Numbers 5–6, May–June), but this practice should be avoided as much as possible.
Issue date
    Weeklies should carry specific dates, not days. The dates should be in ascending or descending order: 12 January 1985 or 1985 January 12 (see section 13.22). Monthlies should carry the month and year. Bimonthlies should carry paired names of months but single issue numbers (for example, Number 1, January–February 1985). Issues of lower frequency should carry the span of months represented (for

example, January–March 1985, for a quarterly, not "Winter 1985" or "Spring 1985").

International Standard Serial Number (ISSN)
See section 1.4. The ISSN should appear on the upper right-hand corner.

Location of the table of contents (page numbers) if the table of contents is not on the front or back cover or the first three pages

The name of the publisher and the sponsoring organization

Additional information may be useful on covers of particular issues.

Index
The cover of the issue with the volume index should state the pages of the index.

Change of title
The previous title should be carried on the covers of all issues of the volume following the volume in which the change was made. Also see section 1.35.

Changes in trim size, frequency of issues, irregularities of issues
See sections 1.36, 1.37, and 1.38.

Supplements and special issues
See section 1.26.

In 1986 efforts were under way to test the utility and acceptability of a bar code (6,7) that would be placed horizontally on a journal's front cover (lower left corner) to carry the ISSN, issue identification, and title code in Code 128 bar. The code would speed the accession of the journal's issues in libraries [fn2].

COVER FORMAT

1.9 The information on the cover (see section 1.8) should appear in the same location, fonts, and type sizes in every issue. Avoid features and locations that might lead to obscuring of, or confusion about, these elements of information from, for example, advertising. The issue number and month should not be located where they might be obscured by a mailing label. The covers should not be included in the pagination.

If the title appears in more than 1 language, the title by which the journal is primarily known should be emphasized by size and location. Text that should be included in bound volumes of the journal should not appear on covers.

---

fn2: Additional information can be obtained from the Serials Industry Systems Advisory Committee (SISAC), 160 Fifth Avenue, New York, NY 10010; telephone (212) 929-1393.

THE SPINE: INFORMATION AND FORMAT

1.10   If the spine is flat and wide enough to carry legible type, it should carry this information.

Title, or its standard abbreviation (see section 1.3)
Volume and issue numbers
Pages in the issue if volumes are continuously paged

If the spine is wide enough, these elements should be placed to run horizontally when the issue is standing on a shelf. Otherwise they should run from the top to the bottom so that they can be read from left to right when the issue is lying with the front cover up.

TABLE OF CONTENTS

1.11   Each issue should include a complete table of contents that completely identifies the issue and all its articles and the sections into which they may be grouped.

TABLE OF CONTENTS: LOCATION

A table of contents should be placed within the first 5 pages of the issue even if a table of contents is also carried on the cover, to reduce the risk of its loss if the cover is torn off. The preferred cover location is the front cover. If the cover table is an abbreviated version, the location of the complete table within the issue should be identified, with page number. The desirable location inside is the right-hand page that faces the inside of the front cover.

Tables of contents of past or coming issues should be clearly identified as such and placed so that they are not likely to be confused with the table for the issue.

TABLE OF CONTENTS: BIBLIOGRAPHIC IDENTIFICATION

1.12   The table of contents should carry all information needed to identify the journal and the issue.

Title
    The complete title (and subtitle)
Abbreviated title and the International Standard Serial Number (ISSN)
    The abbreviated title should be in standard form (see section 1.3); the abbreviated title and the ISSN need not appear adjacent to the title but they should be readily seen and not buried within text.
Volume number, issue number, and date of issue
    The issue date for a journal issued weekly, biweekly, or semimonthly should be an exact date; a monthly need carry only the month of issue.

Notice of a change in title or frequency of issue
The notice should include the previous title or frequency.

TABLE OF CONTENTS: INFORMATION ON ARTICLES AND SECTIONS

1.13   All articles in the issue should be fully identified.

Title
Titles should be complete and in the same form as on the title pages of the articles. Articles of more than ephemeral value that appear within the issue in titled sections (see "Sections" below) should be identified by full title, for example, editorials.
Author names
If space permits, their form should be the same as on the articles.
Pages
Only the initial pages of articles need be given if their pages are continuous; if they are not continuous, the initial page of each appearance of the article should be given.
Sections
If articles are grouped within sections, for example, editorials under a section title "Editorials", these sections and their titles should be identified. Short items of ephemeral value need not be individually identified and can be represented simply by section headings such as "News Notes" or "Notices of Meetings"; short items of sufficient value to be indexed in bibliographic databases, such as letters and book reviews, may be usefully represented by title and author unless their number and hence the space to represent them seem excessive. Initial pages should be given for sections whose individual items are not listed.
Special features
Items that may not appear in every issue should be listed when they do; these may include, for example, an information-for-authors section, an errata section, or a volume index; initial pages should be listed.

TABLE OF CONTENTS: FORMAT AND TYPOGRAPHY

1.14   The journal title and other bibliographic information should precede the title, "Table of Contents". The listing of section titles and articles should be in the same sequence they occupy in the issue, even if sections and their articles are boxed for special attention. Columns are the most legible format of article titles, author names, and page numbers, with titles in the first column, author names in the second, and pages in the third; if the number of articles is too large for this format, give titles first, author names second, and pages in a column at the right side; choose typefaces that clearly distinguish between the first 2, such as an upright (roman) typeface for titles and a slanted (italic) typeface for author names.

Colors and type sizes should be such that the contents page can be readily reproduced, even in a reduced size, in *Current Contents* and similar bibliographic publications (2). Black type on white paper should be preferred. Journals with a page width of 6.5 inches (16.5 cm) or greater should set the contents page in type no smaller than 10 points.

THE MASTHEAD

1.15 Every issue should provide in the same location a section describing the journal, its ownership, availability, and other details likely to be needed by authors, readers, subscribers, librarians, dealers, indexers, bibliographers, and archivists. This section is sometimes known as the "officers page" or "the flag".

THE MASTHEAD: LOCATION

The masthead should appear within the first five pages of the issue, preferably on or immediately adjacent to the table of contents. If it appears on the inside front cover or on a page that is not likely to be bound within a volume, such as a page in an advertising section, it should appear on the back of the volume title page or on the next page.

THE MASTHEAD: INFORMATION

1.16 Certain data are minimally needed in the masthead.

Title, subtitle, and the International Standard Serial Number (ISSN)
 If the journal is published with titles in an additional language, or more, or with an acronymic title, such data should be included.
Publisher
 Name and complete address (including TELEX, electronic-mail, and cable addresses); telephone numbers, with area codes.
Issue frequency
Postal data required for mailing at second-class rates
 See section 1.34.
Copyright information
 In addition to the legally required notice of copyright, the masthead should state the publisher's policy on fair-use copying and whether the journal is registered with the Copyright Clearance Center or has some other arrangement for payment of copying royalties.
Subscription rates, single-issue prices, and ordering information
 The address to which orders are to be sent should be stated even if it is the same as that of the publisher. Include information on terms of payment (currency, payment media), number of volumes per year and issues per volume, availability of back issues, and other publication media such as microforms and online computer services. Include a statement of a policy on supplements.

Address-change procedure
    The relevant address should be stated.
Sponsorship
    The name and address of the sponsoring organization if it is not the
    publisher
Advertising management
    Names and addresses of staff persons or agencies supplying informa-
    tion on advertising in the journal

Additional information may be particularly useful to authors, readers,
and librarians if it is not given in the information-for-authors page.

Editors and other staff persons
    Names and addresses of persons receiving manuscripts and other mail
    relevant to editorial functions
Peer-review policy
    A statement on whether the content of the journal is selected at least
    in part on the basis of peer review is likely to be useful to authors.
Indexing and abstracting
    Identify the print and computer services that index the journal and
    make its abstracts and text available to libraries and other users.

If any of this information appears elsewhere on the page (for example,
the title of the journal), it need not be restated in the masthead.

THE MASTHEAD: FORMAT AND TYPOGRAPHY

1.17   If the masthead is on the Table of Contents page, make sure that the
layout of the page and the type faces chosen emphasize the information
most needed by a majority of users of the journal.

PAGES: INFORMATION CARRIED ON PAGES

1.18   Each pair of facing pages (the double-spread of left-hand and right-hand
pages) must carry enough information to identify the journal and the
issue.

Journal title, abbreviated (in standard form, see section 1.3) if necessary
Volume and issue number (or date)

If the trim size and title length permit, this information should appear
on every page.
       Each page should carry in a headline or footline (see section 1.21)
brief identification of the article or journal section in which it lies.

1.19   Each page should be numbered: right-hand pages odd-numbered and left-hand pages even-numbered. Arabic numerals should be used for text pages to be bound in permanent volumes or portions of volumes. For pages preceding text pages, such as a volume title-page and a table of contents, that are to be bound with text pages, lowercase roman numerals can be used to distinguish them from text pages. Advertising and other pages not to be bound as part of a volume can be distinguished from permanent text pages by a distinctively different convention such as an alphanumeric numbering, for example, A1, A2, and so on. For pagination of issues see section 1.31.

Permanent pages of a volume must be numbered consecutively. Thus, for example, the first right-hand text page of Issue 2 must be given the next odd number above the number of the last page of Issue 1.

Cover pages are not numbered.

PAGES: FORMAT AND TYPOGRAPHY

1.20 Adequate blank space must be allowed around the text and any illustrations or tables within the text area to avoid losses when issues are bound into volumes or parts of volumes; binders must always trim a small fraction from each edge of assembled pages to even up the bound edges, and the binding process takes some space from the inner side of pages. Thus the inner, or "gutter", margin should be at least 1 inch (2.5 cm) wide and the top, outer, and bottom margins each at least 0.75 inch (1.9 cm) wide.

Careful thought should be given to the number of type columns to be used on pages. At the trim size of most scholarly journals, a single column is made up of lines of type that are too long for easy reading. The lines in the columns of a 3-column format are likely to be too short unless the type size is small. The choices in the number of columns and other details of page format in scholarly journals should take into account both the need for efficient use of space and the reader's need for ease of reading and ready orientation on a page.

1.21 The preferred locations for the identifiers of the journal, issue, journal section, and article described above in section 1.18 and for the page numbers are in the bottom margin below the text and separated from the text by the space of at least 1 line. In this location the identifiers are known as "the footline". Identifiers placed instead in the top margin are referred to as "the headline" or "the running head". Left-hand page numbers should be below the left lower corner of the text block and the right-hand page numbers below the right lower corner.

1.22 Orient tables and illustrations so they are readable with the text. If a different orientation is needed for a very large table with the format of a horizontal rectangle, the table should be rotated 90 degrees counterclockwise so that its bottom lies against the right margin if on a right-hand page and against the inner margin if on a left-hand page. Be sure that the table (or portion of a table on a single page) and any footnotes do not have dimensions greater than those of the text block.

INFORMATION FOR AUTHORS

1.23 Most journals publish at regular intervals information for potential contributors on scope of content, the kinds of papers sought, manuscript requirements, the editorial mailing address to which manuscripts should be sent, whether papers published by the journal are peer-reviewed, coverage by indexing and abstracting services, and other similarly useful information. The page (or pages) with this information should be in the same location in each issue in which it is carried, with the location identified in the table of contents unless the information is on the covers or the masthead page (see sections 1.15 and 1.16). If such information is not presented in every issue, its availability (the issues in which it appears or the source from which it is available) should be identified in a prominent position (such as table of contents, masthead, or cover) in each issue. The preferable location for information for authors is within the journal rather than on a cover page.

CORRECTIONS

1.24 Publish statements of errors, omissions, and other faults needing correction in the same location in any issue, preferably a prominent location such as a letters section or the table of contents. The location should be stated in the table of contents if it is elsewhere in the journal. The title for such statements, such as "Errata" or "Corrections", should make clear their function; preferably each statement should have a brief title reflecting the content of the corrected item. Statements must include full bibliographic identification of the corrected item, the material corrected, and the correct substitution.

Correction statements appearing in the same volume as the item corrected should be indexed in that volume.

ARTICLES IN INSTALLMENTS

1.25 Articles too long for publication in one issue may have to be divided into 2 or more installments. Such articles ought to be scheduled so that all installments are published in consecutive issues within the same volume; identify each installment with the article's main title followed by designation of the part as "Part 1", "Part 2", and so on. The concluding part should, however, be designated as "Conclusion" rather than a part. If the divisions of content permit, identify the content of each part with a descriptive title following the designation of part. Be sure the same designations appear in the table of contents. Each part should identify, if possible, the location of preceding or following parts.

References and other content usually placed at the end of an article are placed at the end of the concluding part.

Sequential but separate articles forming a series ought to be published within the same volume. They may also carry a series designation (see section 2.4).

SUPPLEMENTS AND SPECIAL ISSUES

1.26   To accommodate a group of articles on one theme, the proceedings of a meeting, or other text that similarly represents content not found in regular issues and meriting unified presentation, some journals occasionally publish a supplement to their regular issues. To save readers possible difficulties in finding supplements and to save libraries the costs of additional binding, cataloging, and shelving, the format of supplements ought to permit their being bound with regular issues. Thus they should have the same trim size and a pagination continuous with the other pages of the volume. To be clearly identified as such, a supplement usually carries pages bound within its own cover; it should have its own title page and table of contents, but the cover's format, design, and identification characteristics ought to be similar to, if not identical with, those of regular issues (see sections 1.8 and 1.9). Continuity with regular issues is supported by identifying a supplement as part of an issue whether or not it is mailed with the regular issue; thus the companion regular issue should be identified on its cover and table of contents as a part of the issue. The regular issue should be identified as Part 1 of 2; the companion supplement as Part 2 of 2. The supplement's papers must be indexed, of course, in the index of the volume.

For supplements not to lie within the sequence of regular issues and hence not to be bound with them, differing requirements in style and format are likely to be appropriate. Such supplements ought to be avoided in favor of supplements of the kind described above, but if they must be published, guidance can be found in the relevant ANSI standard (1).

A single issue devoted to a particular theme (special, or theme, issue) should have the same trim size and other format characteristics as other issues and should use the same sequence of pagination.

VOLUMES

COMPONENTS OF VOLUMES

1.27   Each completed volume should contain 4 components, in this order.

1. Volume title page
2. A table of contents

3. The text of the volume
4. An index to contents of the volume

If the volume bound for library use does not carry an information-for-authors page or section (see section 1.23) or a masthead (see section 1.16) on pages that would be bound within a bound volume, these components should be provided separately for binding with the rest of the volume, with appropriate pagination and the same trim size.

The title page, table of contents, and index should be the end pages of the last issue of the volume, if possible, to facilitate prompt binding of the volume. If they are sent to subscribers later, as a policy of the publisher, that information should appear in the journal's masthead. If these items are not sent to subscribers and must be requested of the publisher, that information with instructions for requests should appear in the masthead.

The title page must be a right-hand page; the table of contents and the index must begin on right-hand pages. Pagination should begin with the title page and continue through the table of contents; it should use a numeral system differing from that of the text pages. A widely used convention for this pagination is lowercase roman numerals: i, ii, iii, iv, v, and so on; to eliminate the use of the increasingly archaic roman-numeral system, a convenient alternative is an alphanumeric sequence such as P1, P2, P3, and so on ("P" for "preliminary").

VOLUME TITLE PAGE

1.28 The volume title page should carry this information.

The complete title (and subtitle if one is used) of the journal
The ISSN (see section 1.4)
The publisher's name and the name of the sponsoring organization (if it is not the publisher)
The name of the editor (unless this information appears in the masthead or on a separate page placed between the title page and the table of contents, perhaps also carrying other staff names and titles)
The volume number and the numbers of its issues
The dates of the first and last issues in the volume

The reverse of the title page is usually blank; it can be used to carry the masthead, the staff names and titles, and other information not provided in the pages of issues bound within the volume.

If the combined thickness of issues bound as a volume would exceed 2.5 inches or 6.5 centimeters and the volume would therefore be more conveniently bound in 2 parts, provide a second title page for the beginning of the second part of the volume. The first-part title page should then carry only the issue numbers and dates (see paragraph above) for the first part, and the second-part title page the same information for the second part.

VOLUME TABLE OF CONTENTS

1.29   The table of contents must carry no less information than that provided in the table of contents for each issue; see sections 1.12 and 1.13. Articles should be listed in the sequence in which they appear in the issues of the volume. Although the table of contents may be revised from the tables of contents of individual issues to remove identification of individual issues and provide a continuous listing uninterrupted by issue dates, readers are likely to find issue separations a convenience.

The first page should be a right-hand page and thus will be page iii or P3 if the sequence and pagination indicated in section 1.27 are followed; if other pages appear between the reverse of the title page and the first page of the table of contents, such as a right-hand page listing the journal's staff (see section 1.28), a higher page number such as page v or P5 will, of course, be needed.

VOLUME INDEX

1.30   The index for the volume should identify articles by subjects and authors. Separate subject and author indexes are easier to consult than an index carrying both listings; separate indexes should be separately titled according to their content.

The index should be included in the last issue or mailed with it; if another policy is followed, it must be stated in the masthead (see section 1.16). Pagination of the index should continue that of the closing pages of the text in the last issue of the volume even if the index pages do not immediately follow the text pages and are separated from them, for example, by advertisements. The index pages must be continuous and not interrupted by advertisements or pages, such as news pages, not to be bound in the volume.

NUMBERING OF VOLUMES AND ISSUES

1.31   Volumes must be numbered sequentially with arabic numerals, beginning with Volume 1. If the title of the journal is changed, do not continue the sequence of volume numbers; designate the first volume under the new title Volume 1 (also see section 1.35). Do not designate volumes in parallel with volume number and duration of publication, such as "Volume 59, 60th Year".

Issues must be numbered sequentially with arabic numerals, beginning in each volume with Issue 1 (or Number 1); do not continue the sequential numbering in the next volume but start the sequence anew.

VOLUMES: PERIOD OF PUBLICATION

1.32   A volume should represent a full calendar year of publication or an even-numbered fraction of a year; thus a monthly journal started in 1999 to have 2 volumes per year with 6 issues per volume should have its first issue designated "Volume 1, Issue 1" and this first issue should carry the date "January".

PAGINATION OF VOLUMES AND THEIR ISSUES

1.33   Successive pages of the journal to be included within bound copies must be numbered sequentially with arabic numerals beginning with 1 for the first page of the first issue of each volume. Although popular magazines usually start pagination anew in each issue, this practice should be avoided in scholarly journals because of the potential for confusion in finding an article in the bound journal.

    Pages not to be preserved in bound copies, such as pages with advertising or news, must be numbered in an unambiguously different system, such as pages designated A1, A2, and so on, the sequence either beginning with the first right-hand page of such pages in the first issue of the volume or with the page in each issue. Note that pages thus paginated which should be included in bound volumes (such as a page with the masthead, pages with a table of contents) will have to be provided in the last issue of each volume with appropriate new pagination (see section 1.27).

STATEMENT OF OWNERSHIP, MANAGEMENT, AND CIRCULATION

1.34   The United States Postal Service requires journals and other periodicals mailed at second-class rates within the United States to file with it, and to publish within the journal's pages once a year, a statement of frequency of publication, ownership, circulation, subscription price, and other information. The post office of second-class entry for the journal should be consulted for current requirements; they are stated in the *Domestic Mail Manual* (8) of the United States Postal Service.

CHANGES AND IRREGULARITIES

TITLE CHANGES

1.35   The title of a journal should not be changed without careful justification, such as change in scope of topics, change in organizational sponsorship, or some other sound reason. If a change must be made, make it at the beginning of a volume and preferably the first volume of a year. Take steps to be sure that a contemplated new title is unique (see section 1.2) and obtain a new ISSN (see section 1.4) well in advance of the change so that it can appear on the cover (see section 1.8), the table of contents (see section 1.12), and the masthead (see section 1.16); the previous title should be displayed preceded by "Formerly", in a visually subordinate size and location, in the same locations (cover, table of contents, and masthead) for 1 year after the change.

If 2 or more journals are combined and the title of 1 is continued, apply the recommendations above for the discontinued titles to the journal with the retained title and continue the volume numbering of the journal that had the retained title. If none of the titles is retained, start a new journal, following the recommendations elsewhere in this chapter for a new journal; for 1 year the journal should carry a notice on the cover, table of contents, and the masthead stating "[New Title] is a new journal representing [number] discontinued journals, [the previous titles]".

If a journal is divided into 2 or more journals and 1 of them continues the title, continue the volume numbering and ISSN for that title; the journal or journals with new titles should follow the recommendations elsewhere in this chapter for a new journal; in each new journal thus derived the cover, table of contents, and masthead should each carry for one year the notation "Continues in part [title of original journal, ISSN]".

In addition to the notices recommended above for title changes, separate announcements of the changes should be mailed to subscribers.

CHANGES IN TRIM SIZE

1.36 Change the trim size of a journal only at the beginning of a volume. Be sure that any portions of the preceding volume supplied after publication of its last issue, such as an index, have the same trim size and format characteristics as that volume.

CHANGES IN FREQUENCY OF ISSUES

1.37 Make a change in frequency of publication, such as a change from monthly to semimonthly, only at the beginning of a volume, being sure to announce the change in a prominent location on the journal, such as its cover, in at least 1 issue preceding the change and in the issue of the change.

IRREGULARITIES AND OTHER CHANGES

1.38 Any interruptions in the appearance or numbering of issues should be noted on the cover and table of contents of the first issue to be published after the interruption, with information on its nature and duration. The numbering of an issue representing 2 or more combined issues should be in accord with the numbers that would have designated them as separate issues.

If an issue is published in 2 or more parts, the part number and the number of parts should appear with the issue number wherever it normally appears (see sections 1.8, 1.12, and 1.18); an appropriate form is, for example, Issue 2, Part 2 of 2. This recommendation applies to supplements (see section 1.26).

JOURNALS IN TRANSLATION

1.39 The title of the translated version should have as closely as possible the same meaning as the original title; the translation title should be changed only when the original title changes. The original title should appear with the translation title in all of its locations.

The translated version should be published, if possible, in volumes and issues corresponding to those of the original. If the translated version is published at less frequent intervals, its identifiers of volume and issue should include identification of the volumes or issues of the original represented by the translated version.

REPRINTS

1.40 All pages of offprints or reprints of articles in the journal should retain the pagination and other page characteristics of the original articles. Reprints of two or more articles brought together for reprinting may carry additional, new pagination that begins with page 1 for the initial right-hand text page, but the original pagination should be retained within parenthesis marks (round brackets).

The title page of each reprinted article must carry sufficient information for a complete bibliographic reference, preferably in the references format used elsewhere in the journal.

ADVERTISING

1.41 Advertising pages should carry sequential pagination continuous with that of other pages also to be discarded when the rest of the journal is bound (see section 1.33). Advertising with content and format resembling that of text pages in the journal should be refused; advertising should be distinctly different in appearance from the journal's text.

REFERENCES

1. Subcommittee 10 on Periodicals: Format and Arrangement. American national standard for periodicals: format and arrangement; ANSI Z39.1-1977. New York: American National Standards Institute; 1978. As of mid-1986 this standard was under revision.
2. Institute for Scientific Information. ISI checklist for journal editors and publishers. Philadelphia: Institute for Scientific Information; 1983.
3. Institute for Scientific Information. Journal contents page design: guidelines. Philadelphia: Institute for Scientific Information; 1983.
4. International Organization for Standardization. Documentation — rules for the abbreviation of title words and titles of publications; Ref No ISO 4-1984(E). Geneva: International Organization for Standardization; 1984. Available from the American National Standards Institute, 1430 Broadway, New York, NY 10018.
5. National Library of Medicine. List of journals indexed in Index Medicus: 1986. Bethesda, Maryland: National Library of Medicine; 1986; NIH publication no 86–267. Published annually.
6. PES. A standard for serials. Choice. 1986;23:1177.
7. Paul SK. Journal and title identifier. CBE Views. 1986;9:40–2.
8. United States Postal Service. Domestic mail manual. Washington: United States Postal Service.

Chapter 2

Articles: General Format and Style

How articles in a scholarly journal are presented determines in large part how readily the journal and its articles are used. Their format and style should be selected with attention to needs for clear and efficient presentation of content; the specifications for format and style, once selected, should be constant from article to article and issue to issue.

The recommendations in this chapter are based in large part on two standards of the American National Standards Institute, *American National Standard for Periodicals: Format and Arrangement* (1) and *American National Standard for the Preparation of Scientific Papers for Written or Oral Presentation* (2) and on recommendations (3) issued by the Institute for Scientific Information.

TITLE PAGE

2.1   The title page is usually the first page of an article seen by readers. Its elements and arrangement should make clear what the article is about, who wrote it, and the journal and issue in which it appears; this information will be particularly useful when the article is seen apart from the journal as a copy or reprint.

Except for articles of specific types that have their own format needs (see sections 3.9 to 3.11, 3.14), a title page should include these elements in this sequence.

1. Article title
2. Author statement (also known as the byline)
3. Author affiliation
4. Abstract of the article with its bibliographic reference
5. Text of the article

19

6. Footline elements: journal title, volume number with issue number (or date), copyright notice
7. Page number

The title page is likely to have a clearer format if its text is not accompanied by figures (illustrations or graphs) or tables.

ARTICLE TITLE

2.2   The title should be as informative of the article's content as possible within a reasonable length. Articles lacking adequately specific titles may be overlooked in bibliographic searches through permuted-term indexes or online searches of bibliographic indexes in which the search is confined to titles.

Terms likely to be indexed, such as terms for anatomical structures, physiologic functions, pathologic diagnoses, diseases, chemicals, drugs, and so on, should be in accord with standard nomenclature (see Chapter 10). Full terms should be used rather than shortened forms even when the latter are acceptable in current jargon.

NOT   Coronary Heart Disease in the Ukraine
BUT   Coronary Artery Heart Disease in the Ukraine

Hyphenated and possessive-form terms may be missed in computer searches of titles if the searcher fails to use a truncated equivalent. Titles with such terms should be rewritten if possible to avoid the hyphenated or possessive construction (see section 10.10 on possessive forms of eponyms).

NOT   Gentamicin-Induced Hypokalemia
BUT   Hypokalemia Induced by Gentamicin *or* Gentamicin Induces Hypokalemia
NOT   Prinzmetal's Angina: A Review
BUT   Prinzmetal Angina: A Review

Avoid using abbreviations in titles. Standard scientific symbols may be used in appositive constructions.

The Hydrogen Ion Concentration (pH) of Tuberculous Pleural Effusions

When an abbreviation must be substituted for a long term or group of terms, an accompanying term or phrase can helpfully indicate what the abbreviation represents.

NOT   MOPP for the Treatment of Hodgkin Disease
BUT   MOPP, a New Chemotherapeutic Regimen for the Treatment of Hodgkin Disease

An abbreviation for a long term or phrase, like the acronym "MOPP", is more acceptable in a title to readers when it is explained in the abstract on the title page (see section 2.8).

For capitalization in titles see section 7.2.

An organism should be identified by its formal scientific name even if its common, or trivial, name is more widely known.

NOT   Panophthalmitis from Infection with the Lyme-Disease Spirochete

BUT   Panophthalmitis from Infection with *Borrelia burgdorfeii*, the Lyme Disease Spirochete

If possible, the most important word, or words, should be placed at the beginning of the title to catch the scanner's eye in a table of contents; omit words and phrases not specifically representing content of the article.

NOT   A Study of the Therapeutic Efficacy of Panmalignomycin, a New Antineoplastic Agent, in Metastatic Malignant Melanoma

BUT   Panmalignomycin for the Treatment of Metastatic Malignant Melanoma

2.3   A subtitle can be added to supplement a properly condensed title.

FOR   A Controlled Double-Blind Study of the Treatment of Chronic Dyspepsia with Powdered Desiccated Mandrake Root

SUBSTITUTE   Treatment of Chronic Dyspepsia with Mandrake Root [title] A Controlled Double-Blind Study of a Powdered Desiccated Preparation [subtitle]

2.4   Sequential but separate articles derived from the same study can have their relations indicated by an initial title element that represents the series and is an element in common for all of the titles followed by elements unique to each article.

Captopril in Idiopathic Hypertension: 1) Effects on Left Ventricular Myocardial Dynamics

Captopril in Idiopathic Hypertension: 2) Effects on Renal Function

Captopril in Idiopathic Hypertension: 3) Effects on Cerebral Blood Flow

In general, the reporting of findings in a single study should not be divided into 2 or more papers, but if the complexity and detail of a study, and hence the probably excessive length of a single paper reporting all of the findings, justify a group of papers, the structure for a series of titles illustrated above is a means of indicating clearly their relation to each other.

Journals should discourage the serial titling of papers that have no more relation to each other than their representing the general line of research in the same laboratory or by the same investigator.

AUTHOR STATEMENT (BYLINE)

2.5   Persons listed as authors should have qualified for authorship by criteria widely accepted in the scientific community (4,5). Ambiguity of author names in indexes and other bibliographic compilations is reduced when authors identify themselves by at least one full name in addition to their family names (surnames).

NOT   R Smith, R Smith, T Jones, and T Jones
BUT   Roberta Smith, Robert Smith, Thomas Jones, and Tina Jones

Journals should ask authors to use their full names consistently from article to article; the request can be made in the journal's information-for-authors page and in letters requesting revisions. The full names of authors may often be found in references to their articles, either cited articles or references in bibliographic indexes.

In some cultures and nations the family name precedes the given name or names (6), notably in oriental and Hungarian names. Unless a journal publishes only articles from those regions, the names of authors on its articles should all be in the standard Western convention of given names followed by family name.

CONVERT   Szent-Gyorgy Albert, Chan Tai-chien
TO   Albert Szent-Gyorgy, Tai-chien Chan

2.6   Consistency should be followed throughout the journal in giving academic degrees after authors' names, and the journal's policy on degrees in the author statement should be made clear in its information-for-authors page. If degrees are stated, only the highest degrees relevant to the content of an article should be listed. Avoid the use of honorific designations. The best argument against academic degrees in the author statement is that the validity of an article should be supported solely by its content and not by authority implied by the academic degrees of its authors. This argument clearly applies to honorific designations, which while often indicative of intellectual attainment may also simply represent distinctions awarded mainly out of political motives or on the basis of unclear scholarly criteria. Academic degrees can, however, indicate varieties of skills that are relevant to the validity of an article and suggest which author (or authors) in a group is mainly responsible for some particular content.

When 2 degrees must be listed for an author, apply these rules.

1. The higher degree comes second; the Doctor of Philosophy follows the Doctor of Medicine.

   Robertus Robot, MD, PhD

2. A degree awarded after the Doctor of Medicine comes second.

   Florenzia Nachtigall, MD, MPH

3. A Doctor of Medicine awarded after the Bachelor of Medicine comes second.

   Timothy Titmuss, BM, MD

Omit occupational designations. Abbreviations for military ranks and organizations and for academic degrees should not be used together; prefer designations for military organizations to those for military ranks.

NOT   Col Whittam Sydebern, MD
BUT   Whittam Sydebern, MC, USAF

Do not use religious titles of address; instead use academic degrees.

NOT   Rev Francis Seizor
BUT   Francis Seizor, DD

Separate full names from academic degrees and academic degrees from each other with commas; do not separate with commas any elements of names following family names (such as *Junior, III*) from family names. Separate successive author names with degrees by semicolons.

Timothy Titmuss, MD; Hunter Howarth IV, MD, PhD; Francis Seizor, DD

AUTHOR AFFILIATION

2.7   The affiliation and address where the work represented by the content of the article was done should be stated on the title page (3) for each author. If the number of authors for articles in the journal rarely exceeds 2 or 3, the addresses should be given in the author statement (see section 2.5). If the number frequently is greater, list the author names with their addresses in a footnote at the lower left-hand corner of the title page. To save space the names of authors with identical addresses can be grouped above the address without regard to the sequence of names in the author statement.

The author name and address for reprint requests should be stated separately from the affiliation addresses.

Affiliation addresses should be complete mailing addresses: name, department or unit, institution, a number-and-street or postal-box designation, city (town), state (province, geographic department), postal code, country.

Occasionally a "present address" for an author may have to be accommodated, particularly in single-author papers.

ABSTRACT

2.8   The text of the article should be preceded by an abstract of the article. If text pages are in a 2-column format, the abstract should be placed at the head of the left-hand column; if they are in a 1-column format, the abstract can be placed in a box at the upper left-hand corner of the block of text or it can run across the width of the text column with its left-hand margin aligned at the left-hand margin of the text.

Whether the abstract is indicative (indicating the nature of the content of the article) or informative (stating in brief form the content of the article) (7), the sequence of its content should closely follow that of the article. The length of abstracts may have to be determined by limitations of the title-page format; in general, the abstracting services that republish abstracts from journal articles do not accommodate abstracts exceeding 250 words.

If an acronymic abbreviation has been used in the title (see section 2.2), the abstract must state what the abbreviation represents immediately before a parenthetic statement of the abbreviation.

> ... treated with a regimen of mechlorethamine, vincristine (Oncovin), procarbazine, and prednisone (MOPP) for ...

Otherwise, abstracts should not contain abbreviations other than standard scientific symbols that are comprehensible when standing alone, such as pH and DNA, or symbols that represent quantities and are used in the abstract with numerical values.

> ACCEPTABLE ... measurements of the pH of tuberculous pleural effusions ...
> ACCEPTABLE ... the best dose was 10 g per day ...
> NOT ... doses are now best expressed in g rather than oz ...
> BUT ... doses are now best expressed in grams rather than ounces ...

The abstract should close with a full bibliographic reference with the standard elements and format stipulated in sections 15.25 to 15.27, as a guide to subsequent authors in correct referencing of the article.

> ... with complete remission in 15 of the 37 patients. This treatment may not be effective in patients with more advanced stages of the disease. [Dorn PT, Ehve JR, Rotenform Q. Panmalignomycin in the treatment of erysipeloid lymphoma. Ann Intern Med. 1995;101:673–9.]

The square brackets indicate that the reference was added by the editor to the authors' abstract.

The text of the abstract must not include citations of references cited in the text of the article or references themselves aside from the reference for the article itself added to the abstract within square brackets (see the preceding paragraph).

Abstracts must not include tables or figures. Most online computer bibliographic databases are not able to transmit abstracts with such content.

FOOTLINES

2.9 In addition to the information to be carried in footlines specified in sections 1.18 and 1.21, the title pages of copyrighted articles should carry a copyright notice.

> © 1984 American College of Teleology   Surgical Methods
> American Journal of Teleology, Volume 13, November 1994   1

TEXT

2.10   The area of type on the page occupied by text (and additional elements within that area such as tables and figures) should be surrounded by sufficient blank space to allow for binding and trimming (see section 1.20).

The main choice in format for the text is among the number of columns of type on a page. The choice should be determined in part by a desire for harmonious proportions of the areas occupied by type and associated tables and figures and by surrounding spaces. There are advantages with double-column and triple-column formats for text: readers are likely to find the shorter lines in the narrower columns to be easier reading, and more options are available for sizes and layouts of tables and figures (also see section 1.22); columns narrower than 12 to 15 picas tend to be hard to read rapidly.

TEXT HEADINGS

2.11   Readers find text divided logically by headings much easier to read than undivided text. Pages of text running on without headings are likely to have a daunting, "gray" appearance. More important, headings carefully devised to represent succinctly but accurately the content of the text that follows assist scanners of the article in quickly grasping its entire content. Such headings also assist close readers by making clear the sequence of content and orienting them as to where they stand in the development of the author's argument.

The typefaces and type sizes selected for headings should take into account needs for quick distinction by readers among levels of headings. First-level headings indicate the main divisions within the text; second-level headings indicate the divisions of text within each main division; and so on. Fourth-level headings are not often needed. The selection of appropriate typefaces and type sizes for successive levels of headings may be helped by consultation with a designer or typographer. An alternation of all-capital and capital-lowercase headings in roman (upright) and italic (slanted) typefaces may be adequate.

First-level headings
　　All small capitals　　　　METHODS
Second-level headings
　　Capital–lowercase　　　　Chemical Analyses
Third-level headings
　　Italic, all small capitals　　*CALCIUM*
Fourth-level headings
　　Italic capital–lowercase　　*Ionized calcium*

Designers can assist in selecting other sequences that may be just as effective.

Note that in general a heading should not be followed by a single lower-level heading.

The placement of headings in relation to the text following them can help the reader in distinguishing among the several levels. In one widely used format, the first-level headings are centered on the vertical axis of the column of type, the second-level headings are started with the left margin of the column of type and the following paragraph is indented normally, and the third-level headings are run into the first line of the following paragraph. For example:

METHODS

Chemical Analyses

Xxx xxxxxxx xx xxxx xxxxx xxx xxxxxxx xxx xx xxxxx xxx xxxxxxxxxxx x xxxxx xxx xxxxx xxx xx xxxxxxxx xxx xxxxxx xx xxxx xxxxx xxxxxx x xx xxxxxxxx x xx x xxxx xxxx.

CALCIUM Xxx xxxxxxxxxx xx xxxxxx xxx xxx xxxxx xxxxx x xxxxxx xxx xxx xxxxxx xx xxx x xx xxxxx x xxxxxxxxx.

Again, a designer or typographer can be helpful in selecting typefaces and arranging them in relation to the following text so as to make clear to the reader the levels of text and their relation to each other.

TEXT CITATIONS OF REFERENCES

2.12   Documents to which readers are referred by the author for support of the text are concisely described and identified by references listed at the end of the text (see sections 2.32 and 15.1). These references must be cited in the text; in the Vancouver style for citations and references described in Chapter 15, the citations are the numbers assigned to the references in the References section (see section 2.32). The citation numbers should be placed in the text within parenthesis marks (round brackets) at the points at which their references are relevant to the text.

In two studies by Brown and Jones (5,6) of the relevance of surgical teleology to patient satisfaction . . .

Sometimes the most relevant place for the citation is immediately after a word such as "described" or "reported" that alludes to publication. Try to avoid placing a citation at the end of a sentence.

Some journals place the citation numbers, in a smaller type size, slightly above the line of text as superscript numbers, but this style has no clear advantage over that described immediately above and has the disadvantage of forcing typists of manuscripts and printers' compositors into additional keyboard operations. Further, superscripts generally cannot be displayed on monitor screens from text transmitted online.

TABLES

2.13 A table is an efficient format in which to present numeric and descriptive data that indicate relations of independent and dependent variables or covariables. Lists of text elements with or without categorical relationships may be presented in tabular format; see section 2.26.

Typically a table includes 5 main components (see Figure 2.1).

1. Table title
2. Column headings (in a horizontal array called the *box*)
3. Row headings (in a vertical array called *the stub*)
4. Field: the data of the table arranged in columns and rows. The intersection of a column and a row is called *a cell*.
5. Footnotes

(The box, the stub, and the field are called the *body* of the table.)

Most tables need no more than 3 rules (lines) to separate components: a rule below the table title and above the column headings (box); a rule below the column headings (box) and above the body; and a rule below the box and above the footnotes. Other than straddle rules under spanner headings (see section 2.20), additional rules are not likely to be needed; table structure can usually be additionally clarified by groupings of rows with intervening spaces.

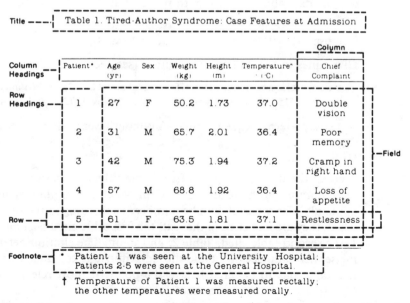

Figure 2.1 A case-summary table illustrating the usual parts of a table and their names.

To avoid unnecessary costs of composition, do not use vertical rules to divide columns of tables.

2.14 Capitalize the title, column headings, row headings, footnotes, and terms and phrases in the field according to the rules for sentences (see section 7.1): capitalize the initial letter of the first word (with exceptions as noted in section 7.1, for example, mRNA, β-Amylase) and any following words normally capitalized in running text, such as proper names, taxonomic names, and brand names. For exceptions to capitalization, see section 2.23.

2.15 In general do not terminally punctuate terms or phrases in any elements of tables; complete sentences and footnotes should, however, end with a period. Internal punctuation should be used as appropriate, for example, commas to separate terms in a series.

2.16 Abbreviations can be used to save space, notably in column headings. If no more than 2 abbreviations are used other than standard symbols such as those for metric units, explain them in specific footnotes; if more than 2 non-standard abbreviations are used, explain them in the first footnote (see section 2.24).

2.17 Dates should be stated in an unambiguous style (see section 13.22); the American numeric convention for 1 September 1978 is 9/01/1978 but the European form for the same date is 01/09/1978. Preferable forms are the sequences year/month/day; or year, abbreviated month name, day; or day, abbreviated month name, year.

> FOR November 5, 1978
> USE 1978/11/5, *or* 1978 Nov 5, *or* 5 Nov 1978

Give times in the 24-hour convention (see section 13.21).

> NOT 3:15 pm Noon, 11/5/78 12:00 pm, 11/5/78 12:01 am, 11/6/78
> BUT 1515 1200, 5 Nov 1978 2400, 5 Nov 1978 0001, 6 Nov 78

Note the preferred sequence, time–day–month–year, when a time is given.

TABLE TITLE

2.18 Precede the descriptive part of the table title with designation of the table number in the form, Table *n*, in which *n* is a number in arabic numerals. The tables should be numbered according to the sequence in which they are first cited in the text, the first table cited becoming Table 1, the second table cited, Table 2, and so on. The citation determining the sequential place of a table should simply cite the table by number; if a table has to be cited before the point of most relevant citation ("passing citation"), use a "see" form.

> USUAL FORM
> . . . we interpret the data on serum calcium (Table 3) to mean that . . .

PASSING CITATION
> . . . the serum sodium values (Table 1), in contrast to those for serum calcium (see Table 3) . . .

Place a colon after the table number and a space before the descriptive part of the table title.

2.19 The descriptive part of the table title should be specific enough to enable readers to understand the table without reference to the text; avoid restating column headings, but summarize them with a phrase.

> NOT Table 1: Serum sodium, potassium, and calcium in patients treated with panmalignomycin
> BUT Table 1: Serum electrolytes in patients treated with panmalignomycin

Use only nouns and noun phrases, with appropriate connectives, in titles; do not use verbs so as to produce titles that are sentences or clauses and thus force conclusions onto readers. Avoid empty initial phrases such as "Comparison of . . .".

Capitalize according to the rules for capitalizing sentences (see sections 2.14 and 7.1). Do not close the title with a period; the table number and the descriptive part of the table title serve together as a title with 2 parts.

TABLE-COLUMN HEADINGS

2.20 The sequence of column headings read from left to right should progress logically if possible, as in the following sequence of events in a hospital admission.

> Patient Symptom Diagnosis Treatment Response Autopsy

Each column heading must apply to all row headings or cells beneath it. The first column heading is above, and identifies, the row headings.

All column headings must be singular so as to apply grammatically to each singular element in a cell.

> NOT Patients Organisms Tests Treatments
> BUT Patient Organism Test Treatment

Use column headings, if possible, that will fit on one line. Abbreviations can sometimes be substituted for 2-line headings, but if they are, they must be explained in a footnote (see section 2.24). When 2 or more column headings belong to the same category, the presentation can be simplified by using a term for that category as a spanner heading; a rule beneath the spanner heading and above the column headings it spans is known as a straddle rule. The spanner heading should summarize the column headings, not restate them.

Hematologic data		
Sedimentation rate	Erythrocyte count	Leucocyte count

Units for the column headings are placed in the line below. Use standard symbols for units (see sections 13.12 to 13.15 and relevant sections in Chapter 16). In small tables some units may be written out rather than being represented by symbols. Note that *number, probability,* and other statistical units should be represented by standard statistical symbols (see section 14.10 and Table 14.2). Thus, *number* is represented by *n*, not by # or "no." or "nbr".

Symbols for units are not capitalized by the rules for sentence capitalization (see section 2.14) but follow the general rules for symbols in text (see sections 13.14 and 13.15 and any relevant sections in Chapter 16). In compound units with only 2 components, use the slant line (/) rather than "per" or indicate the denominator by a power indicator such as −1.

NOT   mmol per L   BUT   mmol/L *or* mmol·L⁻¹

Do not use multipliers, such as × 10⁵, as modifiers for column headings; readers may not always be able to tell whether a multiplier means that the numbers in the column have been multiplied by the multiplier or have to be multiplied by the reader; preferable designations are those that indicate the number of omitted places, such as *"In millions"*.

TABLE ROW-HEADINGS

2.21   The sequence of row headings from top to bottom should represent a logical sequence, such as an alphabetical sequence for states, or an age sequence for patients, or a dates sequence for observations in time on a single patient.

All of the headings should have parallel grammatical forms.

NOT	Standing	BUT	Standing
	Runs		Running
	Sleep		Sleeping

If the row headings describe variables, such as chemical values, for which units must be stated, the units should follow the headings behind commas or within parenthesis marks (round brackets).

Calcium, g/kg body weight *or* Calcium (g/kg body weight)

Row headings should align on their left end ("flush left").

For convenience in reading, tables can be divided internally with section headings; these headings should align flush left, with the row headings aligning flush left but indented.

Men	Americans
Untreated	Native-born
Treated	Foreign-born
Women	Canadians
Untreated	Native-born
Treated	Foreign-born

Capitalize row headings and section headings as specified above (see section 2.14).

TABLE FIELD

2.22 Numeric data in cells should accurately represent the precision of measurement. Numbers representing counts in whole units, for example, number of patients, should be presented without a decimal point.

NOT 139.   BUT 139

Numbers less than 1 should include a zero before the decimal point.

NOT .12 .078   BUT 0.12 0.078

In a column or row of numbers to which the same unit applies, use a decimal point and a number of zeros appropriate to the precision of measurement for data in whole numbers.

NOT	139	BUT	139.0
	0.9		0.9

If all numbers in a column or row to which the same unit applies are whole numbers of 4 digits or less, run the numerals in each number together; if some of the numbers are longer than 4 digits, separate the numerals in groups of 3 as stipulated in the general rule for large numbers in text (see section 13.4).

NOT	4,560	BUT	4560	NOT	4560	BUT	4 560
	399		399		17,277		17 277
	17		17		1,399,211		1 399 211
	2,798		2798		476,321		476 321

Grouping of digits in threes for numbers larger than 9999 rather than separating them with commas reduces the risk of confusion for readers accustomed to the European convention of a comma to represent the decimal distinction rather than the decimal point generally used throughout North America.

Numeric data in a column must be aligned on the decimal point, present or implied, as in the examples above. Roman numerals should be aligned at their right end.

Data in columns made up of paired elements, such as ranges of values, values with accompanying standard deviations or standard errors, and numbers with multipliers, should be aligned on the word or sign dividing each pair.

Ranges indicated by "to"	Values paired by ±	Numbers with multipliers
56 to 371	10.6 ± 0.4	1.6×10^5
9 to 58	9.2 ± 0.1	12.3×10^3
356 to 389	102.8 ± 0.9	0.5×10^5

Cells lacking data because measurements or observations were not made should indicate this lack with an ellipsis mark (3 periods in a row; see section 6.8). In a column with numbers aligned on the decimal point, the right-hand period of the ellipsis mark should align with the right-hand numeral; in a column aligning on a sign as in the examples immediately above, the center period of the ellipsis mark should align with the sign.

123.6	10.6 ± 0.4
. . .	. . .
95.2	102.8 ± 0.9

Cells lacking data because column or row headings are not applicable should be left vacant. Do not use as a cell entry the abbreviation "n. a."; even though it is explained in a footnote, the ambiguity at first glance as to whether it means "not applicable" or "not available" is annoying to some readers. Avoid using symbols such as + and − to indicate, respectively, "present" and "absent"; such symbols can sometimes be misread to mean "increase" and "decrease". Ambiguities can be avoided by using precise terms such as "Present", "Increased".

2.23 Terms or phrases in a column should be aligned on their initial letters, with the location of this alignment determined by aligning the center of the longest term or phrase on the center of the column heading. If a phrase or group of phrases making up the cell entry is too long for the width allotted to the column, the entry should run on in 1 or more additional lines, with the additional line or lines indented from the left-hand alignment of the initial letters by 1 or 2 characters; if such run-on additional lines are needed, spaces between rows may have to be added to maintain uniform spacing between row headings.

Patient	Clinical presentation
1	Convulsions
2	Fever
3	Nausea, vomiting, rash, anxiety

Note that this example follows the general rule for initial capitalization in tables. The rule may be ignored if a table presents a need to distinguish between 2 classes of terms; an example is a table with the names of antibiotics or other drugs in which generic names are not capitalized to distinguish them from brand names, which are capitalized.

A column of normal values, such as for blood-chemistry measurements, should usually be the first column in the field, immediately following the column that makes up the row headings. A column giving totals for data in the row should usually be the right-hand, last column of the field.

The data in cells making up a row should be aligned on the row heading even if it runs into a second line (which should be avoided if possible). A row of normal values, such as for blood-chemistry measurements, should usually be the first row of the field; a row of totals should be the last row of the field.

TABLE FOOTNOTES

2.24 A single explanatory footnote applying to all of a table may suffice for many tables, Such a footnote can, for example, state the conditions under which an experiment was carried out, concisely describe the characteristics of study groups, explain abbreviations, cite references, and state permissions to republish data. Such a footnote should be keyed at the end of the title.

Additional footnotes needed to explain individual components of a table should be keyed to those components. If a footnote applies to all cells in a column, key it at the column heading.

The recommended device for keying footnotes at the relevant points in the table is the square-bracketed symbol [fn] with an arabic number that indicates the place of the particular footnote key in the sequence of keys, as in "[fn1]", "[fn2]", and so on. The footnote key is placed with 1 space after the datum, term, phrase, or table title. The keying after the title should proceed down by rows (including column headings as the first row) and within each row from left to right.

Each footnote should be a separate paragraph that begins with its footnote key, which is immediately followed by a space and the capitalized first letter of the initial word of the footnote statement. Each footnote should end with a period whether or not the period is preceded by a complete sentence. For an example of this recommendation see Table 16.10. A conventional sequence of symbols has been used for many years by many scholarly journals as keys for footnotes: *, †, ‡, §, ||, ¶. If more keys are needed than can be accommodated with these symbols, they have to be supplemented with the same symbols in doubled form, for example, **, ††. These symbols are not available on many typewriters and may be difficult to produce in some word-processing programs; they cannot be displayed via online database systems. The "[fn]" convention recommended above avoids these difficulties and the potential confusion with superscript exponents that can result from using superscript numbers as keys to footnotes, another frequently used system.

If citation numbers for references must be used in 1 or more footnotes to a table, they should follow the sequence of citations that preceded the first mention of the table in the text. If a reference is first cited in a table, the citation and reference number follow the sequence in the text preceding the citation of the table; if that citation is a passing citation, the sequence followed is that immediately preceding the main citation of the table.

NUMBER OF TABLES; TABLE SIZE AND ORIENTATION

2.25   The maximal number of tables that can be accommodated in an article depends on the length of the text, the size of the tables, and the taste of the editor. An excessive number can produce difficulties in layout and visual confusion for readers. The convenient maximal number in a journal for a text of a particular length will depend on the journal's trim size, page format, and other characteristics. In general, difficulties in layout are likely to develop for journals with double-column pages when the number of tables in an article exceeds 1 table per thousand words of text.

An excessive number of tables can usually be reduced by eliminating those not really needed. Disposable tables include tables that are simply lists of items or that carry data readily stated in the text. A second solution is the combining of 2 or more tables, particularly those with closely related data and identical column headings; section headings above appropriately grouped rows can indicate divisions of content of a table that appeared in the tables combined for the single table.

The acceptable width of a table depends largely on the type size used for its headings and data and on the degree of closeness of column headings and columns that is tolerable. A single-column table usually can accommodate up to 65 characters and spaces across its width; a double-column table, up to 130.

A table too wide for one page may be extended onto the facing page; this solution should be avoided if possible, but if it is adopted, the table number must be repeated above the extension of the table on the facing page, with "continued": "Table 2 (continued)". A great convenience for readers is a repetition of the row headings (the stub and its column heading) at the right-hand side of the extension.

A table too tall for a single page can be extended onto the top of the next page, which should be a facing page if possible. Such an extension will have to repeat the column and row headings. As with an excessively wide table extended onto a facing page, the table number should be repeated: "Table 2 (continued)".

Excessively wide tables that are shallow and excessively tall tables that are narrow can sometimes be more conveniently accommodated by exchanging column and row headings, with appropriate relocation of the contents of the field cells. With such rearrangement a wide and shallow table, for example, can be converted into a tall and narrow table readily accommodated in a single column.

For the placement of tables on pages, see section 2.29.

TABULAR LISTS

2.26 Presentation of a sequence of items in the form of a table may be desirable if the list merits visual emphasis. The most valuable use of the tabular-list format is for presentation of a hierarchical list (outline). Numerals and letters typically designating hierarchical levels (divisions) in an outline can be omitted unless such designations are needed for convenience in referring the reader to items in the list from the text; indentations of successive levels usually make clear their differences.

Tabular list without designators of levels	Tabular lists with designators of level	
	Alphanumeric style	**Legal style**
Table 1: Causes of rash	Table 1: Causes of rash	Table 1: Causes of rash
Organic compounds	I) Organic compounds	1. Organic compounds
Hydrocarbons	A) Hydrocarbons	1.1 Hydrocarbons
Lipids	B) Lipids	1.2 Lipids
Inorganic salts	II) Inorganic salts	2. Inorganic salts
Sodium salts	A) Sodium salts	2.1 Sodium salts
Sodium nitrate	1) Sodium nitrate	2.1.1 Sodium nitrate
Sodium vanadate	2) Sodium vanadate	2.1.2 Sodium vanadate
Potassium salts	B) Potassium salts	2.2 Potassium salts
Insect bites	III) Insect bites	3. Insect bites

Designators of level in the legal style should be preferred because of their unambiguous precision when items in lists are referred to frequently in the text. Note in the examples above that the designators in the alphanumeric style are aligned on their parenthesis marks. Alignment follows 2 general rules: 1) designators are aligned on their closing period or parenthesis mark or on the terminal letter or numeral when no terminal punctuation is used; 2) the most left letter or numeral in 1 or more designators of the same level is aligned under the initial letters of the list elements of the next higher level. Note that in the legal style terminal periods are used only in single-number designators (the highest-level designators).

1. Xxxxxxx
  1.1 Xx xxxx
    1.1.1 Xxx xxxxxx
    1.1.2 X xxxxx xxx
    [and so on to]
    1.1.12 Xxxxxx
  1.2 Xxxxxx xx x xxx
  [and so on to]
12. Xxxx xxxxxxxx

In tabular lists without designators of levels, the amount of indentation used to indicate lower-level entries is partly a matter of taste. Two characters should be the minimum of indentation to make visually clear a new level; indentations of more than 4 or 5 characters are usually wasteful of space. Runover lines in any style of tabular list should be aligned to begin with the second or third letter of the first line of the entry.

> Reasons for failing to seek treatment
>   The patient lacks transportation, lives in a very remote region, or does not have access to a reliable source of referral.
>   The patient is not aware of being ill.

If footnotes are needed at the end of a tabular list, they should be separated from the list proper by a partial-width or full-width hairline that begins at the left-hand margin. Use the square-bracketed "[fn]" convention described in section 2.24 for keys in the list to the footnotes.

For the placement of tabular lists on pages, see section 2.29.

FIGURES

2.27 The term *figure* designates illustrative material such as graphs, flow charts, diagrams, photographs, and line drawings. Detailed discussion of style and format requirements for such materials is out of the scope of this manual; useful and authoritative guides can be found in *ASM Style Manual for Journals and Books* (8), *The ACS Style Guide* (9), and in texts on methods of illustration.

FIGURES: SIZE AND PROPORTION

Figures are frequently submitted by authors in sizes and proportions not satisfactory for publication. The size to which a figure should be reduced in publication is determined by the legibility it will retain in the smaller size. The legibility of a graph is usually determined by its lettering and symbols; usually reduction should retain vertical dimensions for symbols and lowercase letters without ascenders or descenders (for example, a, m, s) no less than 2 mm (or 6 points).

The height–width ratio of a figure will be largely determined by its content. The most pleasing ratio usually approximates 2:3; the original of a figure can sometimes be cropped to this ratio without deleting vital content. This ratio is satisfactory for single-column figures whether their major axis is vertical or horizontal; if possible, double-column figures should have a horizontal major axis.

FIGURES: CITATION AND PLACEMENT

2.28   Each figure must be cited at each point in the text to which it is relevant. The citation can usually have the simple form of table designation within parenthesis marks, for example, "(Figure 5)". If a particular aspect of the figure or a point made in its legend (see section 2.30 below) is referred to, the citation should specify the reference, for example, "(see the insert in Figure 2)", or, "(for experimental conditions, see the legend for Figure 3)".

Figures are usually placed on pages in accord with the sequence in which each is first cited, and the successive citations will usually follow the ascending numerical sequence: Figure 1, Figure 2, and so on. Each figure should be placed as close to its first citation as satisfactory formatting of pages permits, preferably on the same page, either immediately below or adjacent to the citation, or on the following page. If a figure has to be cited for a minor relevance in the text before its main point of relevance (a "passing citation"), its page placement near its main point of relevance in the text should take precedence over strict numbering of figures in accord with their first citations.

2.29   The number of figures and tables per page should be held to 1 or 2 so as to minimize the risk of visual confusion for readers. If the number of figures in relation to the length of text is too great for this general rule, some of the figures may lend themselves to being combined into multi-part figures. The possibilities will be determined by such considerations as relations of subject content, the relative scales of lettering, and height–width ratios.

Whether a figure (or table) should be placed on a particular page will be determined mainly by the considerations described in the preceding two paragraphs, but the possible locations on the page have differing visual effects. The visual continuity of an article is determined mainly by its columns of type; therefore priority should be given to locations of figures (and tables) and text that treat text as the "center of visual gravity", or main point of attention, on each page. Two rules follow from this principle. First, in a choice between the top half and the bottom half of a page as location for a figure, place it in the top half, retaining text in the bottom half; the text should be the last element of each page seen by the reader in moving through the article page by page. Second, in a choice between placing a figure adjacent to the inner margin of the page or the outer margin, place it on the inner side of the page, retaining text adjacent to the outer margin where it will be the first element of a left-hand page reached by a reader and the last element seen by the reader on the right-hand page.

Avoid the stacking of figures or tables; it causes visual confusion.

LEGENDS AND FIGURE LABELING

2.30   Each figure must have a legend identifying it by number and describing its content briefly. The figure number is designated in the form, Figure *n*, where *n* is in arabic numerals; place a period after the number and a space between the period and the first letter of the description. Note that this punctuation differs from the colon after a table number (see sections 2.18 and 2.19). The description of the figure may have to include complete sentences or several separate phrases with a period closing each for clear separation, so the same principle determines closing the figure-number designator with a period rather than a colon, which in a table title simply separates 2 coordinate elements.

The legend for the figure should be confined to a brief summary of the main point it makes and any technical details needed by the reader to fully understand the figure. The summary should be, if possible, in phrase form rather than sentence form and omit unnecessary articles such as an opening "The". Extensive explanations of the point made by the figure and descriptions of methods should be in the text rather than the legend, with cross-references such as "See Methods section for details of experimental conditions". References should not be cited in the figure itself but only in its legend.

Titles on figures should be deleted, their content to be represented solely in legends.

The description of the figure may have to include explanations of different lines in a graph, of symbols, of abbreviations, of a feature in a photograph marked with an arrow, and other details. But such explanations should not substitute for mandatory and readily accommodated elements in a graph. Labels for the *x* and *y* axes of a co-variable graph must be on the graph. Labels for lines and keys for symbols can sometimes be fitted into the field of a graph without producing visual confusion and are to be preferred to explanations in the legend; the general principle is that a figure should be as self-explanatory as possible, with the legend adding no more detail than is needed to make unequivocal the main point of the figure. Lines, symbols, and abbreviations needing explanation in a legend can often be efficiently explained by placing them within parenthesis marks immediately after the first mention in the legend of what they represent.

The legend for a multi-part figure should identify and briefly describe each part. The parts can be identified within parenthesis marks. If, for example, the parts have been labeled A, B, and so on, the identifiers in the legend will be the appropriate letters, for example, ". . . electrocardiogram before (A) and after (B) administration of tocainide . . .". Without such labels the parts will have to be identified by location, for example, ". . . electrocardiogram before (top strip) and after (bottom strip) administration of tocainide . . .".

Note that text citations of parts of figures must include the figure number, for example, ". . . (Figure 1A) . . .".

If the original dimensions of a structure illustrated in a figure are made clear by a scale in the figure, the legend need not explain its size or include a statement of magnification. If the figure is a photomicrograph or electron micrograph and readers will need to know the magnification exactly, the magnification stated by the author for the figure will have to be recalculated in accord with the reduction (or enlargement) applied for publication of the figure; for example, a stated magnification of ×500 for a figure reduced in its linear dimensions by one-half will have to be changed for the legend to ×250. If exact dimensions are not important but only the approximate order of magnification, the stated magnification need only be modified to indicate the original statement, for example, ". . . original magnification, ×500 . . .".

The sequence of elements in a legend should be in order of descending importance.

Figure number
Figure description: one or more phrases or sentences
Additional explanations of figure content such as abbreviations not explained in the description
Technical details such as stains, magnification
Statement of permission to reproduce the figure or to adapt data

This order is determined by the relative importance of the legend elements in, first, finding the figure within the article and, second, understanding the content.

ACKNOWLEDGMENTS, APPENDIXES, AND ADDENDA

2.31   Thanks for intellectual assistance, technical help, permissions to use published or unpublished documents, and similar notes are usually placed at the end of the main text of an article under a first-level heading, "Acknowledgments". The minor importance of such text can be indicated by publishing it in a type size 1 or 2 points smaller than that of the main text.

Extensive text distinctly subordinate to the essential content of an article can be efficiently included with the article as an appendix. Such text might be, for example, detailed descriptions of technical methods, extensive quotations from references, or address lists. Large tables of original data from which derived data are presented in the main part of the article can be conveniently presented in appendixes. An appendix should be headed by a descriptive title that starts with the designation of an appendix, for example, "Appendix A: Epidemiologic Methods for Analysis of Death Certificates"; the typeface and type size should be the same as that used in the rest of the article for first-level headings (see section 2.11). The subordinate place of appendix text can be indicated by publishing it in a type size 1 point smaller than that of the main text. Appendixes differ in part from addenda (see below) in being part of the original article rather than a part added at the proof stage.

Text of the same importance in the article as the main body of the text that has to be added in proof usually should be placed at the end of the main text under a first-level heading, "Addendum". References added by citation in the addendum should be assigned reference numbers that follow the original sequence.

REFERENCES AND BIBLIOGRAPHY

2.32   References legitimately cited in the text, tables, and figure legends (see sections 2.12, 2.24, and 2.30) should be listed under the heading "References" at the end of the article in the order in which they are first cited (see section 15.6). "References" should correspond in type size and typeface to those of other first-level headings. Reference numbers and the body of references should be formatted to avoid visual confusion.

NOT 1. Smith J, Jones V. Pulmonary . . . Ann Intern Med. 1922;103 . . .   BUT 1. Smith J, Jones V. Pulmonary . . . Ann Intern Med. 1922;103 . . .

The "References" section should be at the end of the article and follow any such ancillary sections as addenda and appendixes. For details of the style and format for various kinds of references, see Chapter 15.

Documents not cited in the article (and hence not listed in "References") but called to the reader's attention as relevant to the subject of the article should be listed in a separate section headed "Bibliography"; its style and format should be the same as for "References".

REFERENCES

1. Subcommittee on Periodicals: Format and Arrangement. American national standard for periodicals: format and arrangement; ANSI Z39.1–1977. New York: American National Standards Institute; 1978. As of mid-1986 this standard was under revision.

2. Subcommittee on the Preparation of Scientific Papers. American national standard for the preparation of scientific papers for written or oral presentation; ANSI Z39.16–1972. New York: American National Standards Institute; 1972.

3. Institute for Scientific Information. ISI checklist for journal editors and publishers. Philadelphia: Institute for Scientific Information; 1983.

4. CBE Style Manual Committee. CBE style manual: a guide for authors, editors, and publishers in the biological sciences. 5th ed. Bethesda, Maryland: Council of Biology Editors; 1983:1–2.

5. Huth EJ. Guidelines on authorship of medical papers. Ann Intern Med. 1986;104: 269–74.

6. CBE Style Manual Committee. CBE style manual: a guide for authors, editors, and publishers in the biological sciences. 5th ed. Bethesda, Maryland: Council of Biology Editors; 1983:50–53.

7. Huth EJ. How to write and publish papers in the medical sciences. Philadelphia: ISI Press; 1982:77.

8. American Society for Microbiology. ASM style manual for journals and books. Washington: American Society for Microbiology; 1985:77–98.

9. Dodd JS. The ACS style guide: a manual for authors and editors. Washington: American Chemical Society; 1986:115–32.

Chapter 3

Articles: Specific Formats and Style

Articles should have formats appropriate for their kind of content and for the needs of readers. The recommendations in Chapter 2 do not necessarily apply to all articles; variations in format and style should, however, be justified by how well they serve readers.

RESEARCH ARTICLE

3.1   Articles reporting research studies and findings have the elements of critical argument (1) usually set in a structure of chronologic narrative (2). These characteristics determine the sequence of content and the headings that indicate text divisions.

A critical argument poses a question, examines the evidence supporting an answer and the counterevidence that challenges it, weighs their relative strengths, and concludes with the answer best supported. Well-designed research starts with a question or an hypothesis (which is a restatement of a question in positive terms), carries out studies or experiments designed to yield observations or data that may answer the question or support the hypothesis, examines those observations or data and the related evidence for their validity, and concludes with an answer to the question or with support (or no support) for the hypothesis. Most research papers arrange these elements of critical argument as a chronologic narrative.

The most frequently used headings for the main text divisions of research articles (2) are those widely known as the "IMRAD formula": *I*ntroduction, *M*ethods, *R*esults, *a*nd *D*iscussion. These headings correspond to the sequence of ideas and events in a research study but may have to be expanded with lower-level headings or modified, or both, to reflect the content of the article.

RESEARCH ARTICLE: INTRODUCTION

3.2 The Introduction describes the origin of the question the research was designed to answer, or the hypothesis, and states it, preferably explicitly. If the Introduction is short compared to the rest of the text, a first-level heading, Introduction, need not be stated; the opening paragraphs are conventionally the introduction. In 2 circumstances, the heading Introduction should head the opening paragraphs: 1) when the format and typeface used for an opening abstract (summary) of the article do not differ sufficiently from that of the text of the article to prevent visual confusion with the text, or 2) when the introduction is long and needs lower-level headings to clarify its content. But the use of the heading Introduction should be consistent in all research articles in the journal; if the second condition stated above occurs infrequently, it should be ignored and the heading Introduction not used even if lower-level headings are needed in the particular article.

Headings below the first level (Introduction) that divide and clarify a long introduction need not represent fixed usage but can be devised as appropriate to reflect the origin of the question or hypothesis that was the subject of the research; such headings (second-level; see section 2.11) might be "Background", "Previous Studies", "Review of Recent Literature", and so on.

RESEARCH ARTICLE: RESEARCH DESIGN
AND EXECUTION ("METHODS")

3.3 The section on research methods describes the design of the reported research and how it was carried out. The sequence should correspond to that followed in the research: the overall design of the research; definition of subjects of the research (such as diagnostic categories, case selection and assignment, measures of outcome in intervention trials, and so on); descriptions of observational or experimental methods; and methods by which observations were judged for relevance and validity as evidence.

Various first-level headings have been used to head this section, such as "Materials and Methods" or "Patients and Methods". Unless the journal exclusively reports only studies of non-human subjects or only human studies, the preferable heading is Research Design and Methods, a generic heading that readily applies to all research.

Although most Research Design and Methods sections are clear enough with regard to their content and its sequence without second-level headings, a long section may be divided with second-level headings to help readers. Such second-level headings should reflect the content of paragraphs beneath them, for example: Study Design, Selection of Subjects, Assignment of Subjects to Study Groups, Treatment, Measurement of Outcomes, Analytical Methods, Statistics.

If an article has to present a long and detailed account of an unusual study design or an unusual analytical method, that content can be shifted to an appendix to the main text (see section 2.31).

For an article reporting multi-step research, a choice will probably have to be made between structuring it with separate sections on research design and methods and separate Results sections or presenting all design and methods content in a single section with appropriate second-level headings and all findings in a single Results section. An example is an article reporting first an epidemiologic study and then a study of individual case characteristics; 1 option would be to present the epidemiologic study with its own design and methods section and results section, with the same sequence for the cases study.

RESEARCH ARTICLE: RESULTS SECTION

3.4   Short research papers can make the structure of their Results sections clear enough through logical paragraphing and appropriate opening topic sentences in paragraphs. Long Results sections may be clarified with second-level headings that reflect their content and its sequence: for example, Control Group, Treatment Group, Adverse Effects. Occasionally third-level headings are needed to subdivide further sections headed with second-level headings. A Results section, Treatment, might be additionally divided, for example, with third-level headings for sex of subjects, "Men", "Women".

The sequence of content in a Results section should in general place the most important findings first and the remaining findings in descending order of importance with regard to the research's question or hypothesis. Within a section on 1 aspect of the findings, the content should follow a chronologic sequence; thus in an opening Results section on outcomes with a treatment, the outcomes in the control group should precede the outcomes in the treatment group.

Large tables, for example, tables carrying original data from individual subjects that are presented in summary form in the Results section, may be presented in 1 or more appendix tables following the main text.

See section 3.3 for presentation of multi-step research.

RESEARCH ARTICLE: DISCUSSION

3.5   The Discussion section has 2 main functions: assessment of the research findings and relevant literature for their validity and strength for the conclusion reached in the article; and assessment of the conclusion's implications for clinical application or further research. As in the Results section, logical paragraphing and appropriate opening topic sentences for paragraphs may make clear the content and its sequence. Long Discussion sections may benefit from second-level headings that make explicit their content; if this kind of formatting is used, the opening paragraphs usually need not be headed with a second-level heading because by convention a Discussion section usually opens with an assessment of the validity of the study's findings. Thus the first second-level heading might be "Findings in Previously Reported Studies".

RESEARCH ARTICLE: ADDITIONAL SECTIONS

3.6   Most research reports close with additional sections such as Acknowledgments (see section 2.31) and References (see section 2.32). Occasionally appendixes are needed for detailed presentation of unusual methods (see section 3.3) or large tables of data (see section 3.4).

Each appendix or appendix table must have an identifying heading. Appendixes should be headed with a first-level heading, as for the sections in the main text, and the headings should serve as specific titles; successive appendixes should be identified with successive alphabetic or numeric identifiers.

> Appendix A: Method for Automatic Stratification of Cases
> Appendix B: Data from Nine Cases Reported in the Literature

or

> Appendix 1: Method for Automatic Stratification of Cases
> Appendix 2: Data from Nine Cases Reported in the Literature

A citation of an appendix in the main text need not use its full heading; for example, an adequate citation to the first example above would be "(see Appendix A)".

CASE-SERIES ARTICLE

3.7   A frequent type of article in clinical journals reports an analysis of cases, usually a number of cases sufficient for reasonable conclusions on the variety of manifestations in a particular syndrome or disease. A well-written introduction will clearly justify the analysis and indicate the question, or questions, it aimed to answer. If all of the cases have been drawn from the experience of the authors or their institution, the term *case-series article* is appropriate. If some or all of the cases analyzed have been drawn from published reports, the term *case-review article* is appropriate.

A properly conducted analysis of this kind will have proceeded only after explicit decisions on case selection, which may involve diagnostic criteria, age criteria, or other definitions. If a literature search has been carried out for reported cases, both case-selection criteria and the scope of the search will have been defined. Such criteria and definitions should be stated in this kind of article; the section carrying them is analogous to the Research Design and Methods section of a research article (see section 3.3) and should follow the introduction. The section may need first-level headings such as "Case Selection" or "Case Selection and Literature Search".

The section reporting the results of the case analysis corresponds to the Results section (see section 3.4) and can be similarly headed with a first-level heading. Unless this section is short, readers will be well served by its being topically divided with appropriate second-order headings as in a research article (see section 3.4), for example, "Age and Sex", "Ethnic Characteristics", "Presenting Manifestations", "Response to Treatment". If an analysis of literature-reported cases is an integral part of the results, its findings should, of course, be included in the Results section; if literature cases are not integral to the analysis, their characteristics may be more properly considered in the Discussion section following the Results section. Individual case reports may be included in the Results section as examples of types of case characteristics; if so they should be identified as specific cases in the second-level headings, preferably with case identifiers also used in any tabular presentation of case data, for example, "Case 1985-A". Alternatively, individual cases may be described in an appendix rather than in the Results section. Individual case reports can be readily distinguished from the main text, whether in the Results section or an appendix, by setting their text in type 1 point smaller than that of the main text.

A well-conceived case-series analysis will have been designed to answer one or more specific questions. Hence the article reporting it will consider evidence supporting the answer or answers and any counterevidence. As in a research article, these considerations are usually taken up in a Discussion section. A long Discussion section may be divided with topical second-level headings to make its content more readily discerned.

CASE REPORT

3.8   The central point of interest in a case that justifies its being reported is likely to be 1 of 3 kinds: unique or very uncommon clinical characteristics of a known disease, disorder, or syndrome; new information about a pathogenetic mechanism; or an apparently unique case that seems to represent a previously undescribed syndrome. The sections that all 3 kinds of case reports are likely to have in common are the introduction, the case description, and a discussion of the case.

The introduction, which should justify the reporting of the case, should open with a first-level heading, Introduction, only if this heading is standard style for all research and clinical articles in the journal (see section 3.2).

The description of the case should be clearly distinguishable from the rest of the text and hence should be headed with a first-level heading such as Case, Case Summary, Case Description, or some similar designation. Unless the description is long and complex, its narrative sequence and appropriate paragraphing should make clear the usual content: presenting history, past medical history, initial-examination findings, laboratory and other diagnostic findings, and subsequent clinical events. A long description, such as one that must narrate successive episodes of illness and hospitalization, may need second-level headings to make clear the sequence of events.

The discussion section, which should open with the first-level heading, Discussion, has the same function as in a research article (see section 3.5): assessment of the validity and strength of the evidence for and against the conclusion reached, both the evidence derived from the case and that from relevant literature; and assessment of the conclusion for any implications for clinical application or research. Only very long Discussion sections are likely to need second-level headings to make clear their content.

If research findings are the main justification for a case report, a more complex format is likely to be needed: Introduction, Case Description, Discussion of Case, Research Methods, Results, and Discussion. In some case reports of this kind, the Case Discussion may not be needed. The choice of sequence will usually be best determined by the author, but the choice of terms for the headings should be consistent with style elsewhere in the journal. If the research reported is the dominant content, the case description can be subordinated by presenting it in a type size 1 point smaller than that of the rest of the text (see section 3.7).

REVIEW ARTICLE

3.9   There is no standard conventional format generally applicable to review articles such as the "IMRAD" format (see section 3.1). But because reviews are usually long articles, readers benefit from headings that make clear their content and its sequence. The use of a heading for the introduction should be consistent with style elsewhere in the journal. A section describing the scope and methods for the search for relevant literature can be headed Literature Search as in case-series articles (see section 3.7). The subsequent headings will be determined by the content of the successive sections of the text. A review of a disease, for example, may justifiably have a sequence of headings like that in a textbook description of a disease: Etiology, Epidemiology, Pathogenesis, Pathophysiology,

Clinical Manifestations, Diagnosis, Differential Diagnosis, Treatment, Prognosis. In a very long or complex review, second-level headings may also be needed to make more clear the content and its sequence.

EDITORIAL

3.10   Editorials in biomedical journals usually have the character of a short, concise review article or of a polemic; either kind of editorial will, if thoughtfully written, be constructed as a critical argument (3) (see section 3.1). Their brevity determines some differences in format from that of the kinds of articles discussed above.

The title should not seem excessively long or complex for the relatively short text of an editorial; a subtitle, sometimes useful for an article (see section 2.3), should in general not be used.

In most journals editorials are short enough not to need headings to subdivide text.

The author statement (byline) should appear at the end of the text rather than under the title so that the editorial's beginning is not overweighted by the space that usually surrounds an author statement.

The statement of author affiliation should appear under the author statement and should be consistent in content with affiliation statements elsewhere in the journal. The preferred affiliation statement includes all the elements of an address; to maintain the symmetry of the end of a column of text the affiliation with address should be justified to the left margin of the column.

. . . XX XXXXX X XXXXXX XXX XX XXXXXXXX X XXX X XXX XXXXXX XXX XXXXXX XXX.

J Robert Anglewood, MD

Department of Medicine
Wurm Building, Room 3
Transylvania University
Transylvania, New Caledonia 98756

An affiliation statement without the details of an address can immediately follow the author's name, either in run-on style or on successive lines.

. . . XX XXXXX X XXXXXX XXX XX XXXXXXXX X XXX X XXX XXXXXX XXX XXXXXX XXX. — J. Robert Anglewood, MD. Department of Medicine, Transylvania University, Transylvania, New Caledonia

or

. . . XX XXXXX X XXXXXX XXX XX XXXXXXXX X XXX X XXX XXXXXX XXX XXXXXX XXX.

J. Robert Anglewood, MD
Department of Medicine
Transylvania University
Transylvania, New Caledonia

If references are used, the references section should follow the format and style applicable to all articles (see sections 2.32 and 15.10–15.61).

BOOK, SOFTWARE, OR AUDIOVISUAL-PRODUCT REVIEW

3.11 Reviews of books, computer programs (software), or audiovisual products such as audio and video cassettes can, like editorials, have simpler formats than most other articles. Their usual elements of format are, in sequence, the review heading, the text of the review, the author statement, and the author affiliation. Some journals head book reviews with titles indicative of the content of the item reviewed, but many editors might find difficult the coining of such titles so as to make them adequately descriptive but not redundant with the titles of the reviewed items.

The review heading is composed of the same groups of bibliographic elements as a bibliographic reference (see sections 15.34 to 15.40, 15.43) to the book, with a different sequence and usually some additional groups and elements. Because most scanners and readers of reviews are more interested, at least initially, in the subjects of items reviewed than in the identity of their authors, the title of the reviewed item should precede the author statement. See Table 3.1 for a list of the bibliographic groups and their elements as sequenced in a review heading and a comparison with the groups and elements in a bibliographic reference.

Punctuation in the heading follows the same general principles as in bibliographic references: periods at the ends of each bibliographic group and commas separating the elements within each group except for the title group. Elements within a bibliographic group and not closely related should be separated with semicolons. Separate a title from a subtitle (subordinate title) with a colon.

State author names as they appear on the publication and abbreviate authors' given names only if that is how they appear.

Capitalize titles and names in accord with the general rules for capitalization in text (see sections 7.2 and 7.13). (Titles in bibliographic references have only sentence-style capitalization; see sections 7.1 and 15.18.)

A typical bibliographic reference to a book:

Hostler R. Diagnostic methods in the nineteenth century. New York: Siddons and Simon; 1982.

Table 3.1: Bibliographic groups and elements in book review headings compared with the sequence in bibliographic references [fn1]

Book review heading	Bibliographic reference
Title	Authorship
Title [main]	
Title, subordinate	
Title, translated [if needed]	
Edition	Title
Authorship	Edition
Author [single, multiple, collective]	
[names as on title page; unabbreviated]	
Author role indicator [such as *editor*]	
Imprint	Imprint
Place of publication	Place of publication
Publisher	Publisher
Date of publication	Date of publication
Physical description	Physical description
Extent of work [pages, illustrations, tables]	
Medium/packaging	
Size	
Series statement [optional]	Series statement
Notes	Notes
[price]	
Availability [such as address]	
[other data, such as ISBN]	

fn1: For a list and description of bibliographic groups and elements and for an explanation of the principles of punctuation in references, see sections 15.10 to 15.24 and Table 15.1.

Review heading for the same book:

> Diagnostic Methods in the Nineteenth Century. Robert Hostler. New York: Siddons and Simon; 1982. 603 pages, 36 illustrations, 15 tables. $27.00.

3.12   Software (computer program) reviews are built on the same principles. The software equivalent of *edition* is *version*. Descriptions of format (disks) and manuals are placed in the sequence as elements for Physical Description (see Table 3.1).

> Blood Gas Program. Version 5.83. Denver, Colorado: Computerized Pulmonary Services; 1982. Two 5.25-inch, double-density floppy disks; loose-leaf binder, 70-page manual. $1498.00. Available for IBM PC, XT or AT running PC-DOS 1.1, 2.0, 2.1 and for Apple II and IIe.

Additional description, such as a short statement of the software's content and intended audience, can be placed at the end of the heading as part of the Notes group.

3.13   The headings for reviews of video programs, films, slide programs, and audio cassettes are built on the same principles; the elements describing the medium (such as "video cassette") and its format (such as "VHS") are placed in the Physical Description group.

LETTER TO THE EDITOR

3.14   The elements of format for letters are title, text, author designation, author affiliation, and, optionally, references and editor's comments.

A title should precede each letter that stands alone. The general principles governing the content of titles (see section 2.2) apply to letter titles. A balance should be struck between brevity and specificity; letters with titles not including an adequate number of terms to indicate fully their subject content can be missed by searchers in online databases in searches conducted only in titles rather than in text as well.

Letters on the same subject that can be arranged in groups of 2 or more need not carry individual titles but can appear under a collective title that applies to all letters in the group.

The text of letters should follow the style rules for the text of articles, but because of the brevity of letters they do not need headings to indicate divisions of text. Citations of references should follow the general rules (see sections 2.12 and 15.6). If a letter was written as a comment specifically on an article published in the journal, a formal reference to the article should be given in a "References" section to avoid any ambiguity about the article even if the article is identified in the letter by title and issue. If the journal accepts tables and illustrations with letters, the general rules for tables and figures (see sections 2.13–2.30) apply to their presentation with letters. Use a standard opening for all letters such as "To the Editor:", "To the Editors:", "Sirs:" that is appropriate to the journal's staffing and titles.

As in editorials (see section 3.10), the author designation is placed at the end of the text, flush to the right margin of the page column. The author affiliation, with or without complete postal address, is preferably placed flush to the left margin of the page or column. If the letter has 2 or more authors with 2 or more addresses, head each address with the appropriate author's family name.

. . . xx xxxxx x xxxxxx xxx xx xxxxxxxxx x xx xxxxxxxxxx xxxx xxx xxxx xx xxxxxxxx.

Dr. Smith:	C R Smith, MD
Department of Medicine,	T M Jones, MD
Transylvania School of Medicine,	
San Francisco, CA 12345	
Dr. Jones:	
Department of Surgery,	
Transmontane College of Medicine,	
Portland, OR 23456	

References should follow the author designation and affiliation; see sections 2.32 and 15.10–15.61 for format and style of references.

3.15 A letter submitted as a reply to, or comment on, one or more letters placed above it should be introduced by a separating and explanatory notation, in italic (slanted) type to indicate that it is a note by the editor, such as *"In response:"* or *"In reply:"*.

Comments by the editor on a letter should follow the entire letter, including any references. The comments should be in italic (slanted) type to distinguish them unequivocally from the text of letters.

Corrections (also see section 1.24) published as letters should follow the format and style for letters but the titles should open with "Correction:".

> Correction: Name of Dr C R Smith
>
> To the Editor:
> I note that in your 12 January issue, the name of Dr C R Smith was misspelled as "Smythe". He . . .

Corrections that are not letters but are notes from the editor may be conveniently included in the letters-to-the-editor section if its title indicates unambiguously that it includes corrections, for example, "Letters and Corrections".

Some editors may prefer to distinguish between "Corrections" as author corrections and "Errata" as statements of editor or printer error. Either kind of correction should always appear in the same location in the journal (see section 1.24), should be identified in tables of contents (see sections 1.13 and 1.29), and should be indexed in each volume (see section 4.2).

REFERENCES

1. Huth EJ. Critical argument: the basic structure of papers. In: Huth EJ. How to write and publish papers in the medical sciences. Philadelphia: ISI Press; 1982:47–9.
2. Huth EJ. The research paper. In: Huth EJ. How to write and publish papers in the medical sciences. Philadelphia: ISI Press; 1982:50–7.
3. Huth EJ. The editorial. In: Huth EJ. How to write and publish papers in the medical sciences. Philadelphia: ISI Press; 1982:69–71.

Chapter 4

Indexes

Each volume of a journal should include an index (see section 1.30). With the rapidly increasing use of online bibliographic full-text data-bases by searchers who wish to have access to a wide range of journals, indexes to individual journals may become infrequently consulted but even then they may be needed to locate articles indexed erroneously in a database or incorrectly identified in a bibliographic reference.

4.1 A single index can include entries for authors and subjects but readers are likely to find separate author and subject indexes easier to use than a combined index.

Book and journal indexes resemble each other superficially, but because the needs of their users differ, they are built on different principles. A book usually encompasses a discrete subject; its index must identify the locations within it of many details of its content, giving inclusive pages for extended discussions of particular topics; its authors are readily identified from its title page, and the name entries in the index are for names in the text. In contrast, the volume of a journal encompasses many subjects in its often unrelated articles, each of which includes many details. Therefore the subject index, if it is not to be excessively long, must be confined in essence only to identifying articles by main subjects and locating them by initial page. Because of frequent multiauthorship, full entries for articles in the author index should be given only following the name of the first author, with cross-references to that entry from short entries for additional authors. Guidance on the principles, style, and format of conventional book indexes, can be found in standard sources (1–4).

CONTENT TO BE INDEXED

4.2   All articles and other individual items on the pages to be bound as a volume should have entries in the index for that volume. In addition to the usual articles, such as research reports, case reports, reviews, opinion essays, and editorials, the short items that may or may not be identified by separate titles, notably letters-to-the-editor (see section 3.14), reviews of books, software, or audiovisual products (see sections 3.11 to 3.13), and corrections and errata (see sections 1.24 and 3.16), should be indexed. Items that need not be indexed even though they are on pages to be bound include items that are standard and recurrent for the journal, such as a masthead (see section 1.15) at the beginning of the editorials section, and short items with little or no subject value, such as an editor's explanatory note at the beginning of an unusual article.

Items on pages not to be included in the bound volume must not be indexed.

ENTRIES FOR THE INDEXES

4.3   A complete entry for an article or other indexed item must include at least 1 entry in the author index, 1 or more entries in the subject index under 1 or more subject headings, and cross-references, as needed, in each index. Each entry and cross-reference must include a locator: for an entry, the locator is the initial page of the article; for a cross-reference, the locator is the relevant entry elsewhere in the index [fn1].

ENTRIES AND CROSS-REFERENCES FOR THE AUTHOR INDEX

4.4   Each indexed article or other item must be represented in the author index by an entry with the names of all authors, the title, and the initial page. Author names should be presented as in bibliographic references (see section 15.12), with last names and initials, names being separated by commas. The title should be the full title; for book reviews and other similar reviews the title is that under which the review appears or the title of the reviewed item (in italic [slanted] type; see section 6.3) if the review itself has not been titled. The title in any entry for a letter is the title under which the letter appears. The author-name element and the title element are each closed with a period as in bibliographic references (see sections 4.8 and 15.24 and Table 15.2).

> Songsiridej V, Peters MS, Dorr PJ, Ackerman SJ, Gleich GJ, Busse WW. Facial edema and eosinophilia: evidence for eosinophilic degranulation [A]. 503

---

fn1: The term *locator* is also used in descriptions of book indexes, in which locators may be paragraph numbers or indicators other than page numbers.

Paulshock BZ. *Plain pictures of plain doctoring: vernacular expression in New Deal medicine and photography* [BR]. 974

In journals with a variety of articles and other indexed items, designations of the type of item can be added at the end of the title; in the first example above, "[A]" has been added to indicate that the indexed item is an "article" (the journal's designation), and in the second "[BR]" indicates "book review". Such designators should be constant from issue to issue, and a box or footnote at the bottom left corner of the first page of the author index should provide a key to the designators. For capitalization and other style conventions, see section 4.9.

For multiauthor items, list each author after the first as a cross-reference. The convention for the cross-referenced author name is the same as that for the names in the first-author entry (see the paragraph above). The immediately following *"See"* (note italics) indicates the cross-referencing and is followed by the last names of the item's first 2 authors without their initials; if the cross-referenced author is the second author, his or her name is restated. The cross-reference is to the entry by first author for the item elsewhere in the author index.

Peters MS. *See* Songsiridej, Peters

ENTRIES AND CROSS-REFERENCES FOR THE SUBJECT INDEX

4.5   Each indexed article or other item must be represented in the subject index by at least 1 entry that includes either its complete title or a short version, the last name of the author (for multiauthor articles, the last name of the first author followed by "et al."), and the initial page number (or sole page number for articles on only 1 page). The subject entries are listed in alphabetical order under subject headings representing their content. Because most articles cover more than a single subject, most articles have to be represented by more than 1 entry, the additional entries being placed under the various appropriate subject headings.

4.6   For subject headings, use the subject headings published annually in *Medical Subject Headings* (5) by the National Library of Medicine and widely known as MeSH terms. This practice eliminates the synonyms under which articles covering the same subject would be listed and brings them together under the same heading for the convenience of the reader; in addition, the MeSH terms are steadily becoming standard search terms in some strategies for online searching of computer-maintained bibliographic indexes.

Subject cross-references will be needed in 2 circumstances. First, when a subject of an article is represented in the MeSH listing by a cross-reference to the proper MeSH equivalent, the same cross-reference should be used in the subject index to steer readers searching by the cross-referenced term to the MeSH synonym. Second, if 1 or more prominent subjects of an article (such as those represented in the title and the abstract) do not correspond to MeSH terms either directly or by cross-reference in the MeSH listing, those subjects should be represented among the index's subject headings by the terms used for them in the article followed by a *"see"* instruction and the nearest MeSH term that can be selected.

4.7   Entries for book reviews and similar items for which titles of other publications must make up the entry title can be simply listed under "BOOK REVIEWS", which is a MeSH term. If the number of book reviews to be indexed is not excessive, entries can be additionally listed under subject headings relevant to the subjects of the reviewed books. For italicization of book titles, see section 4.9; use the original book titles rather than short versions.

Entries for correction and errata items likewise can be grouped under headings "CORRECTIONS" and "ERRATA" with *"See"* cross-references to these sections under other subject headings.

In journals publishing a variety of article types, descriptions of article types can be placed at the end of the entry title within square brackets (see sections 4.4 and 4.9).

A specimen subject index built on these principles would have the following appearance; for typeface and other format conventions see sections 4.9 and 4.11.

> **BOOK REVIEWS**
> *Atlas of Osteoarthritis* [BR]. Luthra. 823.
> **CERULOPLASMIN**
> zinc-induced copper deficiency [A]. Patterson *et al.* 385.
> **COLONY-FORMING UNITS**
> *see* **STEM CELLS**
> **OSTEOARTHRITIS**
> *Atlas of Osteoarthritis* [BR]. Luthra. 823.
> complications of obesity [A]. Bray. 1052.
> **STEM CELLS**
> primary myeloproliferative disorder and hepatic vein thrombosis [A]. Valla. 329.

Note that short titles used as entry terms are not capitalized (see section 4.9).

PUNCTUATION

4.8   The separation of author names by commas and the closing of each element in the entries in the author and subject indexes is in accord with the principles for punctuation of references; for detailed discussion see section 15.24 and Table 15.2.

The designations of article type, such as A for an article and BR for a book review, are enclosed within square brackets to indicate that they are explanatory elements that have been added editorially to original titles (such as book titles in entries for book reviews) and short versions of article titles; this bracketing convention is described in section 5.31.

CAPITALIZATION AND ITALICIZATION

4.9 Capitalization in index entries should follow the rules for capitalization in running text (see section 7.1), not for initial words of sentences; note, especially, that the initial letter of an entry is not capitalized unless capitalization is needed to indicate the beginning of a title or a proper name.

> *Pneumocystis carini* culture methods [A].
> *Pneumonias and Other Nosocomial Infections* [BR].
> pneumonthorax in elderly men [A].
>
> hydrochlorothiazide pharmacokinetics [A].
> Hydrodiuril bioavailability studies [A].

Note in the second pair of examples that the capitalizing of the brand name drug, Hydrodiuril, indicates that it is a proper noun while the non-capitalizing of "hydrochlorothiazide" indicates that it is a generic, or common, name; see section 10.4 on usage for drug names.

Italicization in index entries is used in accord with the general rules for italicization (see sections 8.2 to 8.11). In the examples in the paragraph above, the formal binomial name of an organism is italicized in accord with one of the conventions for microbial nomenclature (see section 8.2) and the title of a book discussed in a book review is italicized in accord with the convention for representing book titles in running text (see section 8.6).

ALPHABETIZATION

4.10 The sequences of entries in the author index and of subject headings and article entries in the subject index should be determined by alphabetization with the letter-by-letter system (6) in which the letters of an entry or heading, beginning with the first letter, are considered one by one whether or not one or more breaks occur in the sequence because of spaces between terms. This is the system used to sequence entries in dictionaries; it is particularly simple to use in alphabetizing author names and eliminates having to remember the complex rules in the alternative word-by-word system.

> adrenal cortex
> adrenalectomy
> adrenal gland
> adrenalone

Discussions of the word-by-word system can be found in standard general style manuals (2,4).

Prefixes that serve as locants and positional and stereoisomer descriptors in chemical names (see sections 16.26 and 16.27 and Table 16.6) are ignored for alphabetization; the Greek and Latin multiplying prefixes such as "di-" and "bis-" (see section 16.25) are not. Do not use the articles "the", "a", and "an".

> amoxicillin
> cAMP
> amphetamine
> D-amphetamine

The Merck Index (7) is a good guide for alphabetization of chemical names. Note that Greek letters written out as a word are taken into account in the alphabetization.

> alopecia areata
> alpha 1-antitrypsin
> alpha particles
> alphaprodine

In alphabetizing the entries for names of authors, use the last names as they appear on the article and ignore the complex rules in book indexing that lead to indexing "von Hoff" under "H" and grouping together Irish and Scottish names beginning with "Mac" and "Mc".

FORMAT OF INDEXES

4.11   Because of their length, indexes should be set in as small a type size as seems acceptable to readers. Alphabetic groups of entries (the "A", "B", and so-on groups) should be separated by 2 or 3 lines of space to simplify reading.

Indentations from the left margin of the column for runover lines and for short versions of titles under the subject headings help to clarify the structure of the indexes.

Some variations in typefaces for elements of indexes can make the various elements stand out; this is the basis for the use of boldface for the subject headings in the examples in section 4.7.

REFERENCES

1. CBE Style Manual Committee. Indexing. In: CBE style manual: a guide for authors, editors, and publishers in the biological sciences. 5th ed. Bethesda, Maryland: Council of Biology Editors; 1983:113–23.
2. Indexes. In: The Chicago manual of style. 13th ed. Chicago: University of Chicago Press; 1982:511–557.
3. Longyear M, ed. Making the index. In: The McGraw-Hill style manual: a concise guide for writers and editors. New York: McGraw-Hill; 1983:285–299.
4. Indexes. In: Webster's standard American style manual. Springfield, Massachusetts: Merriam-Webster; 1985:253–287.
5. National Library of Medicine. Medical subject headings 1985. Bethesda, Maryland: National Library of Medicine; 1985; NIH publication no. 85–265. Published annually as Part 2 of the January issue of *Index Medicus*.
6. CBE Style Manual Committee. CBE style manual: a guide for authors, editors, and publishers in the biological sciences. 5th ed. Bethesda, Maryland: Council of Biology Editors; 1983:122–3.
7. Windholz M, ed. The Merck index. Rahway, New Jersey: Merck; 1983.

Chapter 5

Punctuation

Marks of punctuation clarify meaning and make easier the reading aloud of text and other printed matter. In scientific writing, the first function is far more important. Thus a decision to use or not use a punctuation mark should hinge mainly on how the mark would support the logic and sense of the text. The rationales of punctuation are discussed thoroughly in Partridge's little masterpiece, *You Have a Point There* (1); he comments, ". . . English — or if you prefer, British and American — punctuation is predominantly constructional or grammatical or logical . . .".

5.1   Three principles can guide the writer in deciding whether to place a punctuation mark at a particular point.

1. Always use punctuation marks called for by firmly established, internationally accepted conventions of style.
2. When in doubt, use a mark; it will probably reduce ambiguity of meaning.
3. When meaning is clear because of a format that clearly and logically isolates elements of text so as to support its meaning, omit punctuation that might otherwise be needed.

Punctuation marks are considered here in a sequence determined by their uses in relation to sentences. The marks for the ends of sentences — period, question mark, exclamation point — come first. They are followed by the marks for breaks within sentences: colon, semicolon, comma, dash, parenthesis marks, square brackets, apostrophe, and hyphen. Ellipsis points, quotation marks, and the slant line are referred to here but discussed in detail in other chapters. All of these marks also serve, of course, functions other than punctuation of text.

Many minor details of punctuation that rarely have to be considered in medical and other scientific writing are discussed in standard manuals of style: *The Chicago Manual of Style* (2), *The McGraw-Hill Style Manual* (3), and *Webster's Standard American Style Manual* (4). Punctuation specific to documents published by the United States Government Printing Office is described in its own style manual (5).

PERIOD (FULL STOP)

5.2   The period has 3 main functions: closing sentences; marking section, paragraph, and list designators; and closing bibliographic groups in references.

The mark we call the period is also used for other functions: decimal point (see section 13.4); raised period or center dot (multiplication sign; see section 14.6); superscript dot (see section 16.60 and Tables 16.19 and 16.20); ellipsis mark (in a group of 3; see section 6.6); and, in a row ("leader"), to lead the eye from a left-hand element of text to a right-hand element in such formats as tables of contents, indexes, and lists.

The period is referred to in British usage as the *full stop. Period* is the preferred term because the question mark and the exclamation mark also serve to mark complete, or full, stops at the ends of sentences. Partridge (1) comments: "Of ... *period* and *full stop*, the former is preferred by most scholars and printers, the latter by most other people. Nobody will go to heaven for using *period*, nor to hell for using *full stop.*" Because the term *period* still refers in literary analysis to "a complex sentence of which the meaning remains in suspense until the completion of the sentence" (6), the term *period mark* might be used. But because this meaning is so rarely used away from discussions of literary style, *period* for the mark seems adequate.

PERIOD: CLOSURE OF SENTENCES

5.3   The period closes 3 kinds of sentences.

1. Declarative sentences.

   Weights did not change during the drug trial.

2. Imperative sentences not needing rhetorical emphasis.

   Stop the drip when the blood pressure begins to rise.

3. Incomplete sentences conceptually acceptable in the context of complete sentences.

   If we did not have antibiotics, where would we be? Back in medieval medicine. We could, of course, treat infections with surgery.

Note that the last use also applies to statements in vertically arrayed lists when the statements can be read as completions of a portion of the sentence introducing the list and the list is not punctuated in its entirety as a single sentence.

> The student physician needs at least three devices.
> > A stethoscope, preferably a diaphragmatic type. [read as "The student physician needs a stethoscope . . ."]
> > A reflex hammer. [read as "The student physician needs a reflex hammer."]
> > [and so on]

Also see the punctuation for the list at the beginning of this section.

PERIOD: SECTION, PARAGRAPH, AND LIST DESIGNATORS

5.4   Designators heading sections of text or identifying elements in a tabular list in legal style (see section 2.26) may be closed with a period when the designators are single letters or numbers and are not closed with a single parenthesis mark. If the designators contain 2 or more elements (as in the designator for this section, "5.4", place a period between the elements.

a. Xxxxxx xx or	a) Xxxxxx xx	1. Xxxxxx xx
b. Xxx xxxx	b) Xxx xxxx	1.1 Xxx xxxx
c. Xx xxxxx	c) Xx xxxxx	1.1.1 Xxxxxxxx
		1.1.2 Xxxx
		1.2 Xxxx xxxxxx

The period is sometimes used to close a text heading that is followed by text on the same line (a "run-in" heading); see section 2.11. A period will not be needed in this location if the typeface of the heading and the space between the heading and the beginning of the text clearly distinguish the heading from the text.

PERIOD: MARK FOR ABBREVIATIONS

5.5   The period is widely used in the United States to close abbreviations, particularly those ending in lowercase letters, but this style is not recommended in this manual and the British style is preferred (see section 11.3).

PERIOD: CLOSURE IN BIBLIOGRAPHIC REFERENCES

5.6   The period closes a bibliographic group in bibliographic references (see section 15.24 and Table 15.2).

> Smith TH, Brown S, Jones ES. Endoscopic treatment of . . .

QUESTION MARK

5.7   The question mark serves as a full stop to close interrogatory sentences and in some other functions.

QUESTION MARK: CLOSURE OF SENTENCES

The question mark closes 2 kinds of interrogatory sentences.

1. Direct questions.

   What is the best antibiotic for treatment of pneumococcal pneumonia?

2. Declarative sentences serving as a question in the rhetorical context.

   This is the time to cut back on Medicare funding?

The question mark also closes a declarative sentence that ends with an interrogatory element even if that element is not enclosed by quotation marks.

Again and again the house officer asks, why are we not paid more when our services earn so much for the department of medicine?

QUESTION MARK: FUNCTIONS WITHIN TEXT

Uncertainty about a datum can be indicated by a question mark immediately following it.

Girolamo Fracastoro (1483?–1553) was in effect the conceptual father of the notion of infectious disease.

See section 16.36 and Table 16.14 for the question mark indicating uncertain identification of a chromosome or chromosomal structure.

EXCLAMATION MARK

5.8   The exclamation mark, also referred to in some style manuals (2,4) as the exclamation point, need be used only rarely in scientific writing; it can be used as a full stop to close a sentence and indicate forceful statement or great surprise whether the sentence is declaratory or interrogatory.

This country has had enough of governmental attempts to define quality practice!

Haven't we had enough of governmental interference in medical practice!

The only common scientific use of the exclamation mark is to indicate a factorial number in equations or other mathematical statements.

$$3! = 1 \times 2 \times 3$$

COLON

5.9   The functions of the colon can be divided into 3 groups: the annunciating functions, the coupling functions, and the special conventions [fn1]. In its annunciating functions the colon sits just short of serving as a full stop; it tells readers in effect that they have not come to the end of the sentence but must pause and be aware that an important and concluding component is about to be delivered. In its coupling functions the colon serves simply to couple elements that must be tied together for complete meaning but that are thus identified as separate to emphasize their individual meanings. In the special conventions the colon has been assigned a specific and arbitrary function for a particular content.

COLON: ANNUNCIATING FUNCTIONS

5.10   Within a sentence the colon can mark a pause less complete than a full stop (period, question mark, or exclamation mark) to announce to the reader that what follows has great weight in completing the full meaning of the sentence. This announcement serves 3 main groups of uses.

1. To introduce a long or notably formal quotation (without quotation marks) or statement (declaratory or interrogative sentence).

   A compassionate physician never forgets Peabody's most memorable aphorism: One of the essential qualities of the clinician is interest in humanity, for the secret of the care of the patient is in caring for the patient.

2. To introduce a following word, phrase, or clause that illustrates, defines, or elaborates on, the meaning of the preceding part of the sentence.

   The government's handling of medical insurance can be summed up in one word: disaster.

3. To introduce a list.

   The complete clinical encounter has three components: the interview, the examination, and the closing dialogue that takes up with the patient the next steps in care.

Note that if the list is immediately preceded by a verb the sequence should not be interrupted by a colon.

---

fn1: This classification is in part an adaptation of Partridge's thirteen uses (7) of the colon: annunciatory, explanatory, appositive, equipoised, parallel, antithetic, compensatory, interpolative, substitutive, cumulative, conclusive, promotional, and non-punctuational. Partridge concedes that many of these uses are similar; the differing nuances seem hardly worth preserving for scientific writing. His "explanatory" and "appositive" uses can, for example, be logically covered by "annunciatory".

NOT   The three components of the encounter are: the interview . . .
BUT   The three components of the encounter are the interview, the exam-
        ination, and . . .
OR   The three components of the encounter are the following: the inter-
        view, the examination, and . . .

(The first of the 2 alternatives is preferred; the second represents a structure more likely to be needed for a longer and more complex listing.)
If the list is to be formatted in a vertical array of its parts to emphasize
visually the components (see section 2.26), the colon is used as in the
example above if the remaining punctuation for all elements is also proper
for a complete sentence.

The complete clinical encounter has three components:
    the interview,
    the examination, and
    the closing dialogue.

But if the list is complex and its components need their own punctuation, close the introductory sentence with a period, punctuate the components appropriately, and let the format make clear the relations in
meaning of the components to the introductory sentence and to each
other.

The thorough clinician will go through a complete clinical encounter in
three steps.
    a) He will take a history, paying careful attention to everything the
       patient says, for important clues may lie in little details.
    b) He will examine the patient efficiently, omitting no potentially import-
       ant maneuvers but wasting no time on looking for diagnostically
       antiquated signs.
    c) He will conclude with a dialogue sensitive to all of the patient's needs:
       an answer, some comfort, and clear instruction.

Also see section 5.3.

COLON: COUPLING FUNCTIONS

5.11   The colon serves 4 coupling functions.

1. Coupling 2 independent clauses closely related in structure and content (even if antithetical) and equal in weight of meaning.

   Respect the patient's privacy: respond to the family's need to know.

   (Most contemporary writers would probably prefer the semicolon in
   this example; the colon is, however, the more commanding division
   of such a sentence.)

2. Coupling elements of titles such as book titles (see section 15.24 and
   Table 15.2), chapter titles (see section 2.2), and table titles (see section 2.19).

The Independent Practitioner: Practice Management for the Allied Health Professional

Chapter 2: Hemodynamic Methods

Table 3: Hemodynamic functions in ten asymptomatic patients

3. Coupling components of a time datum in the 12-hour system (but see section 13.21) and of an elapsed-time datum, and seconds to the rest of the datum in the 12-hour and 24-hour systems.

1:55 PM . . . at precisely 7:12:49 AM . . . at exactly 2319:36 . . . . . . the stopwatch read 8:17:33 . . .

4. Coupling the elements of a ratio or proportion.

. . . the ratio of women to men was 3:1 when they . . .

. . . the suicidal patient ingested at least 2 or 3 kilograms of 5:10:5 fertilizer.

COLON: SPECIAL CONVENTIONS

5.12 The colon is used in 3 special conventions.

1. Within bibliographic groups in bibliographic references as a delimiter (see section 15.24 and Table 15.2).

Smith A. The interview: a new method. Clin Med. 1998;76:11–2.

2. In biblical references between chapter and verse designators (see section 15.55).

Major surgery was first described in Genesis 2:21.

3. To symbolize a chromosomal break (see section 16.36 and Table 16.14).

DOUBLE COLON

5.13 The double colon is used infrequently in scientific writing. In genetics it symbolizes a chromosomal break and reunion (see section 16.36 and Table 16.14).

SEMICOLON

5.14 The semicolon stands between the colon and the comma as a mark of pause and linkage. Partridge (8) stated its strength nicely: "Stronger, more decisive than the comma, the semicolon is slightly weaker, slightly less decisive than the colon, and considerably weaker than the period; it is, however, both slightly stronger and noticeably more elegant than the dash".

The semicolon is used most frequently to separate clauses.

1. Two or more coordinate clauses whether or not joined by a conjunctive adverb such as *however*, but generally not clauses joined by a simple conjunction such as *and*.

   The patient was first treated in the emergency room; shortly, however, she had to be transferred to the intensive care unit.

   We proved our first hypothesis; our second hypothesis was more difficult to support

   NOT   The nurse removed the sutures; and the patient was discharged.
   BUT   The nurse removed the sutures, and the patient was discharged.

   (Note in section 5.11 the use of the colon to separate 2 coordinate clauses of equal weight and similar structure. Also note that very short clauses may be separated by commas; see section 5.17.)

2. Two or more clauses of which at least 1 is internally punctuated with the comma or dash and even if they are connected by a conjunction.

   The nurse removed the sutures; the patient, disregarding his physician's advice, insisted on being discharged.

   The nurse, acting on an order from the surgeon, removed the sutures; and the patient, disregarding the surgeon's advice, insisted on being discharged.

3. Two clauses, the second of which is structurally parallel but grammatically elliptical.

   In women the most important etiologic factor is natural or surgical menopause; the second, inadequate dietary calcium.

The semicolon separates the elements of a series when the elements need their own internal punctuation.

   In 1989, outbreaks of animal rabies were reported from three rural towns: West Branch, Pennsylvania; Whistle Post, Iowa; and Lone Cypress, Texas.

The semicolon has 2 technical uses.

1. Delimits some elements of bibliographic groups in bibliographic references (see section 15.24 and Table 15.2).

   Jones R. Shigellosis. Rev Hosp Infect. 1956;2:1-3.

2. Symbolizes human chromosomal breaks (see section 16.36 and Table 16.14).

COMMA

5.15 After the period, the comma is probably the most frequent mark of punctuation. The large number of rules in style manuals for its use reflects the difficulties in defining its use. Despite the sense of inexperienced punctuators that the comma serves mainly to mark points of pause for reading aloud, most of its uses serve to help in conveying meaning by clarifying the relation of sentence elements to each other.

Generously long sections on the comma can be found in several of the general manuals of style (2–4); that in *The McGraw-Hill Style Manual* (3) is notably helpful for its look at the comma in terms of functions. Partridge's chapter on the comma (9) pays close attention to the relation of comma uses to qualities of literary style.

The comma has 4 groups of uses: delimiting the end of an introductory element of a sentence; separating elements for clear meaning; bracketing some elements; and special scientific uses. Some of these uses represent similar or identical functions.

THE INTRODUCTORY COMMA

5.16 The comma can serve to mark the end of an element at the beginning of a sentence and thereby signal that the main part of the sentence is about to begin.

1. A long subordinate phrase or clause that precedes the principal clause.

   When two treatments appear to be about equally efficacious and safe, great weight should be given to the patient's preference.

2. Transitional words and phrases such as *finally, meanwhile, after all.*

   To be sure, we have no really effective treatment for obesity.

3. Short words of emphasis or address.

   No, state insurance is not the answer.
   Doctors, you all need malpractice insurance regardless of your specialty.

A short introductory element need not be followed by a comma if the omission would not confuse the reader and a sense of quick flow in the sentence is desirable.

Note that opening absolute phrases must be followed by a comma.

Other possibilities for pain relief having been exhausted, cordotomy was recommended to the patient.

THE COMMA OF SEPARATION

5.17 The comma is used to separate various long and short elements within sentences and at the end of sentences.

Independent clauses connected by a coordinating conjunction such as *and, but, or* are separated with a comma.

> The patient was treated with a broad-spectrum antibiotic, but the pneumonia failed to resolve.

The comma may be omitted in such sentences for an effect of rapid flow in the sentence. The comma may be omitted between 2 short independent clauses.

> We tried surgery and we failed.

If the independent clauses contain internal punctuation such as commas, they should be separated by the semicolon rather than the comma (see section 5.14).

Separate compound adjectives by a comma if an *and* would be appropriate in place of the comma.

> After some dissection we reached a necrotic, bleeding tumor.

Do not use a slant line in place of the comma.

> NOT   a low-carbohydrate/low-fat diet
> BUT   a low-carbohydrate, low-fat diet

Words, phrases, and short clauses forming a series of 3 elements or more are separated by commas, including a comma preceding an *and* before the last element.

> Fair, fat, and forty used to be the epigrammatic description of the woman with acute cholecystitis.
>
> Men, women, and children all suffer from the same symptoms in this disease.
>
> The infection usually localizes in the ear, brain, and spinal cord.
>
> I came, I felt, I cut.

Some writers prefer to omit the comma before the conjunction in a series — as in "the ear, brain and spinal cord" — when they decide that no confusion of meaning could result from omitting it, but routine use of this comma saves time from not having to pause to come to a decision.

5.18   The comma is used to separate citation numbers (see section 2.12 and 15.7) but an *and* is not used before the last number; consecutive numbers are represented by their first and last connected by an en dash (1 hyphen in typing).

> NOT   (1, 3, 4, and 9)   BUT   (1,3,4,9)
> NOT   (1, 2, 3, 4)   BUT   (1–4)

In text that must be searchable for specific reference numbers by a computer program, the hyphenated range should not be used; all reference numbers must be given.

NOT   (1–4)   BUT   (1,2,3,4)
NOT   (1–3, 5–7)   BUT (1,2,3,5,6,7)

The comma separates 2 elements in an elliptical construction.

Some patients prefer mineral oil as a laxative; others, milk of magnesia.

Here the comma substitutes for the "prefer" omitted after "others".

THE BRACKETING COMMA

5.19   The function of the bracketing comma is like that of the separating comma, but it is used in pairs within sentences around an element to separate it from the main stream of elements. The writer must be sure that the second comma of the pair is not omitted. Comma pairs are thus used to bracket 4 kinds of elements.

1. Non-restrictive clauses and phrases: their omission would not change the main point of the sentences (see the discussion, *"which; that"*, in section 17.4).

   This method of suturing, tried elsewhere without success, turned out to be the best method.

   The clinical description, which one of our residents found in an obscure nineteenth-century German journal, fit our patient's picture perfectly.

2. Appositive words or phrases following a noun.

   One French city, Paris, was then the real center of European medicine.

3. Interjections, words of address, parenthetical statements.

   Penicillin, alas, was not available in this remote spot.

   Ravdin, and I shall never forget his pudgy figure, was always the first man in the operating suite each morning.

4. Short elements needed for complete meaning but conventionally bracketed when within sentences: examples and their introductory words or phrases, state names with town and city names, year in the month-day-year statement (but not in a day-month-year statement), academic degrees with names. When such elements are at the end of a sentence, only the initial comma is used.

   Some names from nineteenth-century American medicine, for example, Drake and Osler, will always stand out in our minds.

   Experimental centers were first established in Rochester, Minnesota, and Rochester, New York. The first unit was opened on May 5, 1989, and the second on June 16, 1990. (*But*: The first unit was opened on 5 May 1989 and the second on 16 June 1990.)

The first chairman of the department was Robert Smith, Jr, MD, PhD.

COMMA: SPECIAL USES

5.20   The comma is used as a delimiter between subelements of bibliographic groups in bibliographic references (see section 15.26 and Table 15.2).

Smith TH, Brown SH, Jones GI. Endoscopy and the . . .

Letters and numbers identifying the location of an atom or group in a molecule (locants) are separated from each other by commas but unspaced (see section 16.26 and Table 16.6).

1,4-cyclohexadiene   1,2-dichloroethane

Commas separate amino acid residues in an unknown sequence (see section 16.30).

Asp-His-Pro(Leu,Phe,Trp)-Lys

Certain elements in symbolic representation of human chromosomes are separated by commas (see section 16.36 and Table 16.14).

DASH

5.21   The dash has several varieties of which only 2, the em dash and the en dash, are widely used in scientific writing. The em dash is so named because its length in a typeface approximates the width of the capital letter M; the en dash is about half the length of the em dash and slightly longer than the hyphen. In typing, the em dash should be represented by 2 hyphens and the en dash by 1; the copy editor marking a typescript for the printer will distinguish among the 3 signs by appropriate marks. In the remainder of this chapter "dash" refers to the em dash.

EM DASH

5.22   The dash (2 hyphens in typing) is used most frequently to indicate elements in a sentence that express a sharp break in the sentence's line of meaning. Such elements represent a parenthetic thought or, in a stage term, an aside; they usually make an explanatory, defining, summarizing, elaborating, or emphasizing statement, and the statement is one that could be omitted without loss of the sentence's essential meaning.

Osteoporosis — and the diagnosis is hard to make early without expensive equipment — may be the most common disorder among postmenopausal women in the United States.

Smith spent 10 years at Johns Hopkins—they may have been the best years of his professional life—before he took up his post in San Francisco.

The comma and the parenthesis marks serve similar functions, but the 3 marks have differing degrees of strength of interruption. As Partridge (10) puts it, "The dash . . . resembles parentheses, in that, in one important function, it expresses rather more strongly, rather more abruptly, what parentheses express less strongly and much more smoothly". Elements in a sentence set off by 1 or 2 commas usually have less of the parenthetic, or "aside", quality.

The dash can signal the beginning of a summary statement completing a sentence.

Halsted, Kelly, Osler, Welch—they were the "big four" at Johns Hopkins.

The dash is conventionally used to signify the author of a quotation set apart from running text or of a free-standing short text (such as an editor's note).

What is a doctor? A licensed executioner.
—Mazarinade

Publication here of Dr. Smith's letter should not be taken as representing approval of its content by the APA.—The Editor

TWO-EM DASH

5.23   The 2-em dash (4 hyphens in typing) can signify omission of known or unknown letters or words.

The patient gasped, "I have a pain in my——", and fell back dead.

Patient P—— was first seen in the emergency room with chest pain.

EN DASH

5.24   The most common use of the en dash (1 hyphen in typing) in medical writing is to link the numbers representing a range of values such as hours, days, ages, or a sequence of numbered items such as pages in a bibliographic reference and reference numbers in a citation (see section 15.7). The preferred connector, except in bibliographic uses (see section 15.20 and Table 15.2) and some chemical conventions, is the word "to"; see section 13.5

ages 10 to 15   Cases 3 to 7   The clinic hours were 1000 to 1630.

Jones R. Diarrhea and constipation. Scalpel. 1922;103:79–84.

. . . and previous reports (41–56) described . . .

Numeric ranges sometimes include minus numbers, such as temperatures, weight losses, confidence intervals (see section 14.10), financial data; the en dash is readily confused with the minus sign, and use of the "to" eliminates this ambiguity.

... in environmental temperatures in the range -5 to $+27$ °C
CL, -10 to 55%
.... with weight changes of -3.5 to $+7.2$ kg

This style should be preferred for ranges of numerical data by journals with papers reporting such data even if only infrequently. But the en dash convention should nevertheless be used as the convention for linking reference numbers in citations and pages in bibliographic references.

The en dash can serve a hyphen-like function as a connective in a compound or hyphenated modifier.

Columbia-Presbyterian–Brigham combined cases

HYPHEN

5.25 The hyphen serves 2 groups of functions: linkage of word and term elements; linkage of elements of chemical names. For discussion of the first group of functions, see sections 9.14 and 9.15.

The hyphen is used in 5 chemical conventions.

1. Representation of single bonds

   $(CH_3)_2\text{-}CH\text{-}CH_2\text{-}CH(H_2)\text{-}COOH$

2. Designation of the position of an element (see section 16.21)

   C-3 (for the carbon atom at position 3)

3. Linkage of amino acid residues in a known sequence (see section 16.30)

   Leu-Glx-Pro-Ser-Thr-Ala

   (For linkage by commas in an unknown sequence, see section 16.30.)

4. Linkage of nucleotides in polynucleotides (see section 16.31)

   pG-A-C-C-T-T-A-G-C-A-A-T-Gp

5. Linkage between locants (see section 16.26 and Table 16.6) and the term they modify

   1,3-dichloroethane

PARENTHESIS MARKS (ROUND BRACKETS)

5.26 Paired parenthesis marks have 2 main uses: enclosure of parenthetic text (a parenthesis) and enclosure of non-parenthetic text in some specific style conventions.

Paired parenthesis marks are widely called "parentheses" and a single mark, "a parenthesis". But *parenthesis* is a specific term in rhetoric (11): "a word, phrase, or sentence inserted as an aside in a sentence complete in itself". Why not reserve *parenthesis* as a highly specific, and hence clearly useful, term for this definition? Then *parenthesis marks* is itself a highly specific term: marks that mark a parenthesis. Note that the equivalent British term, *round brackets*, has the value of preserving *parenthesis* for its rhetorical meaning.

PAIRED PARENTHESIS MARKS: PARENTHETIC TEXT

5.27 Paired parenthesis marks can be used to mark the beginning and end of text that is not in the main line of meaning of the sentence. Such text may be of a number of different kinds.

The first kind of parenthetic text is digressive statement.

> Osteoporosis (and some other disorders of old age too uncommon to discuss here) is a difficult diagnosis to make in its early stages.

This use is not unlike similar uses of the comma and the dash. A pair of commas holds what it encloses closer to the main line of thought in the sentence; the dash more arrestingly signals to the reader's eye that the enclosed statement is digressive; a parenthesis mark is a less arresting signal and hence in general should be used in pairs more frequently in scientific writing than dashes to mark digressive statements. Note in the example above that the parenthetic statement is grammatically outside the sentence in that the singular predicate "is" does not apply to the plural term "disorders". Also see the comments in section 5.22.

In this use with digressive statements the parenthesis and the marks enclosing it are spaced from the adjacent text; for direct connection to an adjacent element see section 5.28.

In general, a complete sentence within parenthesis marks in a sentence does not open with a capital letter or close with a period, but a question mark or exclamation mark can be used when it is appropriate. A parenthetic complete sentence standing outside of a sentence should have the normal initial capital letter and closing full stop.

There are 2 more kinds of parenthetic text that should be enclosed by paired parenthesis marks.

1. Defining or explanatory text

A scientific name defining a common name (see section 10.5)

> . . . sera of African green monkeys (*Cercopithecus aethiops*) . . .

A brand name specifying a particular product (see sections 10.3 and 10.4)

> . . . in a trial of cimetidine (Tagamet, Smith Kline & French Laboratories) . . .

A nonstandard abbreviation to be used subsequently in the same text (see section 11.2)

> ... patients with the acquired immunodeficiency syndrome (AIDS) in New York and ...

2. Directive text

A citation (see sections 2.12 and 15.6)

> ... in a review (37) by Smith and his associates ...

A cross-reference

> ... and other guides (see the MMWR recommendations preceding this paper; reference 26) ...

For a detailed discussion of punctuation that may be used with paired parenthesis marks, consult *Webster's Standard American Style Manual* (12).

PAIRED PARENTHESIS MARKS: OTHER USES

5.28   Various conventions require enclosure of specified data or other text elements with paired parenthesis marks.

1. Certain bibliographic data in references (see sections 15.31 and 15.32 and Table 15.2)

   > Mastri AR. Neuropathy of diabetic neurogenic bladder. Ann Intern Med. 1980;92(2 Pt 2):316–8.

2. Mathematical elements that must be grouped for implied operations (see section 14.6)

   > $z = k(a + b + c)$

3. Biochemical and other chemical conventions (see section 16.21) Molecular components that must be grouped to define the application of a subscript number

   > $K_4Fe(CN)_6 \cdot 3H_2O$ $(CH_3)_2CHCH_2CH(NH_2)COOH$

   Molecular components that must be grouped within a component of the formula enclosed by square brackets (see section 16.21)

   > 3-[(*p*-chloro)oxy]-1-methylpyrrolidine maleate

   Oxidation numbers (see section 16.21)

   > Pb(IV)

   Unknown sequences of amino acids in polypeptides (see section 16.30)

   > (Asp,His,Pro)

Immunoglobulin notations (see section 16.32)

Gm(1, −2, 3, 4, 5)   IgG(Pr)

4. Symbolization for structurally altered chromosomes (see section 16.36 and Table 16.14)

46,XX,t(4;13)(p21;q32)

5. Specificities of histocompatibility leukocyte antigens (see section 16.48)

HLA-Bw56(w22)

6. Multi-letter symbols representing single physiologic variables (see sections 16.17 and 16.60)

(GFR)   [glomerular filtration rate]
(LVEDP)   [left ventricular end-diastolic pressure]

7. Area codes in US and Canadian telephone numbers

(215) 243-1201

CLOSING PARENTHESIS MARK

5.29   The second parenthesis mark of the paired marks may be used by itself to demarcate numerals or letters introducing elements in a list or a series.

a) The period   1) Syphilis
b) The colon   2) Tuberculosis
c) The semicolon   3) Gonorrhea

Three infections almost wiped out the South Sea populations in the early nineteenth century: 1) syphilis, 2) tuberculosis, and 3) gonorrhea.

This use in a series in running text usually can be avoided with distinctive punctuation; in the example sentence above, semicolons after the first and second enumerated terms would adequately separate the 3 terms.

SQUARE BRACKETS

5.30   Square brackets are used mainly to mark inserted text or letters and for some mathematical and chemical conventions.

The term *square brackets* is more British than American, but it deserves wider use. The term *brackets* for this pair is unsatisfactory because it also serves to cover parenthesis marks and a third type of bracket pair, { }, often called "curly brackets". Partridge (13) prefers *square parentheses* but this term has little currency.

SQUARE BRACKETS: INSERTED TEXT OR LETTERS

5.31   Text may have to be added by the author to a quotation to amplify it or to clarify otherwise obscure elements; the added elements are demarcated with square brackets.

> Cushing (15) commented, "When Osler moved [to Baltimore], he was not risking his future".
>
> The last entry in his diary was "I dined with O[sler] last night and then had a few drinks at the club with P[erkins]".

A closely related use is marking a change in the original form of a word in a quotation to fit it properly into the new context.

In rare instances an editor might feel compelled to add square-bracketed text to an author's original text, but this practice should be avoided and the author asked to make the change instead. In scientific journals the more justifiable editorial addition that should be placed within square brackets is bibliographic information added to clarify a reference (see Table 15.2).

SQUARE BRACKETS: MULTIPLE BRACKETING

5.32   Text within parenthesis marks may need parenthetic bracketing.

> . . . was recommended for the treatment of syphilis (see the MMWR statement [17] issued a year ago) but a later recommendation . . .

Mathematical aggregations may need multiple-bracketing to represent a sequence of operations (see section 14.6).

$$z = k[(a + b) + (c + d)]$$

Unless another convention specifies a different sequence, the general sequence for multiple bracketing in mathematics and chemistry convention is { [( )] }. Note that this is the reverse of the sequence used in text and illustrated at the beginning of this section.

SQUARE BRACKETS: CHEMICAL CONVENTIONS

Use square brackets for chemical concentrations (see section 16.20)

$[Cl^-]$ $[HCO_3^-]$ $[Na^+]$

and for isotopic prefixes (see section 16.21).

$[^{32}P]AMP$ $[^{14}C_2]$glycolic acid

OTHER PUNCTUATION MARKS

QUOTATION MARKS

See Chapter 6: Quotation and Ellipses.

APOSTROPHE

See section 9.23.

PRIME SIGN

5.33   The prime sign is used in chemical notation (see section 16.26) but is often represented in a typescript by the apostrophe. For use of the prime sign in geographic coordinates, see section 13.14.

THE SLANT LINE

5.34   The slant line is also known by other terms: diagonal, shilling mark, slash, solidus, stroke, and virgule. Its main scientific uses are in mathematical notation (see section 14.6) and units of measurement (see section 13.15). It is also used to separate terms in genotypic representation (see section 16.37).

Do not use the slant line as a substitute for the comma (see section 5.17). Avoid using such constructions as "he/she" and "and/or" that are lazy escapes from more precise statement.

AMPERSAND

5.35   The ampersand (&) is sometimes discussed in style manuals as a punctuation mark, but it is more accurately described as a symbol for the word *and*. It should not be thus used in scientific text. The sole exception is retaining it when it is part of the proper name of a company, as in "John Wiley & Sons" (see section 15.21).

REFERENCES

1. Partridge E. You have a point there. London: Routledge & Kegan Paul; 1953:9.
2. The Chicago manual of style: for authors, editors, and copywriters. 13th ed. Chicago: University of Chicago Press; 1982.
3. Longyear M, ed. The McGraw-Hill style manual: a concise guide for writers and editors. New York: McGraw-Hill; 1982.
4. Webster's standard American style manual. Springfield, Massachusetts: Merriam-Webster; 1985.
5. United States Government Printing Office style manual: 1984. Washington: United States Government Printing Office; 1984.
6. Read H. English prose style. New York: Pantheon Books; 1952:43.

7. Partridge E. You have a point there. London: Routledge & Kegan Paul; 1953:52–62.
8. Partridge E. You have a point there. London: Routledge & Kegan Paul; 1953:44.
9. Partridge E. You have a point there. London: Routledge & Kegan Paul; 1953:14–41.
10. Partridge E. You have a point there. London: Routledge & Kegan Paul; 1953:68.
11. Lanham RA. A handlist of rhetorical terms: a guide for students of English literature. Berkeley, California: University of California Press; 1969:72.
12. Webster's standard American style manual. Springfield, Massachusetts: Merriam-Webster; 1985:35–6.

Chapter 6

Quotation and Ellipsis

Some of the recommendations in this chapter depart from conventional American style and draw on British style to simplify the punctuating of quotations.

QUOTATION

6.1   Quotations can be presented in either of 2 styles: run-in or set-off. A run-in quotation is carried entirely within a text sentence, is set in the same type size, and is demarcated with quotation marks. A set-off quotation is presented outside the other text sentences and in a format that distinguishes it as a quotation. The choice in scientific writing between the 2 styles is usually determined by the length of the quotation. Short quotations, such as single words, phrases, or single sentences, should be run-in quotations; longer quotations, likely to be quoted text rather than personal statements, should usually be set-off quotations.

RUN-IN QUOTATION

6.2   A direct primary quotation is demarcated with double quotation-marks; if there is a quotation within it, the internal quotation is marked with single quotation-marks [fn1]. A direct quotation that was a complete statement (one or more sentences) in its original form is preceded by a comma and opens with a capital letter; it closes with its own full stop only if the stop is a question mark or exclamation mark and is needed for the support of sense or force. If the full stop in the original of the quotation was a period or was a quotation mark or exclamation mark that is not needed, the quotation's full stop is omitted and the quoting

---

fn1: The usual British style (1) is single quotation marks for the primary quotation and double quotation marks for the internal quotation.

sentence's full stop alone is used. The quoting sentence's full stop follows the closing quotation mark. (Note that omission of some of the closing part of the original statement quoted can be marked with the ellipsis mark; see section 6.6.)

> When I asked him to name his most important paper, he replied, "I have no idea which is my most important paper, but my most cited paper is that on a modification of the colorimetric method for estimation of serum creatinine".

> As soon as the talk was over, he leapt to his feet and shouted, "That proposal is a proposal for socialized medicine". [In the context of "leapt" and "shouted" the exclamation mark, which was not actually spoken by the speaker, can be omitted.]

Note that in both examples the closing double quotation-mark is placed before the period of the entire sentence. The general rule is that the full stop (period, question mark, or exclamation mark) for the sentence carrying the quotation comes last and is preceded by the closing quotation mark, itself preceded by the quotation's full stop only if that stop is a needed exclamation mark or question mark. This rule draws on British style (1) for the closing of a run-in quotation. It is close to the rule established in 1978 by the American Chemical Society and presented in its 1986 style manual (2); it responds to a plea in the style manual (3) of the American Mathematical Society for a logical use of quotation marks. The merits of this style are discussed in detail by Partridge (4); its logical superiority over the usual American convention is pointed to by the American authors Morris and Morris (5):

> Generations of American typesetters have insisted that the quotes always fall outside periods (commas, too, for that matter) regardless of the sense of the sentence. The theory is that the quotes help fill the small spot of white that would be left if the comma or period came outside the quote. To see the ridiculousness of this argument, you need only read a book or magazine printed in England. The eye quickly becomes used to quotation marks put where they logically belong and you soon become accustomed to that "small spot of white" that is supposed to be so bothersome.

In essence, the American typesetters' preference for keeping the period as close as possible to the end of the last word in the sentence, as it is when a quotation mark is not needed at the close, has been arbitrary and illogical.

The most thorough and logical discussion of the terminal punctuation of a sentence closing with a run-in quotation is that by the Fowlers in *The King's English* (6). Their general rules merit partial quotation here.

1. The true stops should never stand before the second quotation-mark except

> (a) when, as in dialogue given without framework, complete sentences entirely isolated and independent in grammar are printed as quotations. . . .
> 3. The tone symbols [exclamation and question marks] should be placed before or after the second quotation-mark according as they belong to the quotation or to the containing sentence. If both quotation and containing sentence need a tone symbol, both should be used, with the quotation-mark between them.

They discuss at length possible objections to their rules. A new reason for these rules comes from the growing use of computer programs for the manipulation of text by complete sentences for revision or analysis of literary style. These programs can be applied without unnecessary difficulties only if each and every sentence closes with a full stop (period, question mark, or exclamation mark); in such programs a closing quotation mark used as a full stop, as it would be in the American convention, would lead to the amputating of sentences having quotation marks placed internally. American users of this manual are warned that if they are convinced by the logic and value of these simplifying rules and wish to apply them, they will have to insist specifically with their printers on their observance.

When the quotation is not preceded by an introductory word such as *said, replied, answered* and the quotation is syntactically a part of the sentence, the preceding comma should not be used and the initial word of the quotation should not be capitalized.

> He observed tartly that "diagnostic method is the business of the doctor, not the state".

When the quotation comes first, the general rule also applies: the quotation's full stop is omitted and the comma setting off the quotation from the sentence proper follows the rule applied to a closing quotation.

> "I cannot take any more of those pills", said the patient at the next visit.

6.3 Run-in quotations are used most frequently in medical writing not for dialogue and other similar primary quotations but for titles, terms, and translations.

Titles of journal articles, article sections, book chapters, and other such excerpts from longer works (such as encyclopedia entries, individual poems) are demarcated in text with quotation marks. Titles of complete works, such as journals, books, computer programs (software), videocassette programs, films, musical compositions, are italicized (see section 8.6).

> For a good general introduction, I recommend the paper by Sox (73), "Probability Theory in the Use of Diagnostic Tests".
> Osler's most frequently quoted essay is probably "Aequanimitas".

Most of his papers have been published in *The New England Journal of Medicine.*

For scientific word-processing, *PC Magazine* recommended *T³.*

I recommend Woody Allen's film *Interiors* to my first-year students for its compelling portrayal of the complexities of family life.

Note that the capitalization of quoted titles should be that of the title as it appears on the work and not follow the rules for capitalization in bibliographic references (see section 15.18).

6.4 Quotation marks should be used to demarcate proposed new terms and established terms used in a new, unusual, humorous, or ironic sense.

As a name for this constellation of findings we suggest "the acquired immune deficiency syndrome".

One might think of the procedure as a "hemorrhoidectomy" for the esophagus.

The translation of a foreign word or phrase should be demarcated by quotation marks even if the translation is within parenthesis marks.

His favorite motto was *guerir quelquefois, soulager souvent, consoler toujours* ("to cure sometimes, to relieve often, to comfort always").

For italicization of foreign words and phrases see section 8.8.

SET-OFF QUOTATION

6.5 Quotations of long single sentences and longer quotations are most effectively presented as set-off quotations in a column of type indented by 3 or 4 character-spaces from the left and right margins of the main text. The quotation should set in type 1 point smaller than that of the main body of text to distinguish it from the quoting text.

If the quotation is syntactically part of the sentence in which it appears, it can be introduced with a colon (see section 5.10) and quotation marks are usually not needed in such a format.

Every year at the end of his last lecture to the graduating class he made sure that he quoted his favorite passage (47) from Peabody: One of the essential qualities of the clinician is interest in humanity, for the secret of the care of the patient is in caring for the patient.

If the quotation is longer than a single sentence, the introductory statement should close with a period, not a colon; the format and the introduction make clear that the indented text extends the meaning of the introduction but is a quotation.

He always called to the attention of the class the advice (31) of Sir John Parkinson.

The common duty required of a physician lies in the recognition and treatment of disease. If he enlarges his study to cover life as affected by disease, and masters the psychology of the individual sick in body, he will widen his usefulness and reach a fuller life himself as a physician.

Note that in these 2 examples the citation number is within the quoting sentence and not at the end of the quotation itself.

ELLIPSIS

6.6 The omission of words, phrases, or longer portions of text in a quotation from its original form is termed *ellipsis*. The omission is indicated by 1 or more ellipsis marks. The ellipsis mark is often referred to informally as "3 periods".

An ellipsis mark that follows a quoted complete sentence should be preceded by that sentence's period in the usual position close to the last letter of the sentence's last word and the ellipsis mark 1 character space to the right. If the quotation resumes within a following sentence in the source of the quotation, the word at the point of resumption should not be capitalized, but if the quotation resumes at the beginning of a sentence, the usual initial capital letter should be used.

> This was Meier and Cassell's judgment (101).

> The problem . . . is complex and widely variable. . . . gradually losing a loved one to a disease that attacks the mind and spares the body . . . can be overwhelming.

(The original passage quoted: The problem for the family is complex and widely variable. The burden of gradually losing a loved one to a disease that attacks the mind and spares the body, combined with the increasing childlike dependency of the patient on the family, can be overwhelming.)

> This was Meier and Cassell's judgment (101).

> The problem for the family is complex . . . The burden of gradually losing a loved one . . . can be overwhelming.

Note that the ellipsis mark is spaced from adjacent words as if it itself were a word.

Quotations that are themselves incomplete statements should end with a 2-em dash.

> The patient said "I think I am——" and fell back dead.

A quotation with a context that indicates it is not a complete quotation need not begin and end with ellipsis marks.

> Peabody's remarks (47) about "the secret of the care of the patient" should be quoted in every lecture introducing medical students to the art of the medical interview.

An omission in a title should, however, be indicated by an ellipsis mark close to the last quoted element of the title.

> The formats for references specified in the *Uniform Requirements*. . . document are discussed later in this book.

An omission represented by a square-bracketed substitution need not be indicated by an ellipsis mark (see section 5.31).

6.7   An ellipsis mark at the end of a paragraph can be used to indicate the omission of the remainder of a paragraph or the remainder and following paragraphs. This convention is supported by *The Chicago Manual of Style* (7), which, however, points out that in literary works the omission of 1 or more paragraphs or of 1 or more lines of verse may be indicated by 1 line or em-spaced dots.

If some opening part of a new paragraph has been omitted, the ellipsis mark is itself indented to the same extent as other paragraphs so as to make clear that a new paragraph has begun in the quotation.

> The vaccine is safe. . . . Local transient side effects . . . occur in up to 40% of recipients. Systemic side effects are infrequent and rarely severe. . . .
>   [The cost is] approximately $5 per dose . . .

In the original the paragraph about cost followed an omitted paragraph; the square brackets represent a substitution for the opening of the cost paragraph.

6.8   Ellipsis marks are used in tables to indicate the lack of data for cells representing observations not made (see section 2.22).

REFERENCES

1. The Oxford guide to English usage. New York: Oxford University Press; 1983:196.
2. Dodd JS. The ACS style guide: a manual for authors and editors. Washington: American Chemical Society; 1986:18–9.
3. Swanson E. Mathematics into type. Providence, Rhode Island: American Mathematical Society; 1979.
4. Partridge E. You have a point there. London: Routledge & Kegan Paul; 1953:179–82.
5. Morris W, Morris M. Harper dictionary of contemporary usage. 2nd ed. New York: Harper & Row; 1975:503–4.
6. Fowler HW, Fowler FG. The King's English. Oxford: Oxford University Press; 1931:291–9.
7. The Chicago manual of style. 13th ed. Chicago: University of Chicago Press; 1982:294–5.

Chapter 7

Capitalization

In this chapter *capitalization* means designation of the initial letter of a word as a capital letter; for abbreviations with all capital letters, see section 11.2.

Some rules for capitalization are well established, but firm and unambiguous rules are not available for many possible uses of capitals; the recommendations here are offered as general guides.

SYNTACTIC AND TYPOGRAPHIC CAPITALIZATION

7.1 The first letter of the first word in a complete or partial sentence is capitalized whether the sentence is declarative, interrogatory, or imperative.

> The rats were fed with commercial pellets.
>
> What is to be done about the high cost of malpractice insurance?
>
> Add the reagent as soon as cloudiness begins to develop.
>
> Pain. Faintness. A sinking into oblivion. These are the steps into such a death.

An initial lowercase letter in an accepted conventional symbol retains its form even when it is the first letter of a sentence; an alternative structure for the sentence can be used to move the symbol from its initial position.

> pH was measured at 30-minute intervals but the data were lost.
>
> Measurements of pH were made at 30-minute intervals but the data were lost.

A chemical name with a locant prefix that is the first word of a sentence does not begin with a capital letter; locants and other similar prefixes of chemical names (see section 16.26 and Table 16.6) remain in lowercase letters and the root term is capitalized.

> *trans-cisoid-trans*-Perhydrophenanthrene was suspected of being the carcinogen.
> OR   The suspected carcinogen was *trans-cisoid-trans*-perhydrophenanthrene.

Note however that Greek and Latin multiplying prefixes (see section 16.25) are treated as an integral part of the term and capitalized by the general rules for sentences stated above and for titles (see section 7.2).

> Triamine was chosen as the reagent.

The first word of a run-in quotation (see section 6.2) that is itself a complete or partial sentence is capitalized unless the quotation is a syntactical part of the sentence.

> The patient replied, "To die at home is more important to me than a few more weeks of life".
> He had told Cushing that "bleeding will be the big problem".

For capitalization in a set-off quotation with ellipsis, see section 6.5.

Long or notably formal independent clauses that follow a colon may be capitalized by the rule for sentences, but usage is tending away from capitalization immediately after a colon unless it introduces a quotation (see sections 5.10 and 6.5).

For capitalization of table elements (title, column and row headings, text in the field) see sections 2.14, 2.19, 2.20, and 2.23.

The first word in each successive element of an outline or tabular list is capitalized (see section 2.26).

The first word in a term of address, as in a letter-to-the-editor (see section 3.14), is capitalized.

> To the Editor: Sirs:

The vocative *O,* the exclamatory *Oh,* and the first-person pronoun *I* are always capitalized.

> We wish that you were here, O Hippocrates, to see medicine in an HMO!
> Her dying words were, I think, "Oh weh".

Do not capitalize the first word in a subject index unless it is a proper name or term; see section 4.9.

TITLES OF WORKS AND PORTIONS OF WORKS

7.2   The title of a work is capitalized according to the rules specified below when it stands at the beginning of a work such as a book or an article (see section 2.2), forms part of the heading for a review of the work (see section 3.11), or is quoted in text (see section 6.3).

Words in a title that should be capitalized include the first word, the last word, and all nouns, pronouns, adjectives, verbs, adverbs, and subordinating conjunctions.

Words that should not be capitalized include internal articles (the articles *a, an, the* when not at the beginning of the title), coordinating conjunctions (*and, or, nor*), and prepositions (regardless of length).

> Probability Theory in the Use of Diagnostic Tests

> A recommended short introduction is the paper by Sox (48), "Probability Theory in the Use of Diagnostic Tests".

> The Probability Approach to the Use of Diagnostic Tests

> Men and Women without Hope

Do not capitalize locants and other similar prefixes of chemical names in titles; do capitalize the root term. Do capitalize chemical terms that begin with the multiplying Greek and Latin prefixes (see sections 7.1, 16.5, and 16.26).

> Acute Toxicity of *cis*-Dichloroethene

> The Chronic Toxicity of 2,3,5-Tris(1-aziridinyl)-*p*-benzoquinone

Taxonomic names in titles should be capitalized as they are in text (see section 16.4). Thus the species epithet *coli* in the species name *Escherichia coli* is not capitalized in a title.

> Treatment of *Escherichia coli* Infections

Note that the preposition *to* should be capitalized when it is part of an infinitive.

> To Be or Not To Be: A Psychoanalytic Study of Hamlet

In bibliographic references only the initial word of a title is, in general, capitalized (see section 15.18); the 2 exceptions are the initial letters of abbreviated journal titles (see sections 15.18 and 15.26 to 15.34, and Appendix B) and proper and scientific names within the title (see section 15.18).

> Rowson KEK, Rees TAL, Mahy BWJ. A dictionary of virology. Oxford: Blackwell; 1981.

> Brickner PW, Scanlan BC, Conahan B, et al. Homeless persons and health care. Ann Intern Med. 1986;104:405-9.

> Dunn MJ, ed. Proceedings of the Council for High Blood Pressure Research, 1985: Cleveland, Ohio, September 18–20, 1985. Hypertension. 1986;8(6 Pt 2):IIi–II192.

The second component of a hyphenated term in a title should be capitalized if it is a noun or proper adjective or has grammatical weight equal to, or greater than, that of the first component.

The Male-Female Interplay in Staffs of Christian and Non-Christian Hospitals

But do not capitalize the second element if it is a participial modifier of the first element or the components serve together as a single term.

A Review of Sex-linked Genetic Disorders in Man

Mutual Support among Co-workers in an Oncology Staff

Titles of portions of works are capitalized according to the rules for titles of complete works.

... and for details on case selection, see Materials and Methods.

In text, cited titles of portions of the same work are capitalized in accord with their original form; note that they are not surrounded by quotation marks.

For a summary of hematologic disorders with sex-linked inheritance, see Table 1.

For our validation of the radioimmunoassay see Materials and Methods.

But note that portions of a work not referred to by their original forms in the work should not be capitalized.

For a thorough discussion of suitable methods, consult reference 16.

In our discussion section we consider other approaches to validation of the method.

SCIENTIFIC NAMES AND TERMS

Capitalization in text of names and terms in the sciences follows, in general, the principles for capitalization in other fields; see section 7.11 for comment on these principles.

TAXONOMIC NAMES

7.3   A formal scientific, or taxonomic, name of an organism or virus is capitalized when it represents a genus or higher taxon (in ascending order, family, order, class, phylum or division).

Arthropoda	Crustacea
Mus	*Drosophila*
Escherichia	*Retroviridae*

The name of a species is a binomen in complete taxonomic nomenclatures and consists of the generic name and the specific epithet; the specific epithet is not capitalized, and this rule also applies to subspecific epithets in the ternary names of subspecies.

> *Escherichia coli*   *Drosophila melanogaster*
> *Campylobacter fetus* subsp. *venerealis*

For choice of roman or italic typeface for taxonomic names, see section 8.2.

COMMON (VERNACULAR, TRIVIAL) NAMES OF ORGANISMS

7.4   Many plants, animals, lower organisms, and viruses are known by nonscientific names. In general, these names are not capitalized, but components of the names that are proper nouns are capitalized.

mumps virus	Marburg virus
Calmette-Guerin bacillus	glanders bacillus
New Zealand mice	nude mouse

Recommendations on capitalization of vernacular names of plants can be found in the *CBE Style Manual* (1). Long lists with proper capitalization of vernacular plant and insect names can be found in the *United States Government Printing Office Style Manual* (2).

EPONYMIC TERMS

7.5   A proper name that is part of an eponymic term (see section 10.10) retains its initial capital.

the Cushing syndrome	Minamata disease
Tay-Sachs disease	Gram stain
Bunsen burner	Petri dish
Bence Jones protein	the oath of Hippocrates

Terms representing modified proper names or incorporating adjectival forms of proper names are not capitalized.

cushingoid signs	an addisonian crisis
parkinsonism	mendelian genetics

NAMES OF DISEASES AND CATEGORIES

Do not capitalize medical terms that represent categories.

> . . . The exception was case 1 in which we . . .
> . . . tested factor VIII for . . .
> . . . were classified as stage IVB.

Do not capitalize the names of diseases unless they are eponymic; see the preceding part of this section. Diseases are concepts, not specific and unique entities.

> NOT   . . . In the treatment of Pneumococcal Pneumonia, we . . .
> BUT   . . . In the treatment of pneumococcal pneumonia, we . . .

BRAND NAMES

7.6   Brand names for drugs, equipment, and supplies must be treated as proper names (see sections 10.3, 10.4, and 10.11) and capitalized; any idiosyncratic capitalization or punctuation used in the brand name by its proprietor must be maintained.

> Ventolin Inhaler   Tagamet [trade name for *cimetidine*]
> GoLYTELY [an electrolyte solution]   Alka-Seltzer

The proper names of manufacturers are capitalized (see section 7.17).

NAMES OF DISCIPLINES AND SPECIALTIES

7.7   Do not capitalize the name of a scientific discipline or specialty except when it is part of a proper name, as in the name of a specific academic unit.

> . . . the practice of internal medicine . . . (*but* Department of Medicine, Transylvania University)
>
> . . . for training in pathology . . . (*but* Surgical Pathology Unit, Department of Surgery)

NAMES OF NATIONALITIES AND
OF ETHNIC AND RACIAL GROUPS

7.8   Capitalize national, ethnic, or racial names that are derived from proper names for geographic entities. Also capitalize names of relatively homogeneous human groups generally living within a limited and specific distribution. Do not capitalize names representing scientifically ill-defined groups of wide distribution with names having some other basis.

Afro-Americans	blacks	negroes
Hispanics	Spaniards	mestizos
Caucasians	whites	Scandinavians
Japanese	Magyars	Bantus

Adjectival forms of such names are capitalized like the noun form.

> Afro-American dietary habits   an elderly black man
> Japanese families   white families

The *United States Government Printing Office Style Manual* (3) includes a table listing nouns and adjectives for a large number of nationalities.

GEOLOGIC AND GEOGRAPHIC NAMES

7.9   The names of geologic and stratigraphic time units are generally capitalized. The formal names of these units are compound, and both elements of the compound form should be capitalized in formal usage; the second element of the compound name is usually not capitalized in running text and may be omitted.

> the Cenozoic Era (*or* the Cenozoic era)
> the Late Cretaceous Epoch (*or* the Late Cretaceous)

Authoritative guidance on geologic style can be found in *Suggestions to Authors of the Reports of the United States Geological Survey* (4).

Established proper names of geographic and political units are capitalized; well-established popular place names are also capitalized. Variant forms of proper geographic names retain capitals only in the retained formal element.

> Commonwealth of Pennsylvania   the states of New York, Pennsylvania,
> and Delaware   the Rocky Mountains   the Rocky Mountain states
> The Bowery   The Loop   The Left Bank

The proper capitalization of geographic names can be verified in standard reference works on geographic names such as *Webster's New Geographical Dictionary* (5).

ASTRONOMIC TERMS

7.10   The names of celestial objects are capitalized. But note that *earth, sun,* and *moon* are not capitalized when they are used in a non-astronomic context.

> Among the planets, we can be sure only that Earth has pathogenic bacteria; Mars and Venus might have some.
>
> All of us, brothers on earth, are at risk for bacterial infection.
>
> The moon rose behind a city silenced by a plague.

OTHER NAMES AND TERMS

7.11   In general, names and terms are capitalized when they are proper nouns, which are names referring to unique entities such as individual persons, political entities, institutions, and so on. For additional guidance on capitalization, consult *The Chicago Manual of Style* (6) and the *United States Government Printing Office Style Manual* (7), which has a detailed compilation of rules and a comprehensive guide to capitalization particularly helpful on geographic and political terms. Specific rules govern the use of the definite article *the* with proper nouns; consult a comprehensive grammar, for example, Quirk and Greenbaum's *A Concise Grammar of Contemporary English* (8).

PERSONAL AND FICTITIOUS NAMES;
EPITHETS; KINSHIP TERMS

7.12 Capitalize personal names and initials and terms of address used with them.

> Fielding H Garrison   Sir William Osler
> Mr Thomas H Smith   the Hon James A D Waddington

Many non-English names include a particle or definite article, such as *della, du, von, van der, le*; a complex group of rules govern their capitalization (see "Foreign Names", sections 7.8 through 7.14 in reference 6). Because personal names are mainly used in medical writing for reference to published works, the names of authors on cited works should usually be taken as representing the correct forms of the names of those authors as specified by them; some editors, however, impose a house style on an author's preference and the published form may not have been correctly capitalized.

Capitalize fictitious names.

> John Doe   Mary Doe   John Q Public

Capitalize well-known epithets.

> Boston's most famous literary physician was the Autocrat of the Breakfast Table, Oliver Wendell Holmes.
>
> Probably the most widely known quack of eighteenth-century London was Crazy Sally Mapp, Bonesetter of Epsom.

7.13 Capitalize kinship terms when they are not preceded by a modifier; do not capitalize them when they are preceded by a modifier or the articles *a, an,* or *the.*

> The physician I most respected was Father; he would invariably be out of bed in the morning even before my eager brother.
>
> With her birth, he became a father.

TITLES OF PROFESSION, OFFICE, OR STATION

7.14 A title immediately preceding a personal name is capitalized. A title is not capitalized when it follows the name and is linked to a capitalized name by a preposition such as *of* or *for*; in this context it and the following name could be misread as the full formal form of the title. A title following a personal name at a greater distance is not capitalized because in this position it has lost its character as a formal term of address.

> The winner of the election was Dean Sherman Mellinkoff.
>
> The winner of the election was Sherman Mellinkoff, dean of the School of Medicine, UCLA.

The award was accepted for the school by Sherman Mellinkoff, who had served for over twenty years as dean.

Note that when the title follows a personal name but is separated from it and an institutional name by commas, the title is capitalized.

The award went to Sherman Mellinkoff, Dean, the School of Medicine.

Note that a title used not as a formal term of address but as a generic term is not capitalized.

Mellinkoff's term probably exceeded those of all other American deans in this century.

ACADEMIC DEGREES AND HONORS; AWARDS

7.15 Capitalize academic degrees and honors whether stated in full or abbreviated.

Michael Faraday, Fellow of the Royal Society
George Webster, Diplomate of the American Board of Internal Medicine
Albert Kligman, MD, PhD

Capitalize named awards.

Nobel Prize in Physiology or Medicine   Lasker Award

TERMS DERIVED FROM NAMES

7.16 Terms derived from, or including, proper nouns and widely used outside of science are not capitalized.

pasteurized milk   arabic numerals   brussels sprouts
plaster of paris   diesel fuel   india ink   greek letters

For capitalization of eponymic terms containing proper nouns, see section 7.5.

NAMES OF POLITICAL ENTITIES AND DOCUMENTS,
ORGANIZATIONS, INSTITUTIONS, STRUCTURES, AND MEETINGS

7.17 Capitalize the names of all political entities, companies, institutions, societies, meetings, and structures with formal titles. This rule also usually applies to short versions of full names. Note that combined formal names are capitalized as in their individual forms, but informal designations are not.

the United States of America   the United States
Princeton University   Princeton [the university]
the Schools of Medicine and Veterinary Medicine of the University of Pennsylvania
Pennsylvania's medical and veterinary schools
Annual Session of the American College of Physicians

the Declaration of Independence
the Medical Library Assistance Act
Merck Sharp & Dohme   Merck's introduction of the vaccine
the Eisenlohr Wing of the Hospital of the University of Pennsylvania

HISTORICAL AND CULTURAL TERMS

7.18   The practice of capitalization for terms in history and general culture differs widely among popular writers, scholars, and publishers.

Terms for historical periods are capitalized if they have been accepted in general culture or a specific discipline as a convenient tag for major cultural characteristics; adjectival components of such terms are not capitalized unless they are identical with their noun equivalents (see section 7.5).

the Middle Ages   the Renaissance   Renaissance surgery
the Age of Galen   galenic medicine   hippocratic medicine

Archeologic periods are capitalized.

the Paleolithic Age   the Iron Age

Terms for centuries and milleniums are not capitalized.

the twentieth century   the first millenium before Christ

Months, days of the week, holidays, holy days, and days well established in folk traditions are capitalized.

January   Monday   Fourth of July   Hanukkah   Groundhog Day

Terms for cultural movements, scientific developments, ideologies, and concepts are not capitalized, but components of such terms are capitalized if they are unmodified from their form as names.

darwinism   the Morgagni movement   marxism   the Darsee affair
homeopathy   listerian asepsis   jungian psychology
The Cushing school of neurosurgery   cartesian philosophy

Capitalize the specifically bestowed proper names of ships, aircraft, spacecraft, buildings, and bridges.

the USS Mercy   . . . and the flight of Challenger was . . .
. . . had jumped off the Golden Gate Bridge . . .

REFERENCES

1. CBE Style Manual Committee. CBE style manual. 5th ed. Bethesda, Maryland: Council of Biology Editors; 1983:156.
2. United States Government Printing Office style manual: 1984. Washington: United States Government Printing Office; 1984:257-74.

3. United States Government Printing Office style manual: 1984. Washington: United States Government Printing Office; 1984:235-7.
4. Bishop EE, Eckel EB, et al. Suggestions to authors of the reports of the United States Geological Survey. 6th ed. Washington: US Government Printing Office; 1978. A new edition is in preparation.
5. Webster's new geographical dictionary. Springfield, Massachusetts: Merriam-Webster; 1984.
6. The Chicago manual of style. 13th ed. Chicago: The University of Chicago Press; 1982:183-229.
7. United States Government Printing Office style manual: 1984. Washington: United States Government Printing Office; 1984:23-61.
8. Quirk R, Greenbaum S. A concise grammar of contemporary English. New York: Harcourt Brace Jovanovich; 1978:76-80.

Chapter 8

Type Conventions

In its broadest sense *type* means the characters of an alphabet and the accompanying numerals; this is the sense in which *type* is used in this manual. As a term in printing, *type* also means the individual metal units used to print individual characters and the entire group of individual units representing a typeface. A *typeface* is a particular design of alphabetical and numerical characters; a complete typeface usually includes italic and boldface type and small capitals. *Small capitals* are letters in a typeface with the form of capital letters but designed for the height of the letters without risers or descenders, such as *a, c, e*. A good introduction to terms and technology relevant to this chapter can be found in the closing section of *The Chicago Manual of Style* (1); more detail on many aspects of typography can be found in *Practical Typography from A to Z* (2).

8.1 The characters (letters and numerals) usually used for text and tables are roman characters. Some style conventions, scientific and nonscientific, call for departures from the usual characters and specify italic characters, boldface characters, or small capitals. In this manual *roman (upright) type* means the roman characters of a particular typeface; *italic (slanted) type*, the italic characters of a typeface; and *boldface type*, the "bold" (heavy) characters of a typeface. The terms "upright" and "slanted" are used with "roman" and "italic" in accord with nomenclature in *ISO Standards Handbook: Units of Measurement* (3); "upright" includes upright sans serif faces in addition to roman faces, and "slanted" includes sans serif faces tilted to the right. Italic type is often informally called "italics" and boldface type, "boldface". Small capitals are informally called "small caps".

Most of the conventions recommended here are well established and will continue to be used for the print-on-paper versions of journals. But with the growing availability and use of journals through online database services, some of these conventions may eventually have to be modified or, perhaps, abandoned because the needed characters cannot be specified for transmission or cannot be displayed by the usual monitor for microcomputer terminals. Some of the recommendations anticipate this problem.

Note that throughout this manual the use of roman (upright) type for alphabetical, numerical, and related characters is assumed. Needs for other types are specified, but at some points attention is called to the need for a roman (upright) type when confusion might otherwise occur.

ITALIC (SLANTED) TYPE

TAXONOMIC NAMES IN BIOLOGIC DISCIPLINES

8.2   A formal taxonomic name (see section 10.5) for a genus, species, subspecies, or variety must be in italic (slanted) type; some expansions of this general rule are specified below. A taxonomic abbreviation that is part of the name (such as "subsp" for "subspecies", "nom nov" for "nomen novum") is not italicized, nor is an authority name following the taxonomic name proper.

> *Homo sapiens*   *Mus musculus*   *Drosophila melanogaster*
> *Escherichia coli*   *Pseudomonas aeruginosa* subsp *erythrogenes*
> *Protaminobacter ruber* subsp *machidanus* Abe and Kohata

This general rule holds when the genus name is abbreviated.

> *H sapiens*   *E coli*   *P aeruginosa*

The genus name is always capitalized; the species epithet (such as "*musculus*", "*melanogaster*" in 2 of the examples above) that is the second element of the species name (genus name plus species epithet) is not capitalized (also see section 7.3). In bacteriology (see sections 16.1 and 16.7) the taxonomic names of taxa above genus (kingdoms, classes, orders, and families) are italicized and capitalized. In virology family names are capitalized and italicized (if they have been approved by the International Committee on Taxonomy of Viruses).

> *Legionellaceae*   *Herpesviridae*

The rules for italicization apply whether the taxonomic name is in text, a heading, or a title (in roman [upright] type).

> The Biochemistry of *Escherichia* and *Pseudomonas*

When a taxonomic name properly italicized in text is in a title that must be italicized (as when quoted in text), the taxonomic name should be in roman (upright) type.

> . . . wrote his classic monograph, *The Biochemistry of* Escherichia *and* Pseudomonas, in 1953 when he . . .

Note that a taxonomic name used as a common noun or adjective is neither italicized nor capitalized.

> the genus *Rhododendron*
> He contaminated his wound with soil while planting a rhododendron.
>
> *Pneumocystis carini*
> He developed a pneumocystis pneumonia.

For detailed recommendations on taxonomic conventions see Chapter 16: bacteriology, sections 16.1–16.7; mycology, section 16.50; parasitology and entomology, section 16.57; and virology, section 16.63. Additional guidance can be found in the *ASM Style Manual for Journals and Books* (4). For taxonomic conventions in botany, consult the *CBE Style Manual* (5) and the *ASHS Publications Manual* (6).

CHEMICAL NAMES

8.3   Alphabetic prefixes to chemical names or formulas are italicized whether the names are in text or in a title; numerical prefixes are not italicized. Note that alphabetic prefixes must retain their type conventions even if the names in which they serve as prefixes begin sentences or appear in titles, but the root name is capitalized in these positions (see section 7.1). These rules apply to 3 groups of prefixes (see sections 16.26 and 16.27 and Table 16.6).

1. Element-symbol locants

   N,N'-bis(dehydroabiethyl)ethylenediamine dipenicillin G
   S-2-amino-3-fluoropropanoic acid

2. Positional and structural descriptors

   p-aminobenzoic acid   *n*-dichlorobenzene

3. Stereoisomer descriptors

   meso-tartaric acid   *syn*-dichloroethane

Note that the stereoisomer prefixes include *d* for *dextro* and *l* for *levo*. Configurational relations in amino acids and carbohydrates are indicated with small-capital prefixes D and L (see section 8.13).

In polymer nomenclature certain symbols and generic terms within polymer names are italicized; for details consult *The ACS Style Guide* (7).

Note that certain chemical-name prefixes are in roman type. Greek and Latin multiplying prefixes are an integral part of the root name (see section 16.25).

trichloroacetic acid   1,4-bis(trichloromethyl)benzene

The structural prefixes "cyclo" and "iso" are also an integral part of a chemical name.

cycloserine   isobutyl isobutyrate

The best source in which to confirm appropriate conventions for chemical names likely to be used in medical journals is *The Merck Index* (8), but note that the entry names in this reference are all capitalized whether they are proper names or not.

SYMBOLS FOR QUANTITIES

8.4   Letters that serve as symbols for quantities must be in italic (slanted) type. The italicization (and the convention of lowercase or capital letter) applies whether the symbol is in running text, an equation, or a title; note that if the symbol is the inital letter in a sentence the convention still applies (see section 7.1). Italicized symbols in italicized text must remain in italic type, which is in contrast to italicized names (see section 8.2).

Note that symbols for units must be in roman (upright) type (see section 13.16). For comment on the difference between units and quantities, see section 11.1; also see "Rules for the Printing of Symbols and Numbers" on pages 298–301 in reference 9.

Symbols for quantities are in four main groups.

1. Mathematical variables and unknowns whether they are in an equation or text (including an adjectival function in text)

    $x = ay + b$ . . . assigning a value of 16 to b in . . .
    . . . raised to the nth power . . .

2. Physical constants

gravitational constant	G
Michaelis constant	K_m

3. Physical properties measured in biology, chemistry, physics, and other sciences

absorbed dose [ionizing radiation]	D
conductive heat transfer [physiology]	C

molality, solute substance B	m_B
physiological dead space	V_D
potential, electric	V

4. Statistical symbols

correlation coefficient	r
probability	P
sample variance	s^2

Note that superscripts and subscripts modifying such symbols should usually be in roman (upright) type as in several of the examples above; subscripts that are themselves symbols for quantities should be in italic (slanted) type. When such symbols will have to be displayed on a monitor through transmission from text in a database, they must be converted to a written-out format because of the technical limitations on present monitor displays. For example, the full term might be given or the symbol for *sample variance*, s^2, might be converted to read "s sup 2"; at present there are no well-established and widely-accepted conventions for such conversions.

Abbreviations and signs for mathematical operations should be in roman (upright) type: d, !, Σ, and so on.

$$\mathrm{d}x/\mathrm{d}t \qquad p! \qquad \Sigma$$

Abbreviations for mathematical functions, notably the trigonometric functions, should be in roman (upright) type; but a variable stated with the function follows the rule for italic (slanted) type for variables.

$$\cos \qquad \sin \qquad \tan \qquad \tan y$$

SYMBOLS SPECIFIC TO SCIENTIFIC DISCIPLINES

8.5   Gene symbols (gene loci, genotypes) in microbiologic, animal, and human genetics are italicized.

$$ara \qquad araB \qquad onc \qquad gag \qquad myc \qquad Re \qquad v\text{-}myc$$

Note that in some gene symbolic systems a modifier should be in roman (upright) type as in "v-*myc*" above.

Chromosomal aberrations are symbolized for some species by italicized (slanted) letters.

Symbols for physical quantities measured in the biochemical, chemical, pharmacologic, and physiologic disciplines should follow the rules set out in section 8.4; cardiology, section 16.17; enzyme kinetics, section 16.29; pharmacology, section 16.58; pulmonary medicine, section 16.60. Note, however, that this international convention, unfortunately, is not applied in some American journals, particularly in cardiology and pulmonary medicine.

Restriction endonucleases (restriction enzymes) are symbolized by a 3-letter italicized abbreviation made up from the initial letter (capitalized) of the genus name and the first 2 letters of the species epithet.

Escherichia coli	*Eco*
Haemophilus influenzae	*Hin*

Any additional identification for strain should be in roman type, whether closed up or spaced.

Bsu 973   *Eco*P15   *Hin*1056II

The end letter or numeral in the symbol for a bacterial transposon is italicized.

Tn*A*   Tn*3*

Conventions for microbiologic genetics are set forth in great detail in the *ASM Style Manual for Journals and Books* (10). Genetic symbolizations in all of the biomedical disciplines and plant sciences are summarized in the *CBE Style Manual* (5).

GENERAL USES OF ITALIC (SLANTED) TYPE

Italic (slanted) type is used in a number of style conventions applied in many scholarly disciplines; many of these conventions are useful in medical publication.

8.6 Titles of complete works, such as journals, books, computer programs (software), films, musical compositions, and so on, are italicized when they are quoted in text (see section 6.3). Note, however, that they are not italicized in bibliographic references (see sections 15.14 and 15.24). In the possessive form of a title the apostrophe and the *s* are not italicized. When the sense of the text is a pointing to the particular work as outstanding, prominent, or particularly useful, or when the title begins with a generic term like "archives" or "journal", the title may be preceded by "the", which, however, must not be italicized unless it is part of the title.

   . . . disposed of his collection of the *Archives of Neurology.*
   . . . began to bind the volumes of *Neurology.*
   . . . gave up reading *JAMA* and turned to . . .
   . . . recommend the *CBE Style Manual* for details on . . .
   . . . recommend the *The ACS Style Guide* for details on . . .
   . . . the *CBE Style Manual*'s recommendations on . . .

The title of a part of a larger work such as a journal article, a book chapter, an essay in a collection, or a poem in a collection should be demarcated with quotation marks (see section 6.3).

8.7   If legal cases are referred to in text and are italicized in accord with the recommendation of *A Uniform System of Citation* (11), the "v." for *versus* is italicized as well as the names of plaintiff and defendant.

> . . . in reviewing *United States v. Reynolds,* he . . .

For details of legal style, including other uses of italic type, consult "General Rules of Citation and Style" in reference 10. Many of these details are not relevant to medical publishing, but some are in accord with style widely used in fields other than law. For recommendations on bibliographic references to legal documents in medical journals, see sections 15.61 to 15.63.

8.8   Non-English words and phrases not in the standard English vocabulary, general and medical, should be italicized. Words and phrases defined in standard English-language general and medical dictionaries need not be italicized. Do not italicize non-English proper names and widely used abbreviations.

> The physician sees *la comédie humaine* but more of tragedy.
> At one time homeopaths were *les enfants terrible* of medicine.
> . . . was dried in vacuo at a temperature of . . .
> . . . was sensitive in vitro at a concentration of . . .
> . . . and studied at the Allgemeine Krankenhaus in . . .
> . . . and Pierre Charles Alexandre Louis was surely the father of medical statistics.
> . . . as reported by Smith et al (67) and Jones (68).

Note that English equivalents or substitutes for abbreviations from Latin, such as "et al" for "et alii", are to be preferred: not "et al", "e g", "i e"; but "and coauthors", "for example", "that is" (see section 11.2).

A term in a context treating it as such should be italicized.

> Insensitivity is betrayed by the use of *case* for *patient.*

8.9   If the term is quoted as an example (and notably in a context reserving italic type for some specific uses), it can be designated as such by demarcation with quotation marks.

> Insensitivity is betrayed by the use of impersonal terms such as "case" and "schizophrenic".

Proposed new terms and established terms used in a new, unusual, humorous, or ironic sense should be demarcated by quotation marks (see section 6.4).

8.10   Letters of the alphabet used as such should be italicized when they appear in text set in roman (upright) type. An allowable exception to this rule is where the letter is designated specifically as a letter and need not follow the rule for symbols for quantities (section 8.4).

Beeson's textbook gives the details from *a* to *z*.

We designated those cells with the letter T to stand for *thymus*.

8.11 Emphasis on a word or phrase can be indicated by putting it into italic (slanted) type, but avoid overuse of this device. Note that such italicization should be avoided in a context also using italic (slanted) type for any of the other conventions presented in this section. If such emphasis is added within a quotation, an explanation within square brackets should be appended to the quotation (see section 5.31).

The government's scheme for financing care is *a disaster*.

I always told my students that "the secret . . . is in *caring* for the patient" (32) [emphasis added] at all times.

Terms or letters in a figure legend that identify panels of a multipart figure or particular locations in a figure can be italicized to distinguish them from the explanation itself, but a simpler device is enclosing them by parenthesis marks (see section 2.30).

Figure 1. Transmontane School of Medicine from the air: *above left*, the laboratories building; *below right*, the dormitories.

Figure 1. Transmontane School of Medicine from the air: the laboratories building (above left) and the dormitories (below right).

Figure 1. Absorption rates at different doses in the placebo group, *a*, and the treatment group, *b*. [for figure panels *a* and *b*]

BOLDFACE TYPE

8.12 A few style conventions in science use boldface type, but they may have to be changed because of the present impossibility, in general, of displaying boldface characters on the monitors of microcomputers used to access online databases offering full text from journals and books.

The main use of boldface type is in mathematics. The style manual of the American Institute of Physics (13) summarizes the mathematical uses likely to be needed in some journals in the medical sciences.

Boldface is used for three-vectors, dyadics, some matrices, tensors without indices, etc. It is inappropriate for unit vectors . . . , four-vectors . . . , vectors represented by a typical component . . . , and the magnitude of a vector. . . .

An example of the use of boldface type in medicine is in vectorcardiography.

$\mathbf{H}_i \cdot \mathbf{H}_{i+1} = (x_i y_{i+1} - x_{i+1} y_i)\mathbf{k}$, where $\mathbf{k}$ is a unit vector in the z direction.

Also see "Tensors and Vectors" in *Webster's Standard American Style Manual* (12).

Other uses of boldface type in medical publication are also uncommon: designation of serologic specifities in the Wiener Rh-Hr notation for the Rh blood-group system (14); designation of chromosomal aberrations (15) in some mammals. Boldface type may be helpful in distinguishing subject headings in subject indexes from the titles they head (see sections 4.7 and 4.11).

SMALL CAPITALS

8.13   Avoid the use of small capitals if possible. As with boldface type (see section 8.12), monitors for microcomputers accessing online databases cannot, in general, display small capitals.

Small capitals are used as prefixes to chemical names to indicate absolute configuration of amino acids and carbohydrates (see section 16.26 and Table 16.6).

> L-methionine   D-glucose

Modifiers for gas-phase symbols in American systems of symbols for respiratory physiology are small capitals (see section 16.60 and Table 16.19).

For the reason given at the beginning of this section, do not use small capitals but capitals for eras or for the 12-hour divisions of the day (if the 24-hour system is not used; see section 13.21).

> *anno Hegirae, anno Hebraico*   *not* A.H. *but* AH
> *anno Domini*   *not* A.D. *but* AD
> *not* 12:37 A.M. *but* 12:37 AM

Do not use small capitals as abbreviations for "standard error" and "standard deviation"; other conventions are preferred (see section 14.10 and Table 14.2).

GREEK LETTERS

8.14   Greek letters (see Table 8.1) are used in a number of scientific style conventions, but as with italic and boldface types for roman letters, greek letters are generally not being transmitted through online database systems for display on monitors of microcomputers. Therefore journals offering the text from their print-on-paper versions should consider using the names of greek letters in place of the greek letters called for in present conventions. Such a substitution may not be acceptable in the immediate

Table 8.1: Greek letters [fn1]

Name of letter	Capital	Lowercase
alpha	A	α
beta	B	β
gamma	Γ	γ
delta	Δ	δ
epsilon	E	ε
zeta	Z	ζ
eta	H	η
theta	Θ	θ
iota	I	ι
kappa	K	κ
lambda	Λ	λ
mu	M	μ
nu	N	ν
xi	Ξ	ξ
omicron	O	ο
pi	Π	π
rho	P	ρ
sigma	Σ	σ
tau	T	τ
upsilon	Y	υ
phi	Φ	φ
chi	X	χ
psi	Ψ	ψ
omega	Ω	ω

fn1:   Note that the keyboard characters used in word-processing programs to produce greek letters on a printer are not always the roman letter equivalents of the greek letters to be inserted by the printer.

future in some scientific fields, and methods for transmission and monitor display of greek letters may become available.

THE SI PREFIX "MU"

8.15   The SI prefix representing the multiplication factor 10^{-6} is the lowercase greek letter μ ("mu") (see section 13.16 and Table 13.7). This symbol represents "micro" when it is prefixed to one of the SI base units or an equivalent.

microgram   μg   microliter   μL

For display on a monitor this standard convention could be modified by substituting the prefix micro- or "mu-" for the greek letter μ itself.

micro-g   "mu"-g   micro-L   "mu"-L

CHEMICAL NAMES

8.16   Lowercase greek letters in the form of hyphenated prefixes serve in some chemical names as locants and designators of individual compounds in families of compounds (see section 16.26 and Table 16.6).

α-methylbenezeneacetic acid $α_2$-globulin   β-endorphin   γ-sitosterol

Forms of the names in these examples adapted for satisfactory display on monitors contain the names for the greek letters.

alpha-methylbenezeneacetic acid   alpha2-globulin
beta-endorphin   gamma-sitosterol

The lowercase greek letters alpha (α), beta (β), gamma (γ), delta (δ), epsilon (ε), and zeta (ζ) represent globin chains of hemoglobins (see section 16.41).

fetal hemoglobin $α_2γ_2$ hemoglobin Bart's $γ_4$

The heavy polypeptide chains of immunoglobulins are designated by lowercase greek letters corresponding to the roman capital letters used for the immunoglobulin classes (see section 16.32).

IgA   α   IgG   γ

SYMBOLS IN PHYSIOLOGY

8.17   Greek letters are used for some symbols in symbolic systems for respiratory physiology (see section 16.60 and Table 16.19).

SYMBOLS IN STATISTICS

8.18   Some greek letters are used as symbols in statistics (see section 14.10 and Table 14.2). For monitor display these letters should be replaced by the names of the letters.

$χ^2$ chi-squared

REFERENCES

1. The Chicago manual of style. Chicago: University of Chicago Press; 1982:561–683.
2. Romano F. Practical typography from a to z. Arlington, Virginia: National Composition Association; 1983.
3. International Organization for Standardization. Units of measurement. 2nd ed. Geneva: International Organization for Standardization; 1982:23–4. (ISO standards handbook 2).
4. American Society for Microbiology. ASM style manual. Washington: American Society for Microbiology; 1985:28–31.
5. CBE Style Manual Committee. CBE style manual: a guide for authors, editors, and publishers in the biological sciences. 5th ed. Bethesda, Maryland: Council of Biology Editors; 1983.
6. American Society for Horticultural Science. ASHS publications manual. Alexandria, Virginia: American Society for Horticultural Science; 1985:29–30.

7. Dodd JS. The ACS style guide: a manual for authors and editors. Washington: American Chemical Society; 1986:91.
8. Windholz M, ed. The Merck index: an encyclopedia of chemicals, drugs, and biologicals. 10th ed. Rahway, New Jersey: Merck; 1983.
9. Lowe DA. A guide to international recommendations on names and symbols for quantities and on units of measurement. Geneva: World Health Organization; 1975.
10. American Society for Microbiology. ASM style manual. Washington: American Society for Microbiology; 1985:31-6.
11. Harvard Law Review Association. A uniform system of citation. 13th ed. Cambridge, Massachusetts: The Harvard Law Review Association; 1981:2-33.
12. Webster's standard American style manual. Springfield, Massachusetts: Merriam-Webster; 1985:139-40.
13. Hathwell D, Metzner AWK. Style manual for guidance in the preparation of papers for journals published by the American Institute of Physics and its member societies. 3rd ed. New York: American Institute of Physics; 1978:12.
14. CBE Style Manual Committee. CBE style manual: a guide for authors, editors, and publishers in the biological sciences. 5th ed. Bethesda, Maryland: Council of Biology Editors; 1983:200.
15. CBE Style Manual Committee. CBE style manual: a guide for authors, editors, and publishers in the biological sciences. 5th ed. Bethesda, Maryland: Council of Biology Editors; 1983:191.

Chapter 9

Spelling and Word Structure

English does not have simple and rigid rules that govern precisely all possibilities in the spelling and forming of words and terms. At many points, the editor's choice is likely to be determined by needs peculiar to the journal (such as the preferences of readers in its country of publication), by what is recommended by a favorite authority, by a sense of idiom, or by habit. But choices should apply throughout the journal and contribute to consistency of style.

The rules of English spelling and word formation are sometimes logical but often not. Among the most readily available summaries of these rules, the most thorough are in *The Oxford Guide to English Usage* (1) and *Hart's Rules for Compositors and Readers at the University Press Oxford* (2). An American source for a summary of rules for word formation is *Webster's Standard American Style Manual* (3).

SPELLING

AMERICAN AND BRITISH DIFFERENCES

9.1   American and British spelling differ in minor ways. The examples in this section show tendencies in American spelling in the first column, in British, in the second.

One group of differences includes word endings: *-ction* or *-xion*; *-er* or *-re*; *-ize* or *-ise*; *-l* or *-ll*; *-log* or *-logue*; *-m* or *-mme*; *-or* or *-our*; *-se* or *-ce*; *-t* or *-tate*; *-yze* or *-yse*.

connection	connexion
deflection	deflexion
meager	meagre
theater	theatre
rationalize	rationalise

appall	appal
distill	distil
analog	analogue
catalog	catalogue
program	programme
color	colour
honor	honour
license	licence
defense	defence
to orient	to orientate
catalyze	catalyse
paralyze	paralyse

Some of these differences may be carried internally as in the noun forms of the *-ize*, *-ise* verbs, for example, *rationalization* and *rationalisation*. The general rule (1) for the *-ize*, *-ise* formations is that *-ize* is used whenever the suffix would be pronounced "eyes". See reference 1 for preferences for *-ise* over *-ize*. With the *-lyze*, *-lyse* endings, British usage (1) prefers *-lyse* because of its representing the Greek root that also serves in *lysis* and *catalysis*. The American preference for *analyze* and *catalyze* appears to be a tendency to apply the general British rule based on the pronunciation like "eyes", and the British pronunciation of *analyse* in fact closes with the "eyes" sound rather "ice". Most editors using American spelling will not try to remember the exceptions specified in British rules of usage (1) but will trust their sense of American idiom or consult an American dictionary.

Another group of differences includes internal changes when words are derived from stems ending in a silent *-e* by adding *-able* or *-ment*.

like	likable, likeable
sale	salable, saleable
judge	judgment, judgement
acknowledge	acknowledgment, acknowledgement

The American tendency is to drop the silent terminal *-e*, but British usage is not consistent in retaining the *-e*. One authority (2), for example, recommends dropping the *-e* as a general rule (as in *lovable*) but also advises *likeable* and a number of other exceptions. Its plea for retaining the *-e* in formations from verbs ending in *-dge* like *judgement* is based on preserving the soft *-g*, a rational rule, but the American tendency has the value of simplifying decisions.

9.2 A third group of differences includes doubling or nondoubling of consonants.

fulfill	fulfil
skillful	skilful
traveler	traveller

Here is another instance in which British rules ignore etymologic considerations of the kind used to justify *-lyse* instead of *-lyze*.

A fourth group of differences includes words that differ in phonetic representation.

jail	gaol
curb	kerb
mold	mould

In these examples the American spellings of *jail* and *curb* represent closer relations to their French cognates, *geole* and *courbe*.

9.3   The major differences in the medical vocabulary result from the simplifying in American spelling of the British digraphs *ae* and *oe* to *e*.

edema	oedema
esophagus	oesophagus
hematology	haematology
leukemia	leukaemia

Other differences are spellings of some technical words without digraph elements.

aluminum	aluminium

The *-ium* ending here is related to Sir Humphrey Davy's original spelling, *alumium*.

9.4   A journal that has most of its readers of its paper and online versions in regions with scientific publication in American English should use American spelling even in papers from authors submitting typescripts with British spelling. Likewise, a journal with most of its readers in regions publishing scientific literature in British English should use British spelling. This rule is becoming more important with the increasing use of online databases. When variant spellings are carried in a database, its searchers may fail to find documents with terms spelled as variants they have not thought to use in searching.

9.5   The original spelling in titles and proper names mentioned in text or tables or cited in references must be retained. Journals publishing in American English must be sure to retain digraphs in proper names.

. . . infections in leukemia with *Haemophilus influenzae* are . . .

9.6   For American spelling select from any alternative spellings the first choice in one of the standard American dictionaries: *The American Heritage Dictionary of the English Language* (4), *The Random House Dictionary of the English Language* (5), *Webster's Ninth New Collegiate Dictionary* (6), or *Webster's II New Riverside University Dictionary* (7). For British spelling consult *Chambers 20th Century Dictionary* (8) or one of the dictionaries published by Oxford University Press.

For American medical spelling, consult *Dorland's Illustrated Medical Dictionary* (9), *International Dictionary of Medicine and Biology* (10) (which also indicates British spelling), or *Stedman's Medical Dictionary* (11); for British medical spelling, consult *Butterworths Medical Dictionary* (12).

WORDS DERIVED FROM NON-ENGLISH ROOTS

9.7 A choice in spelling may be available for some terms based on roots that represent transliterations from another language. The general rule is select the alternative that poses less ambiguity in pronunciation. The best example is the choice between *c* and *k* in words based on the Greek *leukos* ("white"). The Greek *k* is represented in English words by both possibilities: *leucemia, leukemia; leucocyte, leukocyte.* Here the better choice is *k*; to some readers the *-ce-* in *leucemia* suggests pronunciation with a soft *c* rather than the proper hard *c*. The variant British spelling with the digraph *ae* and the *c* rather than the *k*, *leucaemia*, visually preserves the hard *c*.

Another group of variant spellings are those of words based on the stem *lysis*, of origin in Greek: *paralysis, catalysis.* In their verb forms, American spelling changes the stem to represent its pronunciation: *paralyze* from *paralysis* (also see section 9.1).

The editor's choice among variant spellings should be consistent to reduce the chance that searchers of the text of the journal in a database will miss documents with variant spellings (see section 9.4).

DIACRITICAL MARKS

9.8 Many languages mark individual letters to indicate an accent or a var-

Table 9.1: Diacritical marks frequently used in European-language alphabets based on roman letters

Name	Mark	Example
acute accent	´	é
double acute accent	˝	ő
grave accent	`	è
breve	˘	ŭ
caron	ˇ	ň
cedilla	˛	ç
circumflex	^	â
dot	·	ṁ
macron	—	n̄
ogonek	˛	ę
ring	°	Å
slash (stod)	/	Ø
tilde	~	ñ
umlaut mark (diaeresis)	¨	ü

iety of pronunciation (see Table 9.1). Printers of scholarly journals have typefaces that include the marks, usually as letters carrying the marks. A common noun in the standard English vocabulary thus marked in the language of its origin need not carry the mark, or marks, in English text.

brassiere [English]   brassière [French]

Proper names should carry their original diacritical marks. If the journal's printer does not have typefaces with appropriate marks, omit the marks.

Ramón y Cajal   Sjögren
Ramon y Cajal   Sjogren

For illustrations of the use of these marks with roman letters in European languages, see "Accents" in *Practical Typography from A to Z* (13).

WORD FORMATION

9.9   As with spelling in English, the rules governing word formation are complex, not always easily applied, and not applied in many exceptions. Uncertainty as to how to form a term with a prefix or suffix, or by hyphenation, is usually most quickly dispelled by consulting a standard dictionary (4–11). A notably clear, logical, and thorough discussion of compound-term formation and hyphenation can be found in *Webster's Standard American Style Manual* (3).

PREFIXES

9.10   Most decisions on prefixes are concerned with forming a word by adding a prefix to a stem word. Most formations of this kind eventually become closed compound words in which the prefix is run together with the stem word. Exceptions in which the 2 elements are joined instead by a hyphen are noted in section 9.14. Certain prefixes usually form closed compounds; in general these are prefixes indicating location, number, state, or time, and most of them are not used alone as words.

after-	afterbirth	aftercare
ante-	anteflexion	antepartum
anti-	anticodon	antiemetic
auto-	autoanalyzer	autointoxication
bi-	bimanual	bipolar
bio-	biomechanics	biomedical
co-	coenzyme	corepressor
counter-	countercurrent	counterimmunoelectrophoresis
de-	delouse	demineralization
di-	diphallus	diovulatory
electro-	electropneumograph	electrosurgery

extra-	extrachromosomal	extrapulmonary
hemi-	hemianesthesia	hemiparesis
hyper-	hypernatremia	hyperperistalsis
hypo-	hypopancreatism	hypoventilation
in-	incoordination	inoperable
infra-	infracerebral	infrapsychic
inter-	intermenstrual	interphase
intra-	intracatheter	intraperitoneal
iso-	isoantigen	isoenzyme
macro-	macroamylase	macrocryoglobulinemia
meta-	metaanalysis	metamyelocyte
micro-	micronutrients	microplethysmography
mid-	midbrain	midmenstrual
mini-	minicomputer	minilaparotomy
multi-	multigravida	multinuclear
non-	nonconductor	noninvasive
over-	overcompensation	overlearning
photo-	photodermatitis	photophobia
post-	postmenopausal	postprandial
physio-	physiopathology	physiotherapy
poly-	polyarthritis	polypharmacy
pre-	prealbumin	prediabetes
pro-	proinsulin	promegaloblast
pseudo-	pseudogout	pseudohypoparathyroidism
quadri-	quadribasic	quadrivalent
re-	recombination	replantation
semi-	semicoma	semisynthetic
sub-	subendocardial	subluxation
stereo-	stereoauscultation	stereoradiography
super-	superinfection	supersaturation
supra-	supraocclusion	supraventricular
trans-	transacetylation	transposon
tri-	tribromoethanol	trisomy
ultra-	ultracentrifuge	ultrasonography
un-	unsaturated	ununited
under-	underachiever	undernutrition

These examples illustrate well-established terms, but these prefixes may occasionally appear in newly coined terms as hyphenated prefixes. Unless the closed form might produce confusion in meaning, the hyphen should be omitted and the term converted to a closed compound term as in the examples above. An example of possible confusion is *un-ionized* formed from *un-* and *ionized*, which might be read as the past participle formed from the verb *to unionize*. Such confusion seems highly unlikely in most scientific contexts.

If the prefixes listed above appear in a sequence of terms with the same stem word, do not hyphenate any of the prefixes but give each term in its full form.

NOT . . . under- and overachievers . . .
BUT . . . underachievers and overachievers . . .

As with variant spellings, inconsistent practice in closing up terms with these prefixes or hyphenating them can produce difficulties in searching text on online databases (also see section 9.4).

9.11 Some authors are confused by certain pairs of prefixes; editorial staffs may wish to compile a list of such confused spellings so that the correct form can be verified with the author.

ante-	anti-
en-	in-
for-	fore-
in-	un-

SUFFIXES

9.12 Some alternatives in suffixes occasionally call for decisions on preferred style. One example is the *-log* and *-logue* alternative illustrated in section 9.1. A second example is the alternative choices with the suffixes *-ic* and *-ical*. In many terms the alternative forms attached to the same stem have different meanings; the alternatives are not true alternatives because of the difference in meaning signified by the slightly different suffixes.

economic	economical
historic	historical
statistic	statistical

In such cases the suffix must not be changed unless the author, perhaps unfamiliar with English, has used the wrong form for the context. For some terms there is not an alternative: "chemic" is not an alternative for *chemical* and "metabolical" is not an idiomatic alternative for *metabolic*. In general, when the *-ic* and *-ical* forms do not differ in meaning and the terminal stem is *-ology* or *oscopy*, use the shorter *-ic* form.

etiologic, *not* etiological
histologic, *not* histological
microscopic, *not* microscopical
pathologic, *not* pathological

Used as adjective, *pathologic* is sometimes used to mean "abnormal" with *pathological* used to mean "pertaining to the discipline 'pathology' ". Likewise, physiologic is sometimes used to mean "normal". The adjectival forms of *pathology* and *physiology*, *pathologic* and *physiologic*, should be used only as adjectives referring to the disciplines; adjectives such as *abnormal* and *normal* should be used as adjectives for state of being.

9.13   A number of similar suffixes are frequently confused by some authors and manuscript editors. A journal's editorial staff should establish a list of terms frequently misspelled because of authors' confusions about the correct or preferred suffix.

-ability	-ibility	
-able	-ible	
-ance	-ence	
-ant	-ent	
-ative	-ive	
-cede	-ceed	-sede
-efy	-ify	
-eous	-ous	
-er	-or	
-erous	-orous	
-ful	-full	
-ified	-yfied	
-ous	-us	

The suffixes -*fold*, -*hood*, -*wide*, and -*wise* are attached to their stems; the suffixes -*less* and -*like* are hyphenated when they would form a compound term with a sequence of three letter "els" but are otherwise attached.

threefold	motherhood	worldwide	likewise

. . . a cell-less homogenate . . .   . . . a cell-like structure . . .

HYPHENATION

9.14   The rules for hyphenation are complex and not always easy to apply. There is a trend in English to the forming of new words by attaching once-hyphenated prefixes to form closed compound words and to omitting hyphens in compound modifiers. But retaining hyphens in compound modifiers often helps to keep their meaning clear. The kinds of compound modifiers summarized and illustrated below generally still need hyphens; also see section 9.16 on compound terms.

- Two or more modifiers of the same adjectival noun are hyphenated whether immediately attached to it or not.

    a low- and high-frequency hearing loss
    sodium- and potassium-conserving drugs

- Two or more coordinate adjectives or nouns are hyphenated.

    cost-benefit analysis   the Stevens-Johnson syndrome
    a black-white-Hispanic coalition of patients

(But care must be taken not to hyphenate names that are unhyphenated names of a single person: *Bence Jones protein*, not "Bence-Jones protein".)

- Compound modifiers in which the second element is a past or present participle are hyphenated.

  well-established principles of treatment
  seizure-inducing drugs
  . . . For years he was the well-known professor of . . .

If the first element of a compound modifier is an adverb linked by a hyphen when the modifier immediately precedes a noun, the hyphen is omitted when the modifier is a predicate adjective.

  The principles of treatment are well established.
  He was well known for years as the professor of . . .

- An adverbial element ending in *-ly* is not hyphenated.

  clearly delineated principles of treatment
  widely used diagnostic methods

- Hyphenated compound modifiers not including adverbial or participial elements retain the hyphen when the modifier is a predicate adjective.

  The metabolic yield is rate-sensitive.

- Certain suffixes are hyphenated: *-elect*, *-type*.

  chairman-elect   a Cushing-type syndrome

- Compound modifiers that without hyphenation could be misread are hyphenated.

  a large-bowel obstruction   low-frequency amplitudes

- Compound modifiers with a capitalized second element are hyphenated.

  a psychotic, anti-Japanese outburst   a pro-Reagan faction

- Modifiers with numeric values and units are hyphenated.

  a 5-gram dose   a 5- to 10-gram range of doses

- Written-out compound cardinal and ordinal numbers from 21 to 99 are hyphenated.

  sixty-five cases   the two hundred and fifty-sixth patient

9.15   Decisions on hyphenation become more difficult and rules unclear with multiple modifiers. In general, use hyphenation only to maintain clear meaning. One useful rule is to hyphenate as unit modifiers those elements that when not part of a multiple-element modifier would stand as adjective and noun.

> an unusual tall-man, short-woman group of patients

For hyphenation of chemical prefixes and formulas, see sections 5.25, 16.21, 16.26, 16.30, 16.31, and Table 16.6.

COMPOUND TERMS

9.16   Write out as unhyphenated compound terms those terms that are well established in the medical vocabulary such as terms for methods, chemicals, compounds, diseases, functions.

> amino acid residues   basal cell nevus syndrome
> freezing point determination   sickle cell disease
> sodium chloride excretion

Do not hyphenate a proper name used adjectivally.

> Fisher exact test   Wilcoxon matched-pairs test

Do not hyphenate Latin phrases used adjectivally.

> in vitro methods   a post hoc hypothesis

Do not in general hyphenate letters used in scientific terms as modifiers.

> B cells   S waves   T lymphocyte   LE cells

(But hyphenate these terms when they serve as modifiers: "B-cell lymphoma", "T-lymphocyte functions", "LE-cell rosettes".)

A detailed guide to compounding can be found in the *United States Government Printing Office Style Manual* (14). The closed-compounding, hyphenating, and open-compounding of insect and plant vernacular names is a particularly difficult problem for editors without great experience in entomology or the plant sciences; a thorough and very helpful compilation of such names can also be found in the same source (15).

PLURAL FORMS

9.17   The general rule for forming the plural of a singular noun is add an *-s*.

> hemorrhage   hemorrhages   suture   sutures

When pronunciation of the plural form would be difficult with the simple addition of *-s* as with nouns ending in *-ch*, *-s*, *-sh*, *-x*, or *-z*, an *-es* is added instead. For common nouns ending in -[consonant]*y*, drop the *-y* and add *-ies*.

arterial branch	arterial branches
index	indexes
equity	equities

Most of the exceptions to these general rules are common nouns of early English origin, but there are some other types of exceptions. Some nouns add an ending other than *-s*; some change internally; others have identical singular and plural forms.

ox	oxen
woman	women
goose	geese
mouse	mice
trout	trout
forceps	forceps
series	series
species	species

A proper name must not be changed in spelling in forming its plural; the plural is formed by adding *-s* and the general rules stated above for common nouns do not apply.

... in a world of Toms, Dicks, and Harrys we would ...

A few abstract nouns cannot be plural idiomatically; authors in Spanish-language countries writing in English not infrequently use *information* in the unidiomatic plural, "informations".

9.18 A large group of common nouns in the medical vocabulary are of Greek origin or have been carried into English in their original form from a non-English language written with a roman-letter alphabet. Their plural forms can be determined by specific rules for Greek plurals or rules that apply in the original language; there is a strong tendency now in American usage to form plurals with the general rules stated in section 9.17, but these rules if applied should be applied throughout the journal to maintain consistency of style.

The Latin or Greek ending *-a* changes to *-ae*.

medulla	medullae
papilla	papillae

The French *-eau* and *-eu* add *-x*.

milieu	milieux
rouleau	rouleaux

The Latin *-en* changes to *-ina*.

foramen	foramina
nomen	nomina

The Latin *-ex* and *-ix* change to *-ices*.

index	indices
fornix	fornices

The Greek or Latin *-is* changes to *-es*.

metastasis	metastases

The Greek or Latin *-itis* changes to *-itides*.

enteritis	enteritides
meningitis	meningitides

The Italian *-o* changes to *-i*.

virtuoso	virtuosi

The Greek *-on* changes to *-a*.

criterion	criteria
enteron	entera

The Latin *-um* changes to *-a*.

bacterium	bacteria
medium	media
pudendum	pudenda
serum	sera

The Latin *-us* changes to *-i*.

bronchus	bronchi
fungus	fungi
rhonchus	rhonchi

The choice between forming a plural by the general English rules or by one of the rules summarized immediately above may have to be determined by general usage in the discipline of the journal or the degree of formality it wishes to have in its style.

Table 9.2 recommends some plurals that represent the tendency in medical American English to use the general rules for plurals but includes current preferences in formal medical publishing and forms for which there are no current idiomatically acceptable alternates by reason of need for euphony.

Each journal should compile its own standard list of acceptable plural forms.

9.19   A taxonomic name can be used as an English common noun if not capitalized and italicized (see sections 10.5 and 16.9). The plural form may be formed by the formal rule appropriate to its ending or by the general English rule.

Table 9.2: Recommended forms for some representative plural common nouns in the medical vocabulary

Singular form	Plural form	Singular form	Plural form
abscissa	abscissas	lumen	lumens
alga	algae	matrix	matrixes
ameba	amebas	maximum	maxima
analysis	analyses	medium	media
appendix	appendixes	medulla	medullas
bacillus	bacilli	meningitis	meningitides
bacterium	bacteria	metastasis	metastases
basis	bases	milieu	milieus
calix	calixes	mitosis	mitoses
criterion	criteria	mucosa	mucosas
datum	data	optimum	optima
dialysis	dialyses	papilla	papillas
encephalitis	encephalitides	phylum	phyla
enteritis	enteritides	protozoan	protozoans
foramen	foramens	rouleau	rouleaus
fornix	fornixes	septum	septa
genus	genera	sequel	sequels
hydrolysis	hydrolyses	sequela	sequelas
index	indexes	serum	sera

. . . the biochemistry of *Staphylococcus* is . . .
. . . many staphylococci were found in the . . .

. . . an *Enterobacter* species . . .
. . . his study of the enterobacters . . .

9.20 To form the plural of a year, an example word, or an abbreviation, add *-s.*

the 1960s   . . . too many *parameter*s in the text . . .   PhDs   MDs

If the typeface used in the journal has italic characters readily distinguished from its roman characters, the same rule can be applied to letters used as such, including symbols; otherwise an *-'s* will have to be used instead of the simple *-s.* Example words may need the same treatment.

his *p*s and *q*s   his *p*'s and *q*'s

9.21 The plural form of a compound noun written closed up is usually formed by the general rules for plurals applied to its terminal element.

spokesman spokesmen   teaspoonful teaspoonfuls

The plural form of an open compound noun is formed by making its main element (stem term) plural rather than the modifier.

attorneys-at-law   surgeons general
heirs presumptive   major generals

In a few cases both elements may have to be changed.

a woman doctor　　women doctors

9.22　The plural of an italicized noun, such as a title, is formed by adding a roman -*s* to the last element.

His desk was piled high with unread *New England Journal of Medicine*s.

POSSESSIVE FORMS

9.23　The possessive form of most singular common nouns and proper names, of indefinite pronouns, and of plural nouns not ending in -*s* is formed by adding an apostrophe and an *s*, '*s*.

patient's name　　Osler's library　　one's preferences
men's bias　　the data's complexity

This rule holds even if the word ends in a sibilant, -*s* or -*x*.

the waitress's complaints　　William Carlos Williams's poetry

The possessive form of paired nouns is determined by whether the meaning is joint ownership or individual ownership.

Osler and Halstead's building of the Hopkins faculty
Osler's and Mitchell's libraries

The possessive form of plural nouns ending in -*s* is formed by adding an apostrophe.

doctors' fees　　patients' complaints
the Munros' accomplishments　　the 1960s' turmoil

A few geographic and other proper names have elements with possessive meaning. To verify whether they do or do not have an apostrophied form, consult a geographic dictionary (16) or other similar reference work.

The possessive forms of abbreviations and numerals follow the same general rules as common and proper nouns.

the surprise in 1985's election　　the NIH's annual budget
the CDCs' combined budgets

In formal writing some authors prefer to avoid possessive forms of this kind.

WORD DIVISION

9.24　With the increasing use of computers for typesetting, decisions on word divisions at the end of lines are becoming less frequent. The computer programs generally allow for finer adjustments in spacing between characters and between words than could be made in older systems of composition; the programs include rules for word division and dictionaries for exceptions. But keep in mind that changing a word division or eliminating one can lead to new divisions in following lines as the computer recomposes the paragraph or page.

Even though word divisions will often be avoided by computer programs, some options may be available for needed changes in proof of word divisions judged by the editor to be unacceptable. Some general rules are particularly relevant to scientific publishing.

- Divide words etymologically if possible. Such division will preferably come between 2 stem elements or between a prefix and a stem element. If suffixes or other terminal elements must be carried to the next line, try to keep them intact.

pathologist	patho-	logist
photography	photo-	graphy
stereoradiography	stereo-	radiography
violaceous	viola-	ceous

- Try to avoid carrying an element to the next line that would look like a word with its own meaning.

pathologic	*not* patho-	logic
women	*not* wo-	men

- Divide hyphenated words and compound words after the hyphen and between the 2 elements of the compound word, but avoid breaking chemical names at hyphens connecting initial prefixes that serve as locants (see section 16.26). Long chemical names can be broken by syllables or etymologic roots or after internal hyphens; try, however, to divide long chemical names so that at least 4 or 5 characters are kept on each of the 2 lines.

a blue-black lesion	a blue-	black lesion
cost-benefit analysis	cost-	benefit analysis
databases	data-	bases
2-methyl-2-propenenitrile	2-meth-	yl-2-propenenitrile

- Try to avoid dividing personal names or carrying over appended elements like *FACP, Jr, MD*. If a personal name must be divided, carry over the last component (family name, surname).

Edward C Rosenow, Jr	Edward C-	Rosenow, Jr
Thomas Smith, FACP	Thomas-	Smith, FACP

- Do not divide units from their preceding numeric values.

100 g/L	*not* 100-	g/L
57 mL	*not* 57-	mL

- Try to avoid dividing numbers and, particularly, do not divide a number at a decimal point. If a large number must be divided, maintain 3-numeral groups.

25.67	*not* 25.-	67	*but*	25-	.67
125 679	*not* 125 6-	79	*but*	125-	679

- Do not divide short words.

cutis   iris   rami

Appropriate division points can be found in the entry words of some standard dictionaries (3–8), but these do not always correspond to etymologically justified divisions. In the medical dictionaries, division points may be deduced from the breaks and accents indicated in the phonetic version of a term parenthetically given after the term as entry word, but etymologic divisions should be preferred.

Detailed rules for word division can be found in several standard manuals (17–19).

REFERENCES

1. Weiner ESC. The Oxford guide to English usage. Oxford: Oxford University Press; 1983:1–44.
2. Hart's rules for compositors and readers at the University Press Oxford. 39th ed. Oxford: Oxford University Press; 1983:64–86.
3. Webster's standard American style manual. Springfield, Massachusetts: Merriam-Webster; 1985:82–95.
4. Morris W, ed. The American heritage dictionary of the English language. Boston: Houghton Mifflin Company; 1981.
5. Stein J. The Random House dictionary of the English language. New York: Random House; 1983.
6. Webster's ninth new collegiate dictionary. Springfield, Massachusetts: Merriam-Webster; 1983.
7. Webster's II new Riverside university dictionary. Boston: Riverside; 1984.
8. Kirkpatrick EM, ed. Chambers 20th century dictionary. Cambridge; Cambridge University Press; 1983.
9. Dorland's illustrated medical dictionary. 26th ed. Philadelphia: WB Saunders; 1985.
10. Landau SI, ed. International dictionary of medicine and biology. New York: John Wiley; 1986.
11. Stedman's medical dictionary. 24th ed. Baltimore: Williams & Wilkins; 1982.
12. Critchley M, ed. Butterworths medical dictionary. 2nd ed. London: Butterworths; 1978.
13. Romano F. Practical typography from a to z. Alexandria, Virginia: National Composition Association; 1983:2–4.
14. United States Government Printing Office style manual. Washington: Government Printing Office; 1984:81–116.
15. United States Government Printing Office style manual. Washington: Government Printing Office; 1984:257–274.

16. Webster's new geographical dictionary. Springfield, Massachusetts: Merriam-Webster; 1984.
17. The Chicago manual of style. 13th ed. Chicago: University of Chicago Press; 1982:164-7.
18. Words into type. 3rd ed. Englewood Cliffs, New Jersey: Prentice-Hall; 1974:238-9.
19. Hart's rules for compositors and readers at the University Press Oxford. 39th ed. Oxford: Oxford University Press; 1983:14-6.

Chapter 10

Nomenclature and Addresses

Scientific writing calls for precision as much in naming things and concepts as in presenting data. This chapter takes up major considerations in nomenclature; it includes cross-references to Chapter 16, "Scientific Style in Medical Sciences", for more detail on a number of fields.

Scientific names stand in differing levels of formality and precision, and care must be taken in selecting the right level in different contexts. Careful authors usually will have come to the right judgments in nomenclature, but editors must be sure that the judgments fit the needs of their audiences.

10.1 *Scientific names* is used here to refer to those names that are standard style for various scientific disciplines: the taxonomic names of organisms and, in chemistry, biochemistry, and pharmacology, the standard generic names, systematic chemical names, and brand names that are found in standard reference sources cited below in this chapter. Names that are adequately precise and clear in some fields may be considered imprecise in others. Names that in the plant and animal sciences and in chemistry are considered to lack scientific precision may be adequately precise in clinical medicine; names of this kind are known in some laboratory disciplines as common names, provincial names, or vernacular names; generic drug names and common chemical names are sometimes referred to in the chemical literature as "trivial names".

CHEMICAL NAMES

10.2 Most chemical names in medical publication are common and generic names represented by the entry terms in *The Merck Index* (1). In papers on specifically chemical or biochemical topics, systematic names (such as those used by Chemical Abstracts Service) may be needed; these names call for careful attention to rules for chemical-name prefixes and locants (see sections 5.25, 8.3, 16.25, 16.26, 16.27) and capitalization (see sections 7.1 and 7.2). *The Merck Index* is the best general source in which to verify systematic names, but *USAN and the USP Dictionary of Drug Names* (2) also provides systematic chemical names for drugs in addition to generic names.

10.3   When a specific product is referred to in specifying a reagent in a methods section, in a comparison of brand-named products of the same compound, or in toxicologic papers, the brand name (capitalized; see sections 7.6 and 10.11) should be given, with the name of the manufacturer. If the product is the main subject of the paper, the common or generic name (or names, in a compounded product) should be given at the first mention of the brand name, and within parenthesis marks. For drug names, see section 10.4.

A comprehensive source for brand names likely to appear in toxicologic papers is *Clinical Toxicology of Commercial Products* (3); this source provides indexes for brand names (trade names), ingredients, and manufacturers' names.

A journal should maintain a list of the chemical names most frequently used by its authors in which to verify correct form; use of such a list can reduce the frequency with which an authoritative reference source (*The Merck Index* [1], *CRC Handbook of Chemistry and Physics* [4]) has to be consulted and can help in maintaining consistency of nomenclature throughout the journal. This consistency will raise the probability that online searchers of the journal will find all documents relevant to their needs.

DRUG NAMES

10.4   Drug names include nonproprietary names and brand names. Nonproprietary names include the generic drug names established by national pharmacopeial authorities and the World Health Organization.

Papers on pharmacologic, pharmaceutic, diagnostic, and therapeutic topics should, in general, use generic drug names rather than brand names. If, however, a paper is about specific properties or effects of a brand-named product contrasted with other products of the same generic drug, the brand name (capitalized; see section 7.6) should be used throughout the paper, with parenthetic identification of the drug by generic name in the paper's title and at its first mention in the abstract and the text; the manufacturer should be named at the first mention of the name in the text.

. . . Cytomel (Smith Kline & French) (liothyronine sodium) . . .

If a generic name is used throughout the text but a particular brand of the drug was used in the research or clinical application, the brand name and the name of the manufacturer should be given in the methods section, if the paper has one, or the other notably relevant first mention of the generic name (also see section 10.11).

... liothyronine sodium (Cytomel, Smith Kline & French) ...

Note that generic names, as common nouns, are not capitalized except where appropriate for syntactical or typographic needs (see section 7.1). Do not be misled by the initial capitalization of generic drug names serving as entry terms in reference sources such as *The Merck Index* (1) and *USAN and the USP Dictionary of Drug Names* (2); unfortunately these and some similar sources, including a few dictionaries, do not follow the standard dictionary style of capitalizing entry terms only when they are proper names.

Generic names should be those established by the national pharmacopeial authority of the country in which the journal has its main audience. If a paper, for example, is from the United Kingdom and will be published in the United States, and the generic names for the drug differ in the two countries, the generic name for the United States should be used (with parenthetic statement of the other generic name at its first mention in the text). Attention to this point will reduce the risk that the paper will not be found in an online database by searchers accustomed to the US generic name and hence not including the UK name in the search. In the United States the authority is the USAN Council, formed of representatives from the American Medical Association, the American Pharmaceutical Association, and the United States Pharmacopeial Convention. The United States Adopted Names (USAN) are compiled in *USAN and the USP Dictionary of Drug Names* (2), which must be used in the United States as the standard source for approved generic drug names. *USAN and the USP Dictionary of Drug Names* is invaluable for other drug-name information: systematic chemical names; structural formulas; manufacturers' code designations; International Nonproprietary Names; Chemical Abstracts Service Registry Numbers; brand names; and manufacturers. A useful source for brand names in the United States, particularly those for multicomponent drugs, is *American Drug Index* (5).

An excellent reference work with international coverage is *Martindale: The Extra Pharmacopoeia* (6); its "monographs" (articles for entry terms) indicate the status of generic names in the official pharmacopoeias of a number of countries and the various brand names under which generic drugs, with manufacturer names. A directory of manufacturers gives their full names and addresses. Another reference source with international scope is *Pharmacological and Chemical Synonyms* (7).

In countries without nationally established generic names, the International Nonproprietary Names (INN) established by the World Health Organization should be used as the proper generic names; these are listed in the USAN compilation (2; see second paragraph above).

A drug in an experimental unapproved status and not yet assigned a USAN name may have to be identified by its manufacturer's code number.

Cl-885   ICI-U.S. 457   PAA-3854   R1575

The generic names of radioactive pharmaceuticals should include the name of the carrier compound and the symbol for the radioactive isotope with its atomic weight.

technetium Tc-99m medronate   thyroxine I-131

See section 16.21 and Table 16.5 for the symbols and mass numbers for radioactive isotopes and for comment on the hyphenation in the examples above.

TAXONOMIC NAMES

10.5   The animal, plant, and microbiologic sciences have well-established conventions for the formal and specific names of organisms at the various taxonomic (classification) levels. At the species level, the names are binomens (2-element names) made up of the genus name and the species epithet; the genus name is capitalized and both elements are italicized. The species epithet must not be used by itself. Genus names used by themselves and subspecies names are also italicized, but a modifier before a subspecies epithet, such as "var" for "variety" or "subsp" for "subspecies", or an abbreviation appended to a genus name must be in roman type.

> *Staphylococcus aureus*   *Campylobacter fetus* subsp *venerealis*
> *Pseudomonas* spp   *Drosophila melanogaster* [fruit fly]
> *Malus domestica* [the common apple]
> *Cotoneaster divericata* [a shrub with poisonous fruit]

10.6   After its first mention a species name may be shortened by abbreviating the genus name to a single letter, but if species of more than 1 genus are named the abbreviations chosen must avoid any ambiguity as to genus. Abbreviate, for example, *Staphylococcus aureus* and *Streptococcus bovis* to *S aureus* and *Str bovis* when they appear in the same paper. In clinical papers, a species may be referred to by a common name widely used in medicine, but the taxonomic name must be given with it in the title and the abstract, and at its first mention in the text and in a methods section (see sections 2.2, 2.8, 3.3).

> ... the pneumococcus (*Streptococcus pneumoniae*) ...
> ... the gonococcus (*Neisseria gonorrhoeae*) ...

Common names of this kind are idiomatically preceded by an article, but genus names and species names are not.

> ... clinical importance of the pneumococcus is ...
> ... studies of the metabolism of the gonococcus were ...

but

> ... studies of the genetics of *Streptococcus* were ...

The names of taxa (classification groups at various hierarchical levels; singular, *taxon*) higher than genus are capitalized (see section 7.3). In bacteriology the names of taxa higher than genus are italicized (see sections 8.2 and 16.3); in virology, family names (the level immediately above genus names) are italicized only if they have been approved by the International Committee on Taxonomy of Viruses (see sections 8.2 and 16.63). In other fields the name of taxa above genus should be in the roman type.

> *Legionellaceae*   *Herpesviridae*   Orchidaceae

For further details on taxonomic names see the relevant sections in Chapter 16: bacteriology (sections 16.1 to 16.7), mycology (sections 16.50, 16.51), parasitology and entomology (section 16.57), and virology (sections 16.63 to 16.65).

10.7   The spelling and structure of common and vernacular names in some fields of zoology and the plant sciences are governed by a complex group of rules. A comprehensive list of informal names for plants and insects can be found in the *United States Government Printing Office Style Manual* (8). Many common and vernacular names for animals can be found in standard English-language dictionaries. Further guidance on informal names for plants and animals can be found in the *CBE Style Manual* (9). Rules for the formation and spelling of common names for plants have been summarized by RA Hamilton and republished in a paper by Rudnitski (10).

A convenient compilation of taxonomic names for plants, animals, bacteria, and viruses down to various taxonomic levels (to genera for bacteria) can be found in "Biosystematic Codes" of *Search Guide: BIOSIS Previews Edition* (11). The taxonomic names of many animals used in research can be verified in *Animals for Research* (12) and *Supplement to Animals for Research* (13).

ANATOMIC TERMS

10.8   The internationally standard terms in human anatomy, histology, and embryology are the Latin terms compiled in *Nomina Anatomica* (NA)

(14); the compilations for veterinary anatomy and histology are *Nomina Anatomica Veterinaria* and *Nomina Histologica* (12). These terms are not used widely outside the literature of anatomy but are replaced by anglicized equivalents.

NA	arteria auricularis profunda	NA	ossa carpi
	deep auricular artery		carpal bones

Standard medical dictionaries (16–19) carry both the Latin and English terms and are convenient sources for verification. The Latin terms need not be italicized; they lie within the standard medical vocabulary (see section 8.8).

Note that some of the directional adjectives used to denote position and relationships differ in meaning in human and animal applications because of the differing upright postures.

Human: superior vena cava (the "upper" vena cava)
Animal: cranial vena cava (the vena cava toward the head)

Adverbial forms of the adjectives ending in *-al*, *-ic*, or *-or* are formed by dropping these endings and adding *-ad*.

cephalic   cephalad
dorsal   dorsad

DISEASE TERMS

10.9   The disease and pathologic terms in the Medical Subject Headings vocabulary (MeSH) of the National Library of Medicine (20) form, in effect, a standard terminology for medicine. When circumstances permit an author's substituting a MeSH term for his or her original choice, the MeSH term should be preferred because it is more likely to be used by online searchers in bibliographic and full-text databases and will raise the odds that the paper will be found in such searches. Note, however, that the MeSH vocabulary does not always represent specific disorders and syndromes with specific terms. Further, newly-appearing terms may not be added to the MeSH vocabulary until a term is clearly well established; *acquired immunodeficiency syndrome*, for example, was added only about 18 months after its first appearance in the journal literature.

Specific and descriptive terms for diseases should be preferred to equivalent eponymic terms (see section 10.10 below), which are usually not sufficiently descriptive and may be ambiguous when the eponymic element of the term appears in several eponyms.

NOT   Paget disease
BUT   osteitis deformans *or* pseudo-eczema of the mammary nipple

NOT   Kussmaul disease
BUT   polyarteritis nodosa

Current Medical Information and Terminology (see comment in the next paragraph) (21) extensively cross-refers from eponymic terms to equivalent preferred terms.

Several formal systems of terms for human diseases and their structural expression are used in the United States. *Systematized Nomenclature of Medicine* (SNOMED) (22) includes topographic, morphologic, etiologic, functional, procedural, and occupational classifications and terms as well as terms for diseases. SNOMED is widely used to promote uniformity and, hence, communicability, in case classification, filing, and reporting. Two other classifications of disease terms are also widely used in the United States for case classification and for case-record filing and retrieval: *Current Medical Information and Terminology* (21) and *International Classification of Diseases, 9th Revision, Clinical Modification (ICD-9-CM)* (23). These 2 systems, like SNOMED, serve their purposes in case classification, record filing and retrieval, case reporting, and billing, but like SNOMED may not serve the wider needs of many authors; hence disease terms should not be arbitrarily converted to conform to terms in one of these three systems. The MeSH vocabulary should be preferred. The publications with these 3 classifications can be used, however, to verify many terms in clinical medicine.

Terms for diseases and disease manifestations and for diagnostic and therapeutic procedures are most readily verified in most instances in standard medical dictionaries (16–19). A convenient source for verification of terms for diagnostic and therapeutic procedures is *Physicians' Current Procedural Terminology* (21).

EPONYMIC TERMS

10.10   A large number of compound medical terms include a proper name and hence are known as eponymic terms. The proper names may be those of families, nationalities, patients, places, physicians, or scientists. The terms may be terms for anatomic structures, apparatus, body positions, chemical reactions, chemicals, diseases, factors (biochemical, endocrinologic, hematologic, nutritional), microbiologic agents, procedures and techniques, reflexes, rules, signs, syndromes, tests, theories, units. Some of these terms have used the possessive form of the proper name as in "Hodgkin's disease", "Kussmaul's sign", "Nernst's theory"; others have not, as in those with a proper name not representing a physician or scientist, for example, "Minimata disease" (referring to a Japanese city) and "Hageman factor" (referring to a patient), and those with 2 or more hyphenated names, "Besnier-Boeck-Schaumann disease". Rules governing the use of the proper name in its original form or in its possessive form can be derived from past usage, but for their proper application most manuscript editors would have to know the original use of the proper name; thus in practice, manuscript editors have to know the correct form of the eponymic term or check the author's form in a general medical or eponymic dictionary.

The time has come to abandon the possessive forms of eponymic terms and simplify usage to nonpossessive forms. This style has been used in *Current Medical Information and Terminology* (21) since 1971. Note that the proper idiom for nonpossessive eponymic terms is an appropriate definite article before all eponymic terms except those incorporating the word *disease*.

> the Caplan syndrome   Hodgkin disease   the Babinski sign
> Addison disease   the Master two-step exercise test
> . . . regimens for treatment of Hodgkin disease include . . .
> . . . demonstrated a Babinski sign . . .

This style has also been followed by McKusick (25) in his great catalogs of human phenotypes: "As a rule, the possessive form of eponyms has not been used [by the author]; for example, the Marfan syndrome, not Marfan's syndrome, will be found in the catalogs. The reason is that the eponym is merely a 'handle'; often the man whose name is used was not the first to describe the condition (*America* is a classic example of naming for someone other than the first discoverer) or did not describe the syndrome as it has subsequently become known. As Darwin put it, 'Credit is rarely given to the first one to make a discovery but rather to him who convinces the public'." The passage from which this quotation comes offers, however, some rules for use and non-use of possessive forms, which may be useful to editors who cannot bring themselves to abandon eponyms in the possessive form.

MATERIALS AND METHODS

10.11   Many and various materials and methods are stated and described in the methods sections of papers reporting research. The degree of detail needed will range from brief mention of standard materials and equipment to detailed specification for unusual materials and equipment.

Standard chemical reagents generally need not be identified by brand name and manufacturer; unusual reagents not readily available from a number of potential suppliers should be identified by brand name, manufacturer, and manufacturer's location (city). See section 10.2 on chemical nomenclature.

Drugs need usually be identified only by generic name. In papers concerned with pharmacodynamic or pharmacokinetic research, comparison of commercial products, ineffectual therapy, or adverse effects, brand names should be given in addition and the manufacturer identified by name and city; see section 10.3 on drug nomenclature.

Many biologic materials may have to be identified by taxonomic name, specific type-culture identification (type-culture collection; alphanumeric catalog listing; descriptive title), genetically and physiologically descriptive characteristics, and source (supplier, city): they include viruses, phages, cell lines, hybridomas, bacteria, invertebrate and vertebrate animals.

B10.A(5R)/SgSn (The Jackson Laboratory, Bar Harbor, Maine) [a congenic resistant strain of mouse]

ATCC HB 65, H16-L10-4R5 (American Type Culture Collection, Rockville, Maryland) [a hybrid cell line secreting a monoclonal antibody specific for nucleoprotein of influenza type A virsues]

Designations of animal strains, stocks, hybrids, and mutants and taxonomic names (see section 10.3) and the names of suppliers and their locations can be verified in *Animals for Research* (12) and *Supplement to Animals for Research* (13). A standardized nomenclature is available for outbred stocks of laboratory animals (26). Designations of materials supplied by the American Type Culture Collection (ATCC) can be verified in the ATCC catalogs (27): algae, animal viruses and antisera, bacteria, bacteriophages, cell lines, chlamydiae, rDNA vectors, fungi, human tumor cells, hybridomas, molecularly cloned viruses, mycoviruses, oncogenes, plant tissue cultures, plant viruses and antisera, plasmids, protozoa, rickettsiae, tumor immunology cells, and yeasts.

Standard equipment widely used in laboratory routines need only be named by their common names; unusual equipment not widely available or the performance characteristics of which are critical for the research should be identified by brand name and manufacturer (with city).

The names and locations of manufacturers of reagents and apparatus can usually be verified in an annual compilation published in *Science* (28). Another useful compilation is that in *Trade Names Dictionary: Company Index* (29), which gives names and addresses for manufacturers, importers, marketers, and distributors.

GEOLOGIC AND GEOGRAPHIC NAMES

10.12 Geologic names are used infrequently in the medical literature. The most common names will be found as entry terms in the standard general dictionaries and *McGraw-Hill Concise Encyclopedia of Science & Technology* (30). More detail, including names of provincial stratigraphic series, can be found in *Suggestions to Authors of the Reports of the United States Geological Survey* (31).

Geographic names can be verified in *Webster's New Geographical Dictionary* (32); city, town, and village names can also be verified in the postal-code directories issued by the national postal services in the United States (33), Canada, the United Kingdom, and other countries.

ADDRESSES

10.13   Addresses that must be detailed and specific enough to serve as mailing addresses (such as those for statements of author affiliation; see section 2.7) should include all or some of certain elements.

> In the United States
> Name
> Department or unit
> Institution (with building and room number, or institutional postal route)
> > *Or:* Street number and name (with parenthetical office or suite number, if available)
> City (town), [State as official postal abbreviation] ZIP code
> USA [in addresses to be used outside the United States]

The US postal code (ZIP code) consists of a 5- or 9-digit number (the 9-digit form is hyphenated between the initial 5 digits and the terminal 4) and should be placed after the state ZIP-code abbreviation (see section 11.8) with one space between them. For the ZIP code abbreviations of state names, see Table 11.2; for addresses in which the length of lines must be held to a minimum, additional abbreviations are recommended in the opening pages of the annual ZIP code directory (33).

The Canadian postal code is composed of alphabetic (A) and numeric (N) elements in the form ANA NAN; like the first digit in the US ZIP code, the first letter in the Canadian code stands for a region in Canada. In Canadian addresses for domestic use the postal code should be placed, preferably, on a line by itself or after the abbreviation for the province (separated by a two-character space).

> Dr W M Smith   Dr W M Smith
> 150 Nepean St, Apt 5   150 Nepean St, Apt 5
> Ottawa, Ontario   Ottawa, ON   K2P OB6
> K2P OB6

In addresses to be used by correspondents addressing letters from outside Canada, the postal code should, if possible, occupy the last line of the address by itself or follow "Canada" by several spaces.

> Dr W M Smith
> 150 Nepean St, Apt 5
> Ottawa, ON
> Canada   K2P OB6

GEOGRAPHIC COORDINATES

10.14   In specifying a location by its geographic coordinates, give the latitude first followed, after a comma, by the longitude. In running text *latitude* and *longitude* should be written out; the abbreviations *lat* and *long* can be used in parenthetic statements, footnotes, tables, and figures. The numbers and accompanying symbols for degrees, minutes, and seconds are always closed up.

> . . . and corpses of the Franklin party were found at latitude 52°33′05″ N, longitude 13°21′10″ E.
> *In a table:* lat 52°33′05″ N, long 13°21′10″ E

Avoid breaking such designations at the end of a line if possible (see section 9.24). If a break must be made, divide the coordinate after a symbol for a coordinate unit (such as the degree symbol) and hyphenate at that point.

> 52°-   33′05″ N   13°21′-   10″ E

Other coordinate systems are in use that are not built on the latitude–longitude system; an example is that used with the 1:250 000 topographic maps of the US Geological Survey. These other systems are rarely, if ever, used in medical publishing.

REFERENCES

1. Windholz M, ed. The Merck index. 10th ed. Rahway, New Jersey: Merck; 1983.
2. USAN and the USP dictionary of drug names. Rockville, Maryland: United States Pharmacopeial Convention; [annual publication].
3. Gosselin RE, Smith RP, Hodge HC. Clinical toxicology of commercial products. 5th ed. Baltimore: Williams & Wilkins; 1984.
4. Weast RC, ed. CRC Handbook of chemistry and physics. 66th ed. Cleveland: CRC; 1985.
5. Billups NF, ed. American drug index. 30th ed. Philadelphia: JB Lippincott; 1986. An annual publication.
6. Reynolds JEF, ed. Martindale: the extra pharmacopoeia. 28th ed. London: The Pharmaceutical Press; 1982.
7. Marler EEJ. Pharmacological and chemical synonyms. 8th ed. Amsterdam: Elsevier, 1985.
8. United States Government Printing Office style manual. Washington: Government Printing Office, 1984:257–74.
9. CBE Style Manual Committee. CBE style manual. 5th ed. Bethesda, Maryland: Council of Biology Editors; 1983:156, 187.
10. Hamilton RA. The spelling of common [plant] names. In: Rudnitski S. Choosing and spelling common names for plants. CBE Views. 1982;5:7–10.
11. BioSciences Information Service. Search guide: BIOSIS previews edition. Philadelphia: BioSciences Information Service; [annual publication].

12. Greehouse DD, Cohen AL, eds. Animals for research. 10th ed. Washington: National Academy Press; 1979.
13. Supplement to animals for research. Washington: National Academy Press; 1981.
14. Subcommittees of the International Anatomical Nomenclature Committee. Nomina anatomica, 5th ed; Nomina histologica, 2nd ed; Nomina embryologica, 2nd ed. Baltimore: Williams & Wilkins; 1983.
15. International Committee on Veterinary Gross Anatomical Nomenclature. Nomina anatomica veterinaria, 3rd ed; Nomina histologica, 2nd ed. Ithaca, New York: International Committee on Veterinary Gross Anatomical Nomenclature; 1983. Distributed by Department of Veterinary Anatomy, Cornell University, Ithaca, New York 14853, USA.
16. Dorland's illustrated medical dictionary. 26th edition. Philadelphia: WB Saunders; 1985.
17. Landau SI, ed. International dictionary of medicine and biology. New York: John Wiley; 1986.
18. Stedman's medical dictionary. 24th ed. Baltimore: Williams & Wilkins; 1982.
19. Critchley M. Butterworths medical dictionary. 2nd ed. London: Butterworths; 1978.
20. National Library of Medicine. Medical subject headings [annual]. Bethesda, Maryland: National Library of Medicine; [annual publication].
21. Finkel AJ. Current medical information and terminology: for the naming and description of diseases and conditions in practice and in areas related to medicine. 5th ed. Chicago: American Medical Association; 1981.
22. Systematized nomenclature of medicine. 2nd ed. Skokie, Illinois: College of American Pathologists; 1979.
23. Commission on Professional and Hospital Activities. International classification of diseases, 9th revision, clinical modification (ICD-9-CM). Ann Arbor, Michigan: Commission on Professional and Hospital Activities; 1978.
24. Fanta CM, Finkel AJ, Kirschner CG, Perlman JM, AMA Editorial Staff. Physicians' current procedural terminology. 4th ed. Chicago: American Medical Association; 1986.
25. McKusick VA. Mendelian inheritance in man: catalogs of autosomal dominant, autosomal recessive, and x-linked phenotypes. 7th ed. Baltimore: Johns Hopkins University Press; 1983:xxiv.
26. International Committee on Laboratory Animals. International standardized nomenclature for outbred stocks of laboratory animals. Washington: [distributed by] Institute of Laboratory Animal Resources; 1971. (ICLA bulletin no 30, 1972).
27. American Type Culture Collection. [Catalogs]. Rockville, Maryland: American Type Culture Collection; [publication dates at 4-year intervals]. Catalogs for algae, animal viruses and antisera, bacteria, bacteriophages, cell lines, chlamydiae, rDNA vectors, fungi, human tumor cells, hybridomas, molecularly-cloned viruses, mycoviruses, oncogenes, plant tissue cultures, plant viruses and antisera, plasmids, protozoa, rickettsiae, tumor-immunology cells, and yeasts.
28. American Association for the Advancement of Science. 1986 guide to biotechnology products and instruments. Science. 1986;232(May 30 Pt II):G1–224.
29. Crowley ET. Trade names dictionary: company index. 2nd ed. Detroit: Gale Research; 1979.
30. Parker SP, ed. McGraw-Hill concise encyclopedia of science & technology. New York: McGraw-Hill; 1984.

31. Bishop EE, Eckel EB, others. Suggestions to authors of the reports of the United States Geological Survey. 6th ed. Washington: US Government Printing Office; 1978. A new edition is expected for 1987.
32. Webster's new geographical dictionary. Springfield, Massachusetts: Merriam-Webster; 1984.
33. [Annual] national five-digit ZIP code and post office directory. Washington: United States Postal Service; [annual publication].

Chapter 11

Symbols and Abbreviations

SYMBOLS

11.1   A symbol is an alphabetic character, or 2 or more alphabetic or alphanumeric characters in an unspaced pair or group, or a graphic structure (such as $+$, $=$, $>$, $\neq$) representing a longer term (word or phrase) for a quantity, unit, element, unit structure, operation, or relationship. A symbol may be an abbreviation, such as G for *gravitational constant*, but need not be.

Symbols for quantities and for genes are set in italic (slanted) type even if the accompanying text is also in an italic (slanted) face; subscripts and superscripts modifying symbols should be in roman (upright) type unless they are themselves symbols normally italicized (1,2; also see sections 8.4 and 8.5).

Note that symbols for units of measurement must be in a roman (upright) face (see section 13.15). The distinction between symbols for quantities and symbols for units must be kept clearly in mind. Lowe (2) draws the distinction thus.

> There are two principal types of symbol: symbols for quantities and symbols for units. The two should be carefully distinguished: for example, the symbols for the quantities that are measured by the seven SI base units are l (length), m (mass), t (time), I (electric current), T (thermodynamic temperature), I (luminous intensity), and n (amount of substance), whereas the symbols for the units in which they are measured are m, kg, s, A, K, cd, and mol, respectively.

Also see section 13.15.

Symbols for vectors and tensors should be in italic (slanted) boldface type (see section 8.12).

Note that symbols for mathematical operations such as d for the differential sign and ! as the factorial sign must be in a roman (upright) face.

$$dx/dt \qquad n!$$

A symbol must not be followed by a period unless it comes at the end of a sentence.

For plural forms of symbols and abbreviations, see section 11.4.

ABBREVIATIONS

11.2   Abbreviations are short equivalents of individual words, compound terms, or phrases. They take 2 general forms.

The first form of abbreviations includes short equivalents formed by dropping terminal letters or omitting letters within a word.

Dr   doctor   Fig   figure   ECG   electrocardiogram

The second form of abbreviations includes short equivalents formed from the initial letters of compound terms or the words of a phrase.

USA	United States of America
a.k.a.	also known as
DNA	deoxyribonucleic acid
TPN	total parenteral nutrition
e.g.	*exempli gratia* [for example]

Acronyms are abbreviations that can be read as a word. They are usually formed from the initial letter of each major word in the term.

JAMA   *(J)ournal of the (A)merican (M)edical (A)ssociation*
laser   (l)ight (a)mplification by (s)timulated (e)mission of (r)adiation

An acronym of the second type usually enters the standard vocabulary rapidly and follows all general rules of grammar, syntax, capitalization, and punctuation. Formation of acronymic journal titles is, however, an undesirable practice and should be avoided (see section 1.1).

The extent of use of either form of abbreviation by a journal should be governed by a comprehensive and deliberate policy that has been established by weighing the advantages and disadvantages of abbreviations for the journal's readership. A clear policy reduces the number of decisions the journal's manuscript editors must make in routine work. The policy should lead to consistency of style for abbreviations throughout the journal. No simple rules exist that can be easily applied in establishing a policy on abbreviations but the following points might be weighed.

• Abbreviations of nonscientific terms and phrases should not, in general, be used in the text of scientific writing unless they have been established by a formal convention for specific purposes (such as the ZIP code abbreviations of state names for postal addresses) or are widely accepted abbreviations representing long terms (such as NATO for the North Atlantic Treaty Organization). Abbreviations that represent lazy writing, such as the "a.k.a." given above in the second group of examples, should certainly not be used.

- Abbreviations for Latin phrases or words should be replaced by English equivalents: Not "e.g." for *exempli gratia* but "for example"; not "viz." for *videlicet* but "namely"; not "etc." for *et cetera* but "and so on"; not "et al." but "and others" or "and coauthors" (except in the convention for bibliographic references specified in section 15.13).
- Abbreviations for scientific terms and phrases can be accepted if they are well known to a great majority of the readership and are parenthetically defined by the equivalent terms at first use in the text. Such abbreviations are, however, often a sign of lazy writing, of prose inadequately revised for concise statement: "COLD" for *chronic obstructive lung disease*; "TTP" for *thrombotic thrombocytopenic purpura*. See section 17.1 for comment on this frequent problem in medical prose style.

A journal's policy on abbreviations should be represented in its own style manual by 2 lists: abbreviations (and standard scientific symbols) that are used without explanation; and abbreviations that are acceptable but must be explained by parenthetic statement at their first use in the text of the term each represents.

Abbreviations should not, in general, be used in titles or abstracts (but see sections 2.2 and 2.8).

PUNCTUATION OF ABBREVIATIONS

11.3   Inconsistency in the punctuating of abbreviations has long been characteristic of style in English-language publication, even in scientific journals with consistency in most details of style. But through the past 3 or 4 decades there has been a clear trend to eliminating punctuation for abbreviations. Now appears to be the time to abandon the punctuating with periods of most abbreviations. In rare instances periods may be needed to avoid ambiguity, but even then some minor rewriting can usually eliminate any need for the abbreviation; see the recommendation 3 paragraphs below on optimal use of the period.

Note the view of *The Chicago Manual of Style* (3).

It is often an open question whether or not periods should be used with particular abbreviations. The trend is now strongly away from the use of periods with all kinds of abbreviations that have carried them in the past. In our view this is to the good: anything that reduces the fussiness of typography makes for easier reading.

This is a trend already welcomed by the British lexicographer Eric Partridge over 30 years ago (4); he was thoroughly accustomed, it must be noted, to the then longstanding British style of not using periods after "suspension abbreviations", such as *Mr* and *Dr*, formed by omission of letters within the word.

> . . . from the United States has come a practice that is rapidly growing and that could advantageously become universal. If it did, it would merely fall in line with the very general abandonment of points [periods] in chemistry, physics, electricity . . . [Partridge also points to American practice in abbreviations like TVA, NATO, NIH.] For the initials of all organizations, the omission of points would be – for Americans it already is – an excellent thing. . . . Indeed, I should, except for initials before surnames, retain points only where their omission would cause ambiguity. . . .
>
> . . . .
>
> If ever there was – who doubts that there is? – a strong case for mankind v. useless conventions, the discarding of all but clarificatory points constitutes such a case.

The now widespread use of word-processing programs for scientific writing and its analysis and revision brings another compelling reason to abandon the use of unneeded periods with abbreviations: Some technical operations in word processing and some programs for text analysis function properly only when periods are used solely to mark the ends of sentences; the search term in such procedures can be ". " ("period" and "space"). In view of these considerations, this manual recommends in both this and other chapters that periods not be used, in general, to mark abbreviations.

If periods must used with abbreviations to avoid ambiguity or to allay the anxiety of a habit-bound and nervous editor, close up the conventional spaces between letters of the abbreviation (as recommended in *The ACS Style Guide* [5], which, incidentally, also stands against the use of "periods after . . . abbreviations and symbols").

> e.g.   i.e.   o.d. [outside diameter]

This rule can be applied without disregarding the recommendation in the preceding paragraph because such abbreviations will almost invariably be followed immediately by a comma, which avoids the "period and space" construction.

> . . . in such diseases, e.g., lupus erythematosus.

Conventions calling for an abbreviation, a period, and a space can usually be avoided by writing out the abbreviated word (or words). An example is *versus* in the legal convention for names of cases (see section 8.7).

NOT   *United States v. Reynolds*
BUT   *United States versus Reynolds*

Abbreviations in text of names, such as author initials, should follow the convention for initials in bibliographic references (see section 15.12); the context will make clear the meaning of the abbreviation.

PLURAL, POSSESSIVE, AND COMPOUND FORMS OF ABBREVIATIONS

11.4   Add the letter *s* to an abbreviation to form its plural, but note that symbols for units of measure that are abbreviations are not converted to a plural form when they would be read as plural if written out.

> . . . too many MDs in Florida . . .
> . . . more PhDs are being awarded grants . . .
> 317 mg [even if read as "three hundred seventeen milligrams"]

The possessive forms follow the same rules as those for words (see section 9.23).

> . . . that MD's penchant for malpractice . . .
> . . . many MDs' fears of excessively high premiums . . .

In compound words made of an abbreviation and a word or prefix or suffix, attach the elements with a hyphen.

> . . . a JCAH-approved hospital . . .
> . . . detected anti-DNA antibodies . . .
> . . . some RNA-like molecules . . .

SPECIFIC CLASSES OF ABBREVIATIONS

AGENCIES, DEPARTMENTS, ORGANIZATIONS, SOCIETIES

11.5   Abbreviations formed from the initial letters of the words in formal names are capital letters run together without punctuation.

> ACP   AMA   DHEW   DHHS   FDA   NIH   WHO

Such abbreviations need not be explained at first mention if they are likely to be understood by a great majority of the journal's readership.

COMPOUND COMMON TERMS

11.6   Abbreviations for compound terms likely to be readily understood by the journal's readership after first mention with explanation are formed of initial letters capitalized even though the terms are common-noun terms and thus are not capitalized in their full form.

> DNA   deoxyribonucleic acid
> DRGs   diagnosis-related groups [a plural form]

NSAID   nonsteroidal anti-inflammatory drug
PEFR   peak expiratory flow rate

DEGREES, HONORS, MILITARY TITLES, TERMS OF ADDRESS

11.7   Abbreviations for academic degrees, academic or national honors, military ranks, and terms of address do not need periods because their contexts almost invariably make clear that they are abbreviations.

Abbreviated terms of address are made up of an initial capital letter and one or more conventionally added lowercase letters.

Dr	Doctor	Mrs	"Mistress" [married, "missus"]
Hon	Honorable	Ms	"Mistress" [marriage status not
Miss	"Mistress" [unmarried]		specified]
Mlle	Mademoiselle	Rev	Reverend
Mr	Mister	Sr	Senior, Señor

Note that in accord with British practice (6) these abbreviations do not close with periods. (For comment on the abbreviations for the obsolete social term of address for women, "Mistress", see *The Handbook of Nonsexist Writing* [7].)

Abbreviations of military titles used as terms of address follow the same principles. In military publications in medicine or in addresses of military persons the forms preferred within military organizations (such as those in the second column of the examples immediately below) may be needed (8); such forms will usually be specified in submitted copy. For examples of the two types of abbreviations for military titles (and military organizations) see Table 11.1.

Adm	ADM	Admiral
Col	COL	Colonel
Lt Gen	LTG	Lieutenant General

Most abbreviations for academic degrees and for honors are capital letters; there are some conventional exceptions.

MD   DPhil   DO   FRCP   OBE

See Table 12.1 for a list of academic degrees, honors, and their abbreviations.

GEOGRAPHIC NAMES

11.8   State, provincial, and departmental names should not be abbreviated in article titles, text headings, table titles, and running text. State names in addresses should be abbreviated in accord with the US ZIP Code conventions; see Table 11.2 for the ZIP forms and analogous abbreviations for Canadian provinces. If state, provincial, and departmental names must be abbreviated because of constraints of space, as in tables and lists, use the ZIP and ZIP-type abbreviations.

Table 11.1: Examples of abbreviations for US military titles and organizations

Title or organization	Non-military form	Military form
Admiral	Adm	ADM
Brigadier General	Brig Gen	BG
Captain	Capt	CAPT, CPT
Colonel	Col	COL
Commander	Comdr	CDR
Corporal	Cpl	CPL
Ensign	Ens	ENS
Lieutenant	Lt	LT
Lieutenant Commander	Lt Comdr	LCDR, LTC
Lieutenant General	Lt Gen	LTG
Lieutenant, Junior Grade	Lt (jg)	LTJG
Major	Maj	MAJ
Private	Pvt	PVT
Private, First Class	Pfc	PFC
Sergeant	Sgt	SGT
Vice Admiral	Vice Adm	VADM
US Air National Guard Medical Corps	. . .	MC, ANG
US Air Force Medical Corps	. . .	MC, USAF
US Army Medical Corps	. . .	MC, USA
US Navy Medical Corps	. . .	MC, USN
US Coast Guard	. . .	USCG

Avoid the lazy use of abbreviations like "St" and "Rd" for *street* and *road* in running text.

Country names should be written out in titles and text, but abbreviations for very long names may be used if they are widely known, such as USSR for *Union of Soviet Socialist Republics*. The abbreviation US for the United States of America may be used as part of a compound term, for example, US Government Printing Office, but do not abbreviate *United States* where it stands alone in text as a proper name.

Compass points are abbreviated as capital letters without punctuation. These abbreviations should, in general, be used only for space-saving as in tables, as terminal elements in addresses, or in geographic coordinates in the latitude-longitude system. Statements of compass points in running text or that are part of a geographic term should be written out.

N   north   E   east   S   south   W   west
NNE   north-northeast   NW   northwest   SE   southeast
87°15′11″ N, 79°12′00″ W   51 F Street, NW
19 South Buchanan Street, NE   the Northwest Territories
South Tuscaloosa   New South Wales

DATES AND TIMES

11.9   The names of months and of days of the week should be abbreviated

Table 11.2: ZIP Code abbreviations; analogous abbreviations for Canadian provinces

State, territory, or province	Abbreviation	State, territory, or province	Abbreviation
Alabama	AL	New Brunswick	NB
Alaska	AK	Newfoundland	NF
Alberta	AB	New Hampshire	NH
Arizona	AZ	New Jersey	NJ
Arkansas	AR	New Mexico	NM
American Samoa	AS	New York	NY
British Columbia	BC	North Carolina	NC
California	CA	North Dakota	ND
Colorado	CO	Northern Mariana	CM
Connecticut	CT	Islands	
Delaware	DE	Northwest Territories	NT
District of	DC	Nova Scotia	NS
Columbia		Ohio	OH
Florida	FL	Oklahoma	OK
Georgia	GA	Ontario	ON
Guam	GU	Oregon	OR
Hawaii	HI	Pennsylvania	PA
Idaho	ID	Puerto Rico	PR
Illinois	IL	Quebec	QB
Indiana	IN	Rhode Island	RI
Iowa	IA	Saskatchewan	SK
Kansas	KS	South Carolina	SC
Kentucky	KY	South Dakota	SD
Louisiana	LA	Tennessee	TN
Maine	ME	Trust Territory	TT
Manitoba	MB	Texas	TX
Maryland	MD	Utah	UT
Massachusetts	MA	Vermont	VT
Michigan	MI	Virginia	VA
Minnesota	MN	Virgin Islands	VI
Mississippi	MS	Washington	WA
Missouri	MO	West Virginia	WV
Montana	MT	Wisconsin	WI
Nebraska	NE	Wyoming	WY
Nevada	NV	Yukon Territory	YT

only to save space, as in tables; do not abbreviate them in running text. Table 11.3 lists standardized three-letter abbreviations. See section 13.22 for use of abbreviated names of months in dates.

Abbreviations for the two 12-hour divisions of the day, for eras, and for time zones should be unspaced capital letters without punctuation. The abbreviations are placed where the full term would be in the convention for reading.

4040 BC	4040 before Christ
AH 1327	*anno Hegirae* 1327

Table 11.3: Abbreviations for months and days of the year

Months		Days of the week	
Name	Abbreviation	Name	Abbreviation
January	Jan	Monday	Mon
February	Feb	Tuesday	Tue
March	Mar	Wednesday	Wed
April	Apr	Thursday	Thu
May	[May]	Friday	Fri
June	Jun	Saturday	Sat
July	Jul	Sunday	Sun
August	Aug		
September	Sep		
October	Oct		
November	Nov		
December	Dec		

12:57 PM	12:57 *post meridiem*
AD 1066	*anno domini* 1066
AH 7721	*anno Hebraico* 7721
1:33 AM	1:33 *ante meridiem*

Note however that the 24-hour system should be preferred for designations of times (see section 13.21).

REFERENCES

1. International Organization for Standardization. Units of measurement: ISO standards handbook 2. 2nd ed. Geneva: International Organization for Standardization; 1982;23–4.
2. Lowe DA. A guide to international recommendations on names and symbols for quantities and on units of measurement. Geneva: World Health Organization; 1975:298–9.
3. The Chicago manual of style. 13th ed. Chicago: University of Chicago Press; 1982:376.
4. Partridge E. You have a point there: a guide to punctuation and its allies. London: Routledge & Kegan Paul. 1953:42–3
5. Dodd JS, ed. The ACS style guide: a manual for authors and editors. Washington: American Chemical Society; 1986:24
6. Weiner ESC, comp. The Oxford guide to English usage. Oxford: Clarendon Press, 1983:1–2.
7. Miller C, Swift K. The handbook of nonsexist writing. New York: Lippincott & Crowell; 1980:100–1.
8. United States Government Printing Office style manual. Washington: Government Printing Office; 1984:139.

Chapter 12

Degrees, Honors, and Terms of Address

Journal policies on carrying academic degrees and professional honors after personal names necessarily differ widely. See section 2.6 for comment on degrees and honors in author statements (bylines) on title pages of articles.

ACADEMIC DEGREES

12.1 Academic degrees following names in author statements on title pages of articles and in text should be abbreviated as shown in Table 12.1. Do not punctuate the abbreviations with periods (see sections 11.3 and 11.7). Degrees should be separated from each other and from the preceding name and following text by commas. See section 2.6 for the sequence of degrees of different academic levels. Place abbreviations for honors (such as FRCP, KCB, OBE; see section 12.2) after academic degrees and in order of increasing distinction.

> . . . was represented by Adam Smith, MD, PhD, at the . . .
> . . . offered a course taught by James Jones, MD, MPH, . . .
> . . . was founded by Ferdinand Munro, MD, FRCP, OBE, in . . .

See section 12.3 for comment on academic degrees as terms of address. Do not carry an academic degree after a name preceded by an academic term of address, for example, "Dr Adam Smith, MD".

PROFESSIONAL HONORS

12.2 Many academic and professional societies distinguish levels of membership and honor unusual accomplishments with special designations of which the most common in medicine is "Fellow"; see Table 12.1 for many examples. For reasons discussed in section 2.6 such honors should not

Table 12.1: Academic degrees and professional honors [fn1]

Abbreviation	Term	Abbreviation	Term
AB	Bachelor of Arts	DMD	Doctor of Medical Dentistry
AgrM	Agrégé de Medicine	DO	Doctor of Osteopathy
AgrSc	Agrégé de Science	DOph	Doctor of Ophthalmology
BA	Bachelor of Arts	DPaed	Doctor of Paediatrics
BaO	Bachelor of Obstetrics	DPharm	Doctor of Pharmacy
BCh	Bachelor of Surgery	DPhil	Doctor of Philosophy
BChir	Bachelor of Surgery	DPM	Doctor of Podiatric Medicine
BDS	Bachelor of Dental Surgery	DrMed	Doctor of Medicine
BEc	Bachelor of Economics	DrMed Dent	Doctor of Dentistry
BM	Bachelor of Medicine	DrMedVet	Doctor of Veterinary Medicine
BN	Bachelor of Nursing	DrPhar	Doctor of Pharmacy
BPE	Bachelor of Physical Education	DTM&H	Diploma in Tropical Medicine and Hygiene
BPhar	Baccalaureat en Pharmacie	DU(P)	Docteur de l'Université (de Paris)
BPharm	Bachelor of Pharmacy	DVM	Doctor of Veterinary Medicine
BS	Bachelor of Science Bachelor of Surgery	DVS(Sc)	Doctor of Veterinary Science
BSc	Bachelor of Science	FAAP	Fellow of the American Academy of Pediatrics
BSHE	Bachelor of Science in Home Economics	FACA	Fellow of the American College of Anesthesiologists
BScPharm	Bachelor of Science in Pharmacy		Fellow of the American College of Apothecaries
BSD	Bachelor of Science in Dentistry	FACC	Fellow of the American College of Cardiology
BVSc	Bachelor of Veterinary Science	FACCP	Fellow of the American College of Chest Physicians
CB	Commander of the Order of the Bath	FACD	Fellow of the American College of Dentists
CBE	Commander of the Order of the British Empire	FACDS	Fellow of the Australian College of Dental Surgeons
CC	Companion of the Order of Canada	FACHA	Fellow of the American College of Hospital Administrators
ChB	Bachelor of Surgery	FACOG	Fellow of the American College of Obstetricians and Gynecologists
ChM	Master of Surgery		
CPH	Certificate of Public Health	FACP	Fellow of the American College of Physicians
DBE	Dame Commander of the Order of the British Empire		Fellow of the American College of Prostho-dontists
DDM	Doctor of Dental Medicine		
DDS	Doctor of Dental Surgery		
DEd	Doctor of Education		
DHyg	Doctor of Hygiene		
DM	Doctor of Medicine		
DMD	Doctor of Dental Medicine		

Table 12.1: (*continued*)

Abbreviation	Term	Abbreviation	Term
FACR	Fellow of the American College of Radiologists	FRCPI	Fellow of the Royal College of Physicians of Ireland
FACS	Fellow of the American College of Surgeons	FRCP&S Canada	Fellow of the Royal College of Physicians and Surgeons of Canada
FACSM	Fellow of the American College of Sports Medicine		
FAPHA	Fellow of the American Public Health Association	FRCS(C)	Fellow of the Royal College of Surgeons of Canada
FCRA	Fellow of the College of Radiologists of Australia	FRCSEd	Fellow of the Royal College of Surgeons of Edinburgh
FDSRCS	Fellow of the Royal College of Surgeons in Dental Surgery	FRCVS	Fellow of the Royal College of Veterinary Surgeons
FFARCS	Fellow of the Faculty of Anesthetics, Royal College of Surgeons	FRS	Fellow of the Royal Society
FFDRCSI	Fellow of the Faculty of Dentistry, Royal College of Surgeons in Ireland	FRSH	Fellow of the Royal Society of Health
		FRSTM	Fellow of the Royal Society of Tropical Medicine and Hygiene
FICD	Fellow of the Institute of Canadian Dentists	JD	Doctor of Jurisprudence
		JuD	Doctor of Law
FICS	Fellow of the International College of Surgeons	KBE	Knight Commander of the Order of the British Empire
FIMLT	Fellow of the Institute of Medical Laboratory Technology	KCB	Knight Commander of the Order of the Bath
FRACP	Fellow of the Royal Australasian College of Physicians	LDS	Licentiate in Dental Surgery
		LicMed	Licentiate in Medicine
		LLB	Bachelor of Laws
FRACS	Fellow of the Royal Australasian College of Surgeons	LLD	Doctor of Laws
		LM	Legion of Merit Licentiate in Medicine Licentiate in Midwifery
FRCOG	Fellow of the Royal College of Obstetricians and Gynecologists	LMS	Licentiate in Medicine and Surgery
FRCPA	Fellow of the Royal College of Pathologists of Australasia	LMSSA	Licentiate in Medicine and Surgery of the Society of Apothecaries
FRCP(C)	Fellow of the Royal College of Physicians of Canada	LRCP	Licentiate of the Royal College of Physicians
FRCPEd	Fellow of the Royal College of Physicians of Edinburgh	LRCS	Licentiate of the Royal College of Surgeons
		MACVS	Member of the Australian College of Veterinary Surgeons

Table 12.1: *(continued)*

Abbreviation	Term	Abbreviation	Term
MaO	Master of Obstetrics	MRCSEd	Member of the Royal College of Surgeons of Edinburgh
MB	Bachelor of Medicine		
MBE	Member of the Order of the British Empire	MSc(Med)	Master of Science in Medicine
MCh	Master of Surgery		
MChD	Master of Dental Surgery	MScN	Master of Science in Nursing
MD	Doctor of Medicine		
MDS	Master of Dental Surgery	MSP	Master of Science in Pharmacy
MMSA	Master of Midwifery of the Society of Apothecaries	MVSc	Master of Veterinary Science
MPH	Master of Public Health	PhD	Doctor of Philosophy
MRCP	Member of the Royal College of Physicians	PhG	Graduate in Pharmacy
		ScB	Bachelor of Science
MRCPath	Member of the Royal College of Pathologists	ScD	Doctor of Science
		SM	Master of Science
MRCPEd	Member of the Royal College of Physicians of Edinburgh		

fn1: For an additional listing see "Appendix 1" in reference 1.

be used in author statements (bylines) or in the text of scientific papers. Some scientific societies publishing a journal may require that the journal's author statements on title pages include its own honor designations. Such honors can be properly used with the names of their bearers in news notes of a society and in biographical essays and obituaries.

. . . the portrait of Michael Faraday, FRS, hung in . . .

Another category of honors that may have to be represented in biographic papers, obituaries, and historical essays is titles of distinction awarded by governments to honor great national service or especially meritorious accomplishments, such as "Knight Commander of the Order of the British Empire" (KBE) and "Legion of Merit" (LM). Such abbreviations should always come last in a series of abbreviations for academic degrees and professional honors.

TERMS OF ADDRESS

12.3   Persons with doctoral degrees or distinguished positions in the clergy, government, or military forces are frequently addressed with a term derived from a degree or position: "Doctor", "the Reverend", "the Honorable", "General". Such terms should not be used with personal names in the text of articles representing current or historical scientific reporting or discussion.

> . . . and studies of Hodgkin disease by Rosenberg (14) showed . . .
> . . . was Yalow's main contribution to . . .

Such term of address are often appropriate in news articles and other articles with a social or political, rather than scientific or historical, context.

> . . . and Dr Smith was elected Secretary for a fifth term.
> . . . and General Jones accepted the award for his society.

Such usage should, however, follow a preceding identification of the person thus addressed by full name and full statement of the relevant academic degree or title of position.

> . . . sole candidate for Secretary was E F Smith, MD, PhD.
> . . . awardee was Lieutenant General R P Jones.

The general term of respect used to address members of the clergy, "Reverend", should not be used in text with only a family name; it should be preceded by "the" and followed by a full name or a "Mr" or "Ms" before the family name.

> the Reverend Thomas Smith   the Reverend Ms Gilliland

The same rule applies to the term of respect often used to address persons with government positions, "Honorable".

> the Honorable Mary Smith   the Honorable Ms Smith

Terms of address identical with the title of a clerical post or excerpted from a military title may be used with only the family name.

> Father Brown   Monsignor Jones   General Jones

For capitalization of titles of profession, office, and station, see section 7.14.

REFERENCE

1. Walton I, Beeson PB, Bodley Scott R, eds. The Oxford companion to medicine. Oxford: Oxford University Press; 1986:1484–90.

Chapter 13

Numbers, Units of Measurement, and Time

13.1 The terms *numeral* and *numerals* refer in this chapter and elsewhere in this manual to arabic numerals except where roman numerals (see section 13.10) are specified.

A *numeral* is a written, printed, or spoken symbol that itself or with other numerals represents a number. The arabic numerals are 0, 1, 2, 3, 4, 5, 6, 7, 8, and 9.

A *number* is a statement in one numeral or more, or in the equivalent term (*numeric term*), reporting a count, measurement, or position in a sequence. A *cardinal number* is a number representing the quantity (count or measurement) of items, as a whole number or fraction, in the same class, specified or not: "1", "2", and so on; "1 man", "2 men", and so on; "1 foot", "2 feet". An *ordinal number* is a number representing the position, or order, in a sequence of items of the same class: "5th", "99th"; "5th dose", "99th dose".

NUMBERS IN TEXT

13.2 Style for numbers in text has been shifting in scientific literature from numeric terms ("fifty", "two hundred three", "one thousand sixty-four") to numerals (50, 203, 1064), probably in large part for ready comprehension of large numbers; this shift is also leading to some savings in text length. Numeric terms are still preferred to numerals to a great extent in the humanities and general literature, but choices between the 2 forms are specified by complex rules (1).

Two general rules have been widely used to specify numeric terms or numerals for numbers. The first, used chiefly in nonscientific literature, specifies numeric terms for whole numbers 1 through 99 ("one", "two", and so on) and numerals for whole numbers 100 and higher. The second, which has been widely used in the biomedical literature, specifies numeric terms for whole numbers 1 through 10 and numerals for higher numbers. The great use in medical literature of quantitative data that are most efficiently presented with numerals often makes the applying of such rules arbitrary and time-consuming. The recommendations in this chapter for the style of cardinal and ordinal numbers aim to simplify usage for authors and editors by reducing the number of decisions on style for numbers; they are also based on the premise that most numbers in the medical literature represent exact counts or measurements with scientifically definable precision.

CARDINAL NUMBERS IN TEXT

13.3   Cardinal numbers in the text of scientific papers, including numbers smaller than 11, should, in general, be presented with numerals, not as numeric terms.

> . . . onset of pain 3 weeks before admission . . .
> . . . found 10 dogs infected with . . .
> . . . identified 23 species as pathogens.
> . . . responsible for death in 217 cases.
> . . . multiplied by the factor 2.5167 yields . . .
> . . . the toxic gases killed 2897 inhabitants of . . .

When a number includes one that is part of a modifier and is preceded by another number, be sure that the number which is part of the modifier is connected to its noun with a hyphen.

> . . . needed 2 15-inch catheters for . . .
> . . . seeped out of 23 150-pound bales of . . .

If a number is the first element of a sentence or title, use the term rather than numerals or rewrite the sentence or title, if possible, to move the number from its initial position. If a number immediately follows a colon, use its numeric form.

> Ten patients were seen in the 1st week of . . .
> In the 1st week of August 1984, 10 patients were seen . . .
> The treatment failed in 7 patients: 5 men and 2 women.

Large numbers (above 1 000 000) that represent approximations or estimates can be stated in a combined numeral–term form or the exponential form of scientific notation.

> Among Canada's 26 million inhabitants are . . .
> . . . invested $3.5 million in research for . . .
> . . . a bacterial population of 1.6×10^8 . . .

When a number is an approximate or estimated number that is short in numeric form, preface it with a qualifying modifier (such as "about", "close to", "approximately") or substitute an equivalent term.

. . . pigmentation first became apparent about 10 years ago . . .
A century later the Library found itself serving . . .

Very small numbers are usually most efficiently stated in exponential notation.

. . . calculated the constant to be 1.6789×10^{-6}.

In papers without reported or cited numeric data (for example, editorials, essays, book reviews) cardinal numbers should be stated as numeric terms except where conventions require numerals: times and dates (see sections 13.20 to 13.22), money (see section 13.8), addresses (see section 10.13), latitude and longitude (see section 10.14), numeric constants. In such kinds of papers, numeric values accompanied by units of measurement can be in numeric-term form rather than in numerals when the numeric statements are incidental details in a nonscientific text.

Any physician would drive a thousand miles for that kind of vacation.

For numbers in tables see section 2.22.

CARDINAL NUMBERS: SPACING AND PUNCTUATION

13.4   The numerals forming numbers with 4 digits or less must be run together; the numerals of numbers with more than 4 digits should be spaced in groups of 3. This rule applies to digits on either side of a decimal point.

7247	23	5	12 676	1 223 557	328
0.0003	10.564 321	1.2267	10 777.078 34		

The main exception is in tables (see section 2.22) in which numbers with more than 4 digits and numbers with less must have their digit groups aligned.

4 560	0.003 100
17 277	10.446 229
1 399 211	6.397 061

These recommendations are in accord with those of the International Organization for Standardization (2) and the American National Metric Council (3).

A decimal point is not used with whole numbers 1 and larger unless it is needed to indicate a precision of measurement to a magnitude smaller than a unit value of 1.0.

NOT   . . . 10. men and 3. women . . .
BUT   . . . 10 men and 3 women . . .

The rat retained enough fluid to raise its weight by 15.0 g.

A decimal fraction smaller than 1.0 should have a 0 (zero) preceding its decimal point even when the numeric value of the variable cannot exceed 1.0 (as with probability values and regression coefficients).

$p > 0.05$ $r = 0.78$

The decimal point in the European convention is represented by the comma rather than the period (full stop). This convention does not cause any ambiguity about the magnitude of numbers in numeric form when their digits are spaced in accord with the 3-digit convention described above in this section.

Additional exceptions to the 3-digit convention for spacing are numbers with other specific styles. Examples include numbers in binary notation (0s and 1s without spacing), motor-vehicle license numbers, social security numbers, insurance policy numbers, credit card numbers.

11001001   LBX-515   1234 56 7890   KB-F567-J2-1234

13.5 Compound numeric terms for numbers in the range 21 to 99 are hyphenated (also see section 9.14).

twenty-three   forty-seven   eighty-nine

In a numeric range, connect the 2 numbers with the word "to". The sometimes-used alternative is connection with an en dash (see section 5.24), but because numeric ranges in scientific papers not infrequently must include minus values, the connective *to* avoids the ambiguity between the en dash and the minus sign. Such ranges include, for example, lowest and highest weights, lowest and highest temperatures, lowest and highest prices. If a unit of measurement is designated for numbers in the range, the unit need be stated only for the second number; if a symbol is conventionally attached unspaced to a numeric value, it must be attached to both numeric values.

The weight range 5 to 10 kg had the highest mortality.
The extremes of temperature were −5 to 50 °C.
The charges in the hospitals were in the range $5.00 to $8.00.
Note the poor illustrations on pages 49 to 76.
The mortality rates were 52% to 78%.
. . . found in the northern latitudes 40° to 65°.

If a number is part of a compound adjective and is thus hyphenated, place a hyphen after the first number of the range (for example, 5- to 10-gram dose; see section 13.15).

An exception to the general rule of connecting the numbers of a range with *to* is the connecting of first and last reference numbers in a citation (see section 15.7) and first and last page-numbers in a bibliographic reference (see section 15.20).

FRACTIONS

13.6 In most scientific writing, fractions are used either to indicate an approximate portion, as in "one-half of the patients were seen in the ambulatory-care clinic", or to designate values in partial units in a non-metric system of measures, as in "1/2 inch".

Fractions indicating approximate portions serve as descriptors rather than precise quantitators. Thus they should be styled as numeric terms rather than numerals and hyphenated to preserve their unity; in the rare instances of written-out fractions with numerators or denominators greater than 20, connect the numerator and the denominator with a hyphen and let the suffix of the denominator signal the end of the fraction.

> . . in two-thirds of cases . . .
> Occupancy was only three-quarters of that expected.
> eleven-sixty fourths

Fractions designating a measured quantity including partial unit-values in a nonmetric system of measurement can be in the conventional 1-line form of numerator and denominator separated by a slant line (diagonal, slash, solidus, stroke, virgule; see section 5.34). The preferred form in scientific papers in which nonmetric units must be used is that of decimal fraction, with only 1 or 2 significant places given to indicate the appropriate low degree of precision.

> 1/2 inch   0.5 inch   1 1/2 feet   1.5 feet

Note that the zero must be given to the left of the decimal point (see section 13.4).

PERCENTAGES

13.7   Percentage statements in scientific papers should be in numeric form, in accord with the recommendations for cardinal numbers in text (section 13.3). The percent sign is attached unspaced to the number it modifies and must be repeated for percentage values in a statement of an inclusive range.

> 52%   71.5%   . . . mortalities of 45% to 65% were . . .

In nonscientific text, percentage statements are likely to represent gross approximations and thus should be replaced by numeric terms instead of numerals; see the recommendations in section 13.3. When authors insist on percentages and will not accept numeric-term fractions as substitutes, style the percentages in numeric terms rather than numerals.

> . . . half of the nation . . .   ("fifty percent of the nation")

Note that the term *percent* refers only to the symbol % that is attached to a number to signify a percentage; the term *percentage* denotes a statement of a fraction with 100 as the implied denominator.

> Mortality was calculated as a percentage. (*not* "was calculated as a percent.")

In nonscientific style, *percent* is usually written as a compound term, *per cent*; in scientific style, the run-together style is to be preferred as reflecting the function of the percent sign as a scientific symbol.

In text for online retrieval, the percent sign, %, will be converted to the word *percent*.

MONETARY DATA AND UNITS

13.8   In accord with the general rule for cardinal numbers in scientific text (see section 13.3), statements in text of amounts of money should be in numerals with appropriate modifying symbols rather than in numeric terms. Symbols (including abbreviations serving as symbols) for basic monetary units (dollar, franc, mark, pound, yen, and so on) precede, and are attached to, the number for the amount.

$49.95   F45.00   £6.75   Y3200

The context of a monetary statement will usually imply the country of the monetary unit; any ambiguity about the implied country should be dispelled by prefixing the unit symbol with a modifier indicating the country. For the basic monetary units of major countries, their symbols, and the modifiers that indicate country, see Table 13.1; additional lists of monetary units and symbols can be found in *Webster's Ninth New*

Table 13.1:   Monetary units and symbols for some countries of the free world

Country	Unit	Symbol	Modified symbol
Australia	dollar	$	A$
Canada	dollar	$	C$
Denmark	krone	Kr	DKr
Finland	markka	Mk	FMk
France	franc	F	
Germany (Federal Republic of Germany)	deutsche mark	DM	
India	rupee	Rs	
Ireland	pound	£	Ir£
Italy	lira	L	
Japan	yen	Y	
Mexico	peso	Mex$	
The Netherlands	guilder	Fl [florin]	
New Zealand	dollar	$	NZ$
Norway	krone	Kr	NKr
Spain	peseta	Ptas [singular, Pta]	
Sweden	krona	Kr	Skr
Switzerland	franc		SF
United Kingdom	pound	£	
United States of America	dollar	$	US$

Collegiate Dictionary (4) and the *United States Government Printing Office Style Manual* (5).

> . . . price of C$100.00 (US$69.00) seems excessive for . . .
> . . . annual expenditures of A$10 million covered . . .

Symbols for principal fractional monetary units usually follow, and should be attached to, the numbers they modify; such symbols are needed infrequently in scientific writing and are most likely to be used in historical contexts.

> . . . in 1860 cost only about 10¢ . . .
> . . . average miner earned only £1 12s 5d per . . .

Approximate small amounts should be given without the decimal point; a large amount can be given in numerals with a numeric term. A decimal point implies an exact amount and must be followed by appropriate numerals for the amount.

> . . . were charged $5 to $10 for . . .   The price is $10.00.
> . . . appropriated $115 million for research on . . .

ORDINAL NUMBERS

13.9   Ordinal numbers generally follow the rules for cardinal numbers.

In scientific papers ordinal numbers should take the form of numerals with suffixes derived from the last 2 letters of the number written as a numeric term: $-st$, $-nd$, $-rd$, $-th$. This rule is in accord with that for cardinal numbers (see section 13.3).

> . . . the 1st operation . . .   [first]
> . . . the 2nd child . . .   [second]
> . . . the 3rd biopsy . . .   [third]
> . . . the 4th episode . . .   [fourth]
> . . . in his 21st year . . .   [twenty-first]
> . . . above the 90th percentile . . .   [ninetieth]

If an ordinal number is the first word of a sentence, use the numeric-term form or rewrite the sentence to move the number to within the sentence.

> First-born children have advantages over their siblings.
> Among siblings, the 1st-born child has advantages.

In nonscientific text with only low-order ordinal numbers, the numbers can be in the form of a numeric term.

> An oration on Osler as a bibliophile was the first choice of the delegates.
> He matriculated at Verona in his twenty-first year.

Note that an ordinal number which is a numeric term in a proper name must retain that form.

. . . the outbreak started in the First Ward and spread . . .
. . . and survey in the Thirty Years' War . . .
. . . hospital was moved to the Fifth Avenue site . . .

ROMAN NUMERALS

13.10 The use of roman numerals is decreasing, a desirable trend, but they are still used in some well-established conventions: terms for anatomic, embryonic, and histologic structures (such as cranial nerves, aortic arches, bronchial segments), cancer stages (see section 16.54), coagulation factors (see section 16.44), electrocardiographic leads (see section 16.14); designation of generations in family pedigrees (see section 16.40); oxidation numbers in chemistry (see section 16.21); and personal names that must be distinguished from antecedent names with the same given and family elements.

cranial nerve V [the trigeminal nerve]
B IX [the lateral basal segmental bronchus]
state IIIB   factor VIII   lead III
subject 3 in generation II   Solomon Rosenstern III

Dates of publication were often stated in roman numerals well into the 19th century; in bibliographic references to such books or journals, convert such dates to their equivalent in arabic numerals, bracketing the date to indicate that its original form was not in arabic numerals (see Table 15.2).

NOT   Philadelphia: Lea and Jones; MDCCCXXIII.
BUT   Philadelphia: Lea and Jones; [1823]

Preliminary pages in a book (such as title page, table of contents) are often numbered with lowercase roman numerals; such designations must be retained in bibliographic references to avoid ambiguity of reference to such pages or those in the book numbered with arabic numerals (see section 15.20).

Avoid the use of roman numerals in the titles of papers in a series; see section 2.4 for the preferred use of arabic numerals.

13.11 The rules for constructing, and hence interpreting, numbers built of roman numerals are stated succinctly in the *United States Government Printing Office Style Manual* (6): "A repeated letter repeats its value; a letter placed after one of greater value adds to it; a letter placed before one of greater value subtracts from it; a dashline over a letter denotes multiplied by 1000". See Table 13.2 for the basic roman numerals and examples of numbers and dates (years) built from them.

Table 13.2: Roman numerals, examples of roman numbers and dates, and arabic-numeral equivalents

Roman	Arabic	Roman	Arabic	Roman	Arabic
I	1	XX	20	C	100
II	2	XXIII	23	CXXIV	124
III	3	XXV	25	CXLII	142
IV	4	XXIX	29	CL	150
V	5	XXX	30	CC	200
VI	6	XL	40	CCC	300
VII	7	XLV	45	CD	400
VIII	8	XLVI	46	D	500
IX	9	XLIX	49	DC	600
X	10	L	50	DCCC	800
XI	11	LI	51	CM	900
XII	12	LIX	59	CMXC	990
XIV	14	LX	60	M	1000
XV	15	LXX	70	MD	1500
XVII	17	LXXX	80	MDCCXIX	1719
XIX	19	XC	90	MDCCCII	1802
				MCMLXXXVI	1986

UNITS OF MEASUREMENT

13.12   Through the past decade, the preferred use of units of measurement has been changing rapidly, and change will continue through at least the next decade. English units are vanishing even in the English-language world of medicine, while the metric units of the International System of Units (SI) are rapidly becoming the standard units in medicine and its related disciplines. SI units for body dimensions (height and length, mass [weight]) should now be standard usage. The degree Celsius, although not an SI unit, should be used instead of the degree Fahrenheit. SI units for clinical chemistry, hematology, and radiation medicine are rapidly being adopted as standard; the schedule of the American National Metric Council calls for full establishment by 1988 of SI units in clinical chemistry and hematology as their standard units. Shifts to some SI units in other fields (nutrition and metabolism, physiology, pharmacology and pharmacy) will be slower. Through these transitions, each journal, taking into account its potential authorship and its actual readership, may have to modify its policy on units from year to year. Each journal should aim, however, to lead its constituencies as quickly as possible toward the ideal of international uniformity in the use of SI units.

Detailed presentations of basic SI usage and specific usage in medicine are available in a number of publications (7–15); journal offices should have at least some of these in their reference libraries. A comprehensive guide to SI units in clinical chemistry and hematology and to style conventions for SI units is presented in Appendix A.

SI: BASE AND DERIVED UNITS

13.13   The SI includes base units and units derived from them. For the 7 base units and 2 supplementary units (rarely used in medicine), see Table 13.3.

The derived SI units are formed from the base units by multiplication and division. Some of the derived units do not have special names (see Table 13.4).

Some derived SI units have special names and symbols. These symbols are generally used in preference to those that make up a unit in the form that shows its derivation from the base units (see Table 13.5).

Specific rules determine the formation and structure of symbols for derived units and for decimal fractions and multiples of base and derived units (see section 13.15 and Appendix A).

SI AND RELATED UNITS APPLIED IN MEDICINE AND RELATED FIELDS

13.14   Many SI units are already in use in medicine and the closely related fields. Some non-SI but preferred units are also in wide use. Both classes of

Table 13.3:   SI base and supplementary units

Unit	Symbol for unit	Quantity measured
Base units		
ampere	A	electric current
candela	cd	luminous intensity
kelvin	K	thermodynamic temperature
kilogram	kg	mass
metre	m	length
mole	mol	amount of substance
second	s	time
Supplementary units		
radian	rad	plane angle
steradian	sr	solid angle

Table 13.4:   Some SI derived units without special names

Unit	Symbol for unit	Quantity measured
cubic metre	m^3	volume
metre per second	m/s (*or*, $m \cdot s^{-1}$)	velocity
metre per second squared	m/s^2 (*or*, $m \cdot s^{-2}$)	acceleration
mole per cubic metre	mol/m^3 (*or*, $mol \cdot m^{-3}$)	substance concentration
square metre	m^2	area

Table 13.5: Derived SI units with special names

Unit	Symbol for unit	Derivation	Quantity measured
becquerel	Bq	s^{-1} (*or*, $1/s$)	activity (radionuclide)
coulomb	C	A·s	electric charge; quantity of electricity
farad	F	C/V	capacitance
gray	Gy	J/kg	absorbed dose of ionizing radiation
henry	H	Wb/A	inductance
hertz	Hz	s^{-1} (*or*, $1/s$)	frequency
joule	J	N·m	work; energy; quantity of heat
lumen	lm	cd·sr	luminous flux
lux	lx	m^{-2}·cd·sr	illuminance
newton	N	m·kg·s^{-2}	force
ohm	Ω	V/A	electric resistance
pascal	Pa	N/m^2	pressure
siemens	S	A/V	conductance
tesla	T	Wb/m^2	magnetic flux density
volt	V	W/A	electrical potential; potential difference
watt	W	J/s	power; radiant flux
weber	Wb	V·s	magnetic flux

units are presented in Table 13.6; note that most of the customary units in column 4 of this table are not equivalents of the units in column 2.

SI UNITS: RULES FOR FORMATION, STYLE, AND USAGE

13.15 Terms for the units that represent decimal fractions and multiples of SI base units (other than the kilogram) are formed by adding specified prefixes to the terms for the base units; the symbols for the units thus formed are likewise formed by prefixing the base-unit symbols (other than the kilogram) with specified prefix symbols. For example, *kilometre*, the term for the unit of 1000 metres, is formed from *metre* by prefixing to it the term representing "1000", *kilo*. Note, however, that units of mass other than the gram and the kilogram are formed by attaching prefixes to *gram*, not to *kilogram*. The names of the SI base units other than the kilogram (see Table 13.3) and the derived SI units (see Table 13.4) do not carry prefixes. The use of decimal multiple and fractional units should be confined to those units representing multiplication by steps of 10^3 or 10^{-3} (see Table 13.7).

The SI unit symbols are placed after the numbers stating the values of measurements in those units and separated by one space. Terms for metric units mentioned in running text without a number representing a measurement should be written out.

The patient's temperature was 40.2 °C and his pulse rate . . .
The temperature unit for this hospital is the degree Celsius.
. . . was 1.65 m tall.   . . . unit for height is the metre.

Table 13.6: SI and related units applied in the medical sciences

Quantity	SI or related unit	Symbol	Customary unit	Application
Length	kilometre	km	mile	Distance
	metre	m	yard, foot	Distance in visual acuity, body linear dimension
	centimetre	cm	inch	Body and organ linear dimension
	millimetre	mm	inch fraction	Organ linear dimension
	micrometre	μm		Cell linear dimension
Surface area	square centimetre	cm²	square inch	Surface area
	square metre	m²	square foot	Body surface area
Mass ("weight")	kilogram	kg	pound	Body mass ("weight"),
	gram	g	ounce	laboratory measure-
	milligram	mg	ounce fraction	ment, drug doses
	microgram	μg		Laboratory measurement
Temperature	degree Celsius	°C	°F	Body temperature, laboratory measurement
Time	day	d	day	Time in clinical record
	hour	h	hour	Time in clinical record
	minute	min	minute	Duration of procedure, of symptoms
	second	s	second	Duration of procedure, reaction time
Volume	litre	L	quart	Amount of fluid or gas, container capacity
	millilitre	mL	cubic centi-metre, fluid ounce	Formula portion, body fluid measurement
Power	watt	W	horsepower	Mechanical power, ergometry, exercise test
Energy	joule	J	kilocalorie,	Energy: kinetic,
	kilojoule	kJ	calorie	metabolic
Catalytic activity	katal	kat	International unit	Enzyme activity
Pressure	pascal	Pa	millimetre of	Pressures: blood,
	kilopascal	kPa	mercury; inch of water	cerebrospinal fluid, ocular
Frequency	hertz	Hz	cycle per second	Frequencies: hearing, radio, radiation
Substance concentration	mole/litre	mol/L	milligram per 100 millilitres milliequivalent per litre	Body fluid components
Dose equivalent	sievert	Sv	rem	Radiation protection

Table 13.6: (*continued*)

Quantity	SI or related unit	Symbol	Customary unit	Application
Absorbed dose	gray	Gy	rad	Absorbed dose of ionizing radiation
Activity	becquerel	Bq	curie	Radionuclide activity
Exposure		C/kg (air)	roentgen	Radiology

A number and a unit term used together as an adjective should be linked by a hyphen.

> a 15-gram dose   a 15-g dose

Note that the symbols for the degree, the minute, and the second as used by themselves, for example, in geographic coordinates (see section 10.14) or trigonometric statements, are attached to numeric values without spacing.

> 40°17′23″   . . . gradient of 25° and an altitude of . . .

13.16 SI units must always be in roman (upright) type even when they appear in text set in italic (slanted) type.

> *Editor's note: The value referred to in Dr Smith's letter should have been 1.23 m, not 1.32 m. We apologize to him for this error.*

Table 13.7: SI prefixes, prefix symbols, and the recommended factors they represent [fn1]

Factor	Prefix	Symbol
10^{18}	exa	E
10^{15}	peta	P
10^{12}	tera	T
10^{9}	giga	G
10^{6}	mega	M
10^{3}	kilo	k
10^{-3}	milli	m
10^{-6}	micro	μ
10^{-9}	nano	n
10^{-12}	pico	p
10^{-15}	femto	f
10^{-18}	atto	a

fn1: Note that the multipliers of 10^{3} and greater are all capital letters except for the letter k representing *kilo*, the capital letter K being reserved for *kelvin*.

Most of the SI symbols are in lowercase letters except for those representing unit terms derived from proper names (for example, P for *pascal*, Gy for *gray*) and the symbol L (capital letter "ell") for *litre* (see Tables 13.3, 13.4, and 13.5). Note that the terms based on proper names are not capitalized, but *Celsius* and its symbol are capitalized within the compound term *degree Celsius* and its symbol °C. Note that the degree sign ° precedes without a space the capital letter C for *Celsius* so that the two elements serve together as a single symbol like the compound symbols in the SI. As with the SI units, the symbol for *degree Celsius* follows the numeric value after one space.

The prefix symbols also must be in roman (upright) type and immediately precede unit symbols without spacing; compound prefixes are not allowed.

kPa   mm   MHz   g, *not* "mkg" for "millikilogram"

The symbols represent both singular and plural forms of the unit terms, and the letter s must not be added to the symbols even if the unit would be read aloud as the plural form ("six grams" for "6 g"); periods do not follow symbols unless the position of a symbol calls for a following period, for example, the end of a sentence.

The daily dose was 6 g, taken as 2 g three times a day.
The daily dose was 6 g.

Do not combine symbols and terms: MHz, not "megaHz".

13.17   Designate the product of 2 or more units by a center dot ("raised period") between units without spacing; the dot must be above the line to distinguish it from the decimal point.

N·m ("newton times metre")
m·s⁻¹ ("metre times second to the minus one")

Note that this recommendation departs from that of the International Standards Organization (2), which calls for the "times sign", ×, when the decimal point is a period rather than a comma. Avoidance of the "times sign" seems preferable because it can occasionally be confused with the letter X and the center dot (raised period) allows for a clearer format.

A compound unit with a divisor can be formatted in 3 ways: vertical fraction (stacked fraction), in-line fraction with a slant line separating numerator and denominator, or in-line multiplication with negative exponents for denominator units.

$$\frac{m}{s} \qquad m/s \qquad m·s^{-1}$$

Do not, however, use more than one slant line in more complex compound units. Appropriate use of the multiplier center-dot, slant line, and, in very complex units, parenthesis marks can prevent the ambiguity likely to be produced by more than one slant line in a compound unit.

$$m^2 \cdot kg \cdot s^{-2} \cdot A^{-2} \qquad m^2 \cdot kg/s^2 \cdot A^2 \qquad not \ m^2 \cdot kg/s^2/A^2$$

13.18 The spelling variants *meter* and *liter* for *metre* and *litre* may be preferred by journals with readership mainly in the United States; this usage is endorsed by two American authorities (3,9).

Plural forms of unit names generally follow the customary rules for plurals (see section 9.17), but the plural forms for *lux, hertz,* and *siemens* (all ending with a sibilant) are the same as these singular forms.

gram	grams
metre	metres
henry	henries
hertz	hertz

For a tabular summary of style rules for SI units, see Table A.4 in Appendix A.

ENGLISH UNITS

13.19 The English units of measurement in the avoirdupois and apothecaries systems should be used in only 2 contexts: in papers on topics in the history of science or medicine; and in dual presentation of values in scientific papers during a transition to exclusive use of SI units. If abbreviations must be used to save space, as in tables or parenthetic values following values in SI units, follow the conventions stipulated in the preceding sections and do not place periods after abbreviations for units (see Table 13.8 for abbreviatons).

TIME AND DATES

13.20 Values for periods of time not including fractions of seconds should be given in number and unit-symbol form. If the value is for only 1 unit, space the number and the unit symbol as with SI units. If the value calls

Table 13.8: Abbreviations for some English units of measurement

Weight		Length		Area		Volume	
grain	gr	inch	in	square inch	in²	fluid ounce	fldoz
ounce	oz	foot	ft	square foot	ft²	pint	pt
pound	lb	yard	yd	square yard	yd²	quart	qt
ton (short)	tn	rod	rd	square rod	rd²	gallon	gn
		mile	mi	square mile	mi²		

for more than 1 unit, run the numbers and symbols together as in the convention (16) for other sciences such as astronomy reporting exact times and intervals. The respective symbols (3) for *year, month, week, day, hour, minute,* and *second* are y, mo, w, d, h, min, and s. Among these symbols, s is an SI symbol and d, h, and min are acceptable (3,8,9) for use with the SI; note, however, that d, for *day*, is the same as the SI symbol d for the prefix *deci*, but the 2 uses are not likely to be confused in the context of time.

> 1 y   3 mo   12 h   12h3min   1h5min3s

Values including fractions of seconds should be written with decimal fractions.

> 3.21 s   5min14.17s

For values of time do not use the symbols for *minute* and *second* specified in sections 10.14 and 13.15 for geographic coordinates (latitude and longitude) or values of angular measurement.

13.21 Times of the day should be given in the 24-hour system (astronomical system), with 0000 representing midnight at the beginning of a day and 2400 representing midnight at the end of the same day; thus 0000, 21 June 1986 is the same point of time as 2400, 20 June 1986. Because the third and fourth digits represent minutes and not decimal fractions of an hour, the symbol h should not be used with a time of day given in the 24-hour system.

13.22 Dates should be written in either the sequence of year, month, and day or that of day, month, and year. In text the name of the month should be written out. In tables, particularly tables with dates spanning more than 1 year, the preferred sequence is year, month, and day; ambiguity will be avoided if the month is stated in the 3-letter abbreviated form (see Table 11.3) rather than its numeric equivalent.

Text: . . . assassinated on 5 December 1963 as he was . . .

Tables:	1984 Dec 6	84 Dec 6	84/12/6	1984/12/6
	1985 Jan 12	85 Jan 12	85/1/12	1985/1/12

For designations of eras, see section 11.9.

REFERENCES

1. The Chicago manual of style. 13th ed. Chicago: University of Chicago Press; 1982:232–5.
2. International Organization for Standardization. Units of measurement. 2nd ed. Geneva: International Organization for Standardization; 1982. (ISO standards handbook 2).

3. American National Metric Council. Metric editorial guide. 4th ed. Washington: American National Metric Council; 1985.
4. Webster's ninth new collegiate dictionary. Springfield, Massachusetts: Merriam-Webster, 1983:765–6.
5. United States Government Printing Office. United States Government Printing Office style manual. Washington: Government Printing Office; 1984:238–40.
6. United States Government Printing Office. United States Government Printing Office style manual. Washington: Government Printing Office; 1984:171
7. Lowe DA. A guide to international recommendations on names and symbols for quantities and on units of measurement. Geneva: World Health Organization; 1975. (Progress in standardization: 2).
8. Institute of Electrical and Electronics Engineers. American national standard metric practice. New York: Institute of Electrical and Electronics Engineers; 1982. (ANSI/IEEE std 268-1982).
9. American Society for Testing and Materials. ASTM standard for metric practice: E380-85. Philadelphia: American Society for Testing and Materials; 1985.
10. World Health Organization. The SI for the health professions. Geneva: World Health Organization; 1977.
11. The SI manual in health care. 2nd ed. [Metric Commission Canada, Sector 9.10, Subcommittee]; 1982.
12. CBE style manual committee. CBE style manual: a guide for authors, editors, and publishers in the biological sciences. 5th edition. Bethesda, Maryland: Council of Biology Editors; 1983.
13. National Council on Radiation Protection and Measurements. SI units in radiation protection and measurements. Bethesda, Maryland: National Council on Radiation Protection and Measurements; 1985. (NCRP report [number] 82).
14. Lippert H, Lehmann HP. SI units in medicine: an introduction to the International Systems of Units with conversion tables and normal ranges. Baltimore: Urban & Schwarzenberg, 1978.
15. Young DS. Implementation of SI units for laboratory data. Ann Intern Med. 1987;107 [in press]. See Appendix A.
16. United States Government Printing Office. United States Government Printing Office style manual. Washington: Government Printing Office: 1984:166.

Chapter 14

Mathematics and Statistics

Few journals in medicine and the closely related disciplines publish mathematical text and equations with complexities greater than those of algebra, trigonometry, and calculus. The recommendations here are likely to suffice for virtually all journals in the medical sciences; the possible exceptions are highly specialized journals in disciplines like bioengineering, biomathematics, and biophysics. Additional recommendations can be found in two general style manuals. *The Chicago Manual of Style* (1) and *The McGraw-Hill Style Manual* (2). The best manual for detailed guidance in style for, and copy preparation of, mathematical text and equations is *Mathematics into Type* (3), notable for its clear and logical rules for the spacing of symbols and styling of equations. It should be a reference work in every editorial office publishing any papers with mathematical content. Definitions of mathematical characters and specifications for typeface and format can be found in *Units of Measurement* (4) published by the International Organization for Standardization (ISO).

MATHEMATICS

TYPEFACES

Widely used and authoritatively endorsed conventions (4) govern the use of roman (upright) or italic (slanted) type for characters in mathematical statements in text and displayed equations.

14.1   Italic (slanted) type (see section 8.1) must be used for single-letter characters representing quantities whether they serve to represent unknowns, variables with known values, or constants (potential variables with conventionally fixed values) (also see section 8.4). This rule applies to such characters in text, displayed equations, and tables.

When a value of 12 was assigned to b in the equation, . . .

$$a + b = c \qquad x = a - by^3 \qquad (\mathrm{d}f/\mathrm{d}x)_{x=a}\ \mathrm{e}^x$$

Note that the logarithmic base e is in roman (upright) type; e represents a specific number of fixed value, not a variable, and numbers must be in roman (upright) type (see section 14.2 immediately below). Note, too, that f representing *function* is in italic type because it represents a variable with a fixed correspondence to another variable.

The rule for italic (slanted) type also applies to 2-letter symbols representing dimensionless parameters, for example, Fourier number (*Fo*), Mach number (*Ma*), Reynolds number (*Re*).

Authors who wish to be sure that characters properly in slanted (italic) type are thus interpreted by an editor should underline them in the typescript.

If a̲ is assigned a value of . . .

14.2   Roman (upright) type must be used for alphabetic characters serving as superscript or subscript modifiers (in contrast to single alphabetic characters representing quantities as discussed above), as multicharacter abbreviations for physiologic-function terms even when the abbreviation represents a quantity, or as abbreviations for names of mathematical functions or operators.

C_{in}	(clearance of inulin)
SBF	(systemic blood flow)
FE_{Na}	(fractional excretion of sodium)
ln x	(logarithm of x to the base e)
tan y	(tangent of y)
$\mathrm{d}x/\mathrm{d}t$	(derivative of x with respect to t)
lim sup	(limit superior)

Abbreviations of mathematical functions and modifiers occasionally used in medical-science journals can be found in Table 14.1.

Table 14.1:   Abbreviations of representative mathematical terms that must be in roman (upright) type

Abbreviation	Term	Abbreviation	Term
arcsin	arc sine	ln	logarithm to the base e
cos	cosine	log	logarithm to the base 10
cosec	cosecant	max	maximum
cosh	hyperbolic cosine	min	minimum
d	derivative	sec	secant
cot	cotangent	sin	sine
det	determinant	sinh	hyperbolic sine
exp	exponential	tan	tangent
lim	limit	tanh	hyperbolic tangent

Note that abbreviations like "SBF" and "FE" (see the examples in the paragraph immediately above) that stand for quantities are an undesirable convention. They should be replaced by single-character symbols in italic (slanted) type with appropriate modifiers. Unfortunately such multicharacter abbreviations standing for quantities are widely established in American physiology and clinical medicine. Editors should discourage the use of these older conventions and require for their journals the conventions that are widely used in other sciences and that are the chief basis for recommendations in this chapter and some in Chapter 16. It is to be hoped that in the not-too-distant future intellectual leaders in the disciplines perpetuating such abbreviations for physiologic functions will take on the task of bringing their usage into conformity with scientific style widely used in other disciplines. Also see comment in sections 16.17 and 16.60.

14.3 Operational signs (operators) and sigma-class symbols in mathematical functions must be in roman (upright) type: the multiplication sign ($\times$), the minus sign ($-$), the plus sign ($+$), the plus-or-minus sign ($\pm$), the greater-than sign ($>$), the less-than sign ($<$), the identity-with sign ($\equiv$), the equals-approximately sign ($\cong$), the summation sign (Σ), and the integral sign ($\int$).

14.4 The numerals of numbers in statements of quantity and in equations must be in roman (upright) type when, as is usually the case, they are in text set in roman (upright) type. Numbers not in a mathematical context and in text set in italic (slanted) type should be set in the same typeface.

> . . . which led to the equation, $x = 1.267 + 3.2y^3$, and . . .
> *Editor's Note: Also see Chapter 36.*

14.5 Symbols for units of measurement, SI and English, must be in roman (upright) type regardless of whether the text in which they appear is roman (upright) or italic (slanted) type (also see section 13.16).

AGGREGATION, MULTIPLICATION, AND DIVISION

14.6 Mathematical terms that must be aggregated (grouped) in a fraction or an equation or for some other function should be enclosed within marks (*fences* in mathematical terminology) of the conventional sequence: {[( )]}. The parenthesis marks are used for a first-step or innermost aggregation, and so on. The three sets of aggregation marks are likely to suffice for any mathematical text in medicine.

> $(a + b)/(c + d)$ $[a + (b + c)^3]^2$

Note that this sequence of marks is the reverse of that used in text statements that represent a parenthesis within a parenthesis, ([ ]); see section 5.32.

Aggregation is most commonly used by editors to eliminate the ambiguity likely to occur in converting fractions in display style to the in-line style.

$$\frac{2}{a+b} \quad to \quad 2/(a+b) \quad not \quad 2/a+b$$

Multiplication of 2 or more single terms can be represented in 3 styles: center dot ("raised period"), multiplication sign ("times sign"), nonspaced characters.

$$a \cdot b \quad a \times b \quad ab$$

Multiplication with 1 or more aggregated terms is indicated by nonspacing between aggregation signs.

$$a(b+c) \quad (a+b)(c+d)$$

Division can be represented by a display fraction, an in-line fraction, or a negative exponent for a multiplying term.

$$\frac{a}{b} \quad a/b \quad a \cdot b^{-1}$$

In scientific text avoid use of the division sign ($\div$).

SPACING AND PUNCTUATION

14.7 A narrow space must be placed between a term and an operator sign (such as the plus sign, the minus sign); exceptions are the center dot ("raised period") as a multiplication sign and the slant line used as a fraction line in an in-line fraction.

$$a-b \quad ab = 3y \quad a \times b \quad a \cdot b \quad (a+b)/(c+d)$$

Also see the examples in sections 14.1 and 14.6

In a sequence of terms that includes both punctuation marks or operator signs and an ellipsis mark (see section 6.6), the ellipsis mark must be treated as unstated terms and thus preceded and followed by the punctuation or sign.

$$y_1 + y_2 + \ldots + y_n \quad y_1, y_2, \ldots, y_n$$

Sentences that include equations, whether they be in line or displayed, may need punctuation such as a closing period if they are to be read as grammatical sentences (see section 14.8 below).

EQUATIONS

14.8 Simple and short equations should be incorporated within text sentences. An equation presented in this style is called an in-line equation.

The power generated is expressed by $P = p(dV/dt)$ and the . . .

Some notations that would encroach on the interline space can be converted to another notation that does not; for example, the radical sign for square root $\sqrt{a + b}$ can be eliminated by revising the term to $(a + b)^{-\frac{1}{2}}$.

The in-line style may be inappropriate because of the complexity or length of an equation: complex equations may need too much space above and below a line to fit in line; equations may be too long to fit in line without running into the next line, which should be avoided. Clearly an equation such as

$$x(1) = y - 0.000139 + 0.025[x(7) - x(1)] - 0.15x(1)$$

$$+ \begin{cases} \dfrac{6.82x(2)}{2 + 1000x(2)[x(4) - 293]/7} & \text{if } x(4) > 300 \\\\ \dfrac{6.82x(2)}{2 + 1000x(2)} & \text{if } x(4) \leqslant 300 \end{cases}$$

must be presented as a display equation. If an equation must be accompanied by explanation of its terms, both the equation and the explanation will be more comprehensible if the equation and the explanation are presented in a display format rather than in a very long sentence; note in the example below that the entire sentence, which includes the display equation and the explanation, is punctuated with commas and terminated with a period.

. . . and thus the glomerular filtration rate can be calculated by the formula

$$F_g = \frac{UV}{P}$$

in which F_g is glomerular filtration rate in millilitres per second,
U is urine concentration of insulin in millimoles per millilitre,
V is urine volume in milliliters per second, and
P is plasma concentration of inulin in millimoles per millilitre.

14.9 If a paper includes a large number of display equations and the text must refer to them, each equation should be identified by a numeric or alphabetic identifier within parenthesis marks set flush with the right margin of the column of text. In books numeric identifiers are standard style; they are made up of the chapter number, a period, and the number representing the place of the equation in the sequence of all equations in the chapter: the third equation in a chapter 13 would have a right margin identifier, (13.3). Such numeric identifiers may be satisfactory in journal articles if citation numbers (see section 15.6) are superscript numbers rather than the recommended citation numbers within parenthesis marks; a satisfactory substitute for numeric identifiers is an alphabetic sequence of identifers.

. . . and appropriate substitutions for the terms in equation A yield

$$Y_e = (2a + 3b)(5c + 6d) \qquad [B]$$

which in turn can be expanded to a much more useful form . . .

Care must be taken with this style in formatting to avoid any possible confusion between the alphabetic identifiers and terms in equations.

STATISTICS

14.10 The symbols most likely to be needed for statistical statements are given in Table 14.2. These symbols, recommended by the International Organization for Standardization (ISO) (5), are in accord with ISO's general rules for symbols applied in section 14.1. Note that *standard deviation* and *standard error of the mean* are not represented by the two abbreviations "SD" and "SEM", which are inappropriate notation for mathematical symbols, but by s and $s_{\bar{x}}$.

. . . yielded a mean value of 13.2 g/L ($s_{\bar{x}} = 1.2$).

(This example is the equivalent of the statement ". . . yielded a mean value of 13.2 grams per litre with a standard error of the mean of 1.2".) These symbols can also be used at the top of a tabular column to specify its notation; for example, a column of mean values with standard deviations connected by plus-or-minus signs could be headed (below the appropriate heading for unit) with ($\bar{x} \pm s$), which is read as "mean plus or minus standard deviation".

The ISO recommendations (5) do not include a symbol for *confi-*

Table 14.2: Statistical symbols [fn1]

Term	Symbol	Term	Symbol
variable in a population	$X, Y, \ldots$	standard error of the mean	$s_{\bar{x}}$
particular value	$x, y, \ldots$	coefficient of correlation in	r
population size	N	a sample	
sample size	n	number of degrees of freedom	ν
range of a sample	w, R	chi-squared distribution	χ^2
arithmetic mean of a	$\bar{X}$	t-distribution (Student)	t
population		F-distribution	F
arithmetic mean of a	$\bar{x}$	level of significance of a test,	α
sample		type I risk	
variance of a population	σ^2	level of significance of a test,	β
variance of a sample	s^2	type II risk	
standard deviation of a	s	probability	P
sample			

fn1: For symbolization of confidence interval, see section 14.10.

dence interval. Until a symbol is established, the recommended representation is the percentage indicator selected for the interval immediately follo*w*ed by "CI", and the numeric values for the limits of the interval.

. . . resulted in a mortality rate of 62% (95%CI, 42% to 82%).

REFERENCES

1. The Chicago manual of style. 13th ed. Chicago: University of Chicago Press; 1982:351–73.
2. Longyear M, ed. The McGraw-Hill style manual: a concise guide for writers and editors. New York: McGraw-Hill; 1982:107–23.
3. Swanson E. Mathematics into type: copyediting and proofreading of mathematics for editorial assistants and authors. Providence, Rhode Island: American Mathematical Society; 1979
4. International Organization for Standardization. Units of measurement. 2nd ed. Geneva: International Organization for Standardization; 1982. (ISO standards handbook 2).
5. International Organization for Standardization. Statistical methods: handbook on international standards for statistical methods. Geneva: International Organization for Standardization; 1979:287–8. (ISO standards handbook 3).

Chapter 15

Bibliographic Citations and References

15.1   In addition to the original observations they report, most articles in medical journals draw on previously published materials for evidence (1), supporting or contradictory, to be assessed in reaching a conclusion. An honest and careful author indicates at each point in an article where such evidence is relevant (2); at this point is placed the *citation*, which in the system of citation and reference recommended in this manual, is the number of the bibliographic reference given at the end of the article (also see sections 2.12, 2.24, and 2.32). The *reference* is the concise description needed by readers to find the cited item. References in medical journals are most frequently to other journal articles, books, and chapters in books, but other items are also cited, such as government documents, newspaper articles, legal documents, technical reports, software.

"Published materials" includes manuscripts, letters, and other such items that have not been made widely available in replicates, the usual meaning of "publication", but have been cataloged by, and are available for reading, in libraries, archives, and similar depositories. Referenced materials should not include personal communications such as uncataloged personal letters not available to the scholarly public and unrecorded speeches and other similar ephemera unlikely to be available in the future for examination by scholars. Such cited but unreferenced items should be cited only in the text (see section 15.8).

SYSTEMS OF CITATION AND REFERENCE

15.2   The 2 main systems of citation and reference most widely used in the journals of medicine and closely related disciplines are the author-and-year system and the reference-number system.

In the author-and-year system (often called "the Harvard system"), the citation has the form, in general, of parenthesis marks enclosing the author(s) name and year of publication of the cited item; the references format starts with an inverted author name and gives the year of publication after author names(s).

CITATION   . . . the other procedure (Grant, 1937) is often . . .
REFERENCE   Grant FC. 1937. A new method for . . .

The references are listed at the end of the article alphabetized by author family-name (surname). More detailed descriptions of this system, its variants, and other systems used in scientific literature can be found in general and specialized style manuals (3–7).

15.3   In the reference-number system, the citation is the number of the reference cited placed within parenthesis marks (or superscripted in some journals) at the point of citation. The references, at the end of the article, are usually arranged and numbered in the order in which they were first cited in the article; in one variant the references are in alphabetic order, by author name.

CITATION   . . . the other procedure (5) is often . . .
REFERENCE   5. Grant FC. A new method for . . .

Each of the 2 systems has advantages over the other. For readers familiar with much of the literature in a small discipline or in a narrow range of interests, the citation in the author-and-year system is likely to identify quickly the item referred to. But in disciplines like medicine with huge literatures, few readers who are not extreme specialists in the subject of a journal article get such information from the citations. In articles citing large numbers of consecutive references, such as reviews, the citations would produce long lists of author names interrupting the flow of the text. The reference-number system has citations taking little space in the text; the arrangement of references in order of their first citations brings together references of related chronology or importance; and readers looking for references in a long list are likely to find them more rapidly than in the author-and-year system.

15.4   The system recommended here is a reference-number system in the Vancouver style. It acquired its name from Vancouver, British Columbia, the city in which the present International Committee of Medical Journal Editors first met, in 1978, and agreed on the style and format of citations and references that would be acceptable in manuscripts submitted to their journals.

The history (8,9) of the Vancouver agreement and style really runs back to 1968. Augusta Litwer of Seattle, administrative secretary to the eminent nephrologist Belding Scribner at the University of Washington, was tired of reformatting and retyping references whenever one of Dr Scribner's papers was rejected by one journal and submitted to another. Early in 1968 she wrote to the editors of *Annals of Internal Medicine, Journal of the American Medical Association,* and *The New England Journal of Medicine* and asked why they could not agree on a format for references. In response, they and the editors of some other American clinical journals met in Atlantic City in 1968 and 1969 during meetings of the American Federation for Clinical Research and finally agreed to use the *Index Medicus* format for references to journal articles. This agreement was subsequently joined by other journals; the group finally totaled 18. "The spirit of accommodation and compromise that characterized these efforts led to optimism about extending the agreement further to include other matters" (8). Subsequent informal discussion among Dr John F Murray, then editor of *American Review of Respiratory Disease,* Dr Stephen P Lock, editor of *British Medical Journal,* Dr M Therese Southgate, a deputy editor of *Journal of the American Medical Association,* and Dr Edward J Huth, editor of *Annals of Internal Medicine,* led Drs Murray, Huth, and Southgate to organize the January 1978 meeting in Vancouver at which the Vancouver style was born. The agreement reached was that all of the cooperating journals would receive and consider for publication any manuscript meeting its editorial needs and prepared in accord with the requirements for manuscripts and for the citation–reference system specified in the group's original "Uniform Requirements . . ." document (10,11). If a journal in the agreement wished to publish a paper submitted in the Vancouver style but preferred to use another style for publication, it would not require the author to change details of style but would make the changes itself. A large fraction of journals that joined the agreement did go on to use the Vancouver style as their publication style. That the agreement included all of the American Medical Association journals and the 2 leading weekly British journals, *British Medical Journal* and *The Lancet,* as well as the other journals initially represented, was critically important in subsequently bringing what is now 300 or more journals around the world into the agreement.

CITATIONS AND REFERENCES: THE VANCOUVER STYLE

15.5   The Vancouver style and format for citations and references have been specified in the original document (10,11) that established the style and in its second edition (12,13). A new edition will probably be published early in 1988.

The formats for references were drawn up for the Vancouver group by the National Library of Medicine. The Library built the formats on the principles established in *American National Standard for Bibliographic References* (14) (referred to below as "the ANSI standard"). For some savings in space "characters", the formats deviated from the standard in a few details, the most notable of which for the recommendations here was omission of the period called for in the ANSI standard to mark the end of the journal title (the collective title in the title group of reference elements; see sections 15.17 and 15.18 and Table 15.1). Because of the importance that the period marking the close of each bibliographic-element group will have for computer sorting and reordering of reference elements, the recommendations here do place a period at the close of the journal title in a reference; this change is a minor departure from the original Vancouver style but brings it into accord with the ANSI standard. The omission of spaces in the imprint group of bibliographic elements for references to journal articles (date of publication, volume number, pagination; see section 15.20) that was specified by the Library but not by the ANSI standard has been retained.

CITATIONS

15.6 References must be cited (identified) at relevant points within text, tables, and figure legends by arabic numerals within parenthesis marks (round brackets) representing the reference numbers assigned in the references list; the references are sequenced in the references list and assigned numbers in accord with the sequence in which the references are first cited (see sections 2.12 and 2.32).

> . . . the other procedure (5) is often preferred for . . .
> As reported by Smith and Brown (7), the procedure . . .

15.7 The punctuation of 2 or more reference numbers within a citation is determined by their number and consecutiveness.

> Two consecutive numbers: unspaced comma.   (47,48)
> Three or more consecutive numbers: the initial number and terminal number connected by an en dash (or hyphen).   (47–49)
> Two or more nonconsecutive numbers: unspaced comma.   (47,51,54)
> Hyphenated numbers: punctuated as single numbers.   (7,47–49, 51–55,59)

Within a citation the reference numbers must be in ascending order. Note that the connective *to* recommended in section 13.5 for numeric ranges is not used in citations.

15.8 Each citation in text should be placed immediately after the title, term, or phrase to which it is relevant, with a character space before and after the parenthesis marks of the citation to separate it from adjoining text. Do not place a citation within the quotation marks of a quoted title or passage. If a citation must be placed immediately before a punctuation mark closing the part of the sentence to which it is relevant, it is not spaced from the mark. In general, try to avoid placing a citation at the end of a sentence.

> ... contradicted the previous report by Smith and Brown (7) as well as that of ...

> In his chapter "Leucotomy" (8), he noted that ...

> Using our new assay (11) developed for ...

If numbers other than reference numbers appear within parenthesis marks, be sure that they are clearly identified by appropriate elements.

> ... and in at least one case (Case 1) the reaction did not ...

Unreferenced citations of personal communications, unpublished speeches, and materials similarly not available to the scholarly public are placed at their relevant points in the text and also enclosed by parenthesis marks (see section 5.27)

> ... and some unpublished data (Grant FJ, personal communication) suggest that ...

15.9 Citations in tables are usually most appropriately placed in footnotes, but if they are needed in a table field (see section 2.22) in a separate column, be sure to retain the parenthesis marks to avoid any confusion with tabulated numeric data.

Study	Reference
Brown and Jones	(47)
Carrington	(51)

Citations should not be placed within figures; a relevant citation should be in the figure's legend (see section 2.30).

Some journals do not use the citation form specified by the Vancouver style but indicate citations by placing reference numbers as superscripts to text. The Vancouver style seems highly preferable. The typing of manuscripts is speeded by authors, or their typists, not having to take the extra steps to type superscript numbers or mark on-the-line numbers as superscripts. On-the-line citations are much more readily found in search-and-replace procedures of the word-processing programs during revision. Similar advantages and efficiencies accrue in editorial offices and composing rooms. Possible confusion in tables with superscript numbers used as power exponents is avoided.

REFERENCES

REFERENCES: STRUCTURAL PRINCIPLES

15.10 Although this chapter includes examples of the most frequent types of references likely to be needed in articles in medical journals, a few infrequently needed types are not represented. Editors who understand the basic principles set forth in the ANSI standard for references (14) will be able to construct references for publications in any medium that will be in accord with the Vancouver style. The immediately following paragraphs (sections 15.11 to 15.24) are, in essence, a summary of the main principles for the construction of references set forth in the ANSI standard, with the specific requirements for the Vancouver style. Every editorial office should have a copy of the ANSI standard (14) among its reference books to consult on details that have to be omitted here.

REFERENCES: BIBLIOGRAPHIC-ELEMENT GROUPS

15.11   The bibliographic elements for references form 7 groups: authorship, title, edition, imprint, physical description, series statement, and notes. The elements in a reference are usually arranged in this sequence, but not all groups are always represented. Some types of bibliographic elements may be represented more than once in a reference, notably author and title elements. See Table 15.1 for examples of bibliographic data arranged in accord with the 7 groupings. The text accompanying the example references in sections 15.25 to 15.63 indicates how the references are built with the groups and the elements within each group.

Author names, publication title, and other information needed to construct the bibliographic elements of a reference should be taken from the work itself. Titles and author names should be as they appear on the title page (including misspellings and other errors), but author names and publisher names should be condensed as indicated below in the discussions of the authorship group (see section 15.12) and the imprint group (see section 15.20). Some information ordinarily found on a title page such as publication date sometimes may be found instead in another location such as the reverse of the title page or may be substituted for by another datum (such as copyright date for an unspecified publication date).

REFERENCES: THE AUTHORSHIP GROUP OF BIBLIOGRAPHIC ELEMENTS

15.12   The authorship group of elements includes primary author(s) and other author(s) with roles such as editor or compiler specified by an author-role indicator. Personal author names are inverted, family name (surname) placed first and initials for given names second, with a space between the two elements; a comma and a space separates a name from a following name; each name must represent the form in which it appears on the referenced document. Corporate (collective) author names (committees, groups, organizations, governmental agencies) are written out in full in the form in which they appear on referenced documents, but widely known abbreviations such as "US" for *United States of America* and "WHO" for *World Health Organization* may be used as

Table 15.1: The bibliographic elements most frequently needed for references in medical-journal articles arranged by bibliographic groups [fn1]

Bibliographic group	Bibliographic element	Example
Authorship group	Author(s), primary	Personal name
		Corporate (collective) name: author-group, agency, organization
	Author-role indicator	Editor, compiler
Title group	Title, analytic	Journal-article title, article-section title, book-chapter title
	Title, monographic	Book title, journal-supplement title
	Title, collective	Journal title
Edition group	Edition statement	Edition number
	Author, secondary	Translator
	Author-role indicator	Editor
Imprint group	Place of publication	Books and other monographs: city of publication
	Publisher name	Books and other monographs: company agency, organization
	Date of publication	Books and other monographs: title-page date or copyright date
	Volume-identification data	Journals: year of volume, volume number
	Issue-identification data	Journals, magazines, newspapers: issue date
	Extent of work	Book: pages cited
		Journal articles: pages cited
	Report identifier	Agency publications: report number
Physical-description group	Extent of work	Books: page-number total
		Video and audio cassettes: playing time
		Computer software: number of disks
	Packaging method	Books: pages
		Cassettes: format type
		Software: type of disks
Series-statement group	Title, collective	Series title
	Volume-identification data	Volume number in series
Notes group	Availability	Notes on purchase sources

fn1: This table is based on the list on pages 24 and 25 of the ANSI standard on bibliographic references (14).

the first element in the authorship group. When no personal author or corporate author is specified on the title page, use the name of the issuing organization as the author name; do not, however, use the name of a commercial publisher as author name for works, such as dictionaries, compiled by the publisher.

The rules for capitalization of personal names (see section 7.12) and organizations (including committees) (see section 7.17) apply to names in the authorship group, but a lowercase initial letter of a family name that is the first element is capitalized. *Editor* is abbreviated "ed" and *compiler* "comp"; their plural forms are "eds" and "comps". An authorship group closes with a period (full stop).

> You CH, Lee KY, Chey RY, Menguy R.
> The Royal Marsden Hospital Bone-Marrow Transplantation Team.
> US Government Printing Office.
> WHO Expert Committee.
> DuBois E, Cecil R, Jones R, eds.

15.13 List all personal authors when there are 6 or fewer. Of 7 authors or more, list only the first 3 and substitute for the remaining names ", et al".

> Abrams G, Brown H, Candido I, Dent J, Eve K, Frost L.
> Gans M, Hearst N, Iquitos O, et al.

In the example immediately above the comma following "Iquitos O" signals the function of "et al" as an equivalent to an author name. The ANSI standard places "et al" within square brackets to indicate that this is an element which does not appear on the referenced work; this authorship statement would be styled by the standard as "Gans M, Hearst N, Iquitos O [et al].". Authorship of a work at the analytic level (see discussion in the next paragraph) is given in the standard as "[Anonymous]" if an author is not stated on the work.

REFERENCES: THE TITLE GROUP OF BIBLIOGRAPHIC ELEMENTS

15.14 The title group of elements include main titles at the 3 bibliographic levels (*analytic, monographic,* and *collective;* see description immediately below), subordinate titles, and translated titles. The group also includes medium designators such as "Film strip", "Sound recording", "Database", "Videorecording".

15.15 An *analytic title* is the title of an individual document within a monographic- or collective-level work, such as the title of an article in a journal or of a chapter in a book.

15.16 A *monographic title* is the primary title of a work that can stand alone, such as a journal supplement, a book, a report, a videorecording, a complete musical work.

15.17 A *collective title* is the title of a collection or set of physically separate pieces, such as the title of a monographic series, a journal title (the title covering the volumes and issues of a journal).

15.18 In references to multilevel works, the analytic title comes first and is followed, as needed, by the monographic title and the collective title; for example, in a reference to a journal article, the article's title (analytic title) precedes the collective title (journal title). A journal title is abbreviated in accord with the standard abbreviations for elements of journal titles used in *Index Medicus* (see Appendix B).

The initial letter of a title is capitalized; proper and scientific names within the title normally capitalized in text are capitalized by the appropriate rules for capitalization within text sentences (for proper names, see section 7.11; for scientific names, section 7.3). Italicize elements of a title normally italicized in text as a scientific convention (see section 8.2). A subordinate title follows the primary title closed with a colon and a space, and is not capitalized. A title group is closed with a period.

> Coffee drinking and cancer of the colon.
> Functional asplenia: demonstration of splenic activity by bone marrow scan.
> Surgical operations in short-stay hospitals: United States—1975.
> Clinical manifestations of infection with *Escherichia coli*.

Note, however, that each title element in the abbreviated titles of journals is capitalized in accord with the style in *Index Medicus* (see Appendix B).

REFERENCES: THE EDITION GROUP OF BIBLIOGRAPHIC ELEMENTS

15.19 The edition group of elements includes secondary author, author-role indicator, and edition statement. The edition statement includes the number of the edition in the style for ordinal numbers (see section 13.9) followed by the abbreviation "ed" for edition; note that this "ed", which does not follow a name, will not be confused with the abbreviation "ed" for *editor*, which follows a name and a comma. The edition group closes with a period.

> Immunology: an introduction to molecular and cellular principles of the immune response. 5th ed.

REFERENCES: THE IMPRINT GROUP OF BIBLIOGRAPHIC ELEMENTS

15.20 The imprint group of elements includes place of publication, publisher name, date of publication, volume identification, issue identification, location and extent of the work. The "location and extent of work" most frequently applies in medical references to the first and last pages of a journal article or book chapter; the first-page number is given in full in arabic numerals (unless the page numbers are roman as on the preliminary pages in many books), but the final page number is represented by only enough digits to distinguish it unequivocally from the first-page number. Other elements included in this group in the ANSI standard are rarely, if ever, needed in references in medical articles (such as, for example, master, matrix, and acquisition numbers for sound recordings).

New York: Harper and Row; 1974.   [for a book]

New York: Harper and Row; 1974:23–7.   [for the cited pages]

1980;79:311–4.   1979;78:685–93.   1979;78:1998–2003.   [for a journal article]

When the place of publication is a city likely to be recognized internationally, give only the name of the city. If the city must be identified unequivocally or is not likely to be known internationally, fix its location by adding the unabbreviated name of its state, province, or similar political entity. If more than 1 city is given on the title page, give only the first.

Paris   London   London, Ontario   Bethesda, Maryland

15.21 Publisher names are condensed by omitting prefatory articles (notably "The") and closing elements used in common in many publisher names (such as "Incorporated", "Limited", "Book Company", ", Publisher"). Note, however, that a term like "Press" following an institutional name should be retained if the institution may have other publishing functions (as in a university issuing catalogs from its academic offices while also operating a university press). Initials are treated as in author names but without inversion. Retain an ampersand (&) connecting 2 proper names if it is used on the title page.

John Wiley & Sons *becomes* John Wiley
McGraw-Hill Book Company *becomes* McGraw-Hill
Merriam-Webster Inc., Publishers *becomes* Merriam-Webster
The University of Chicago Press *becomes* University of Chicago Press
Oxford University Press *remains* Oxford University Press
W. B. Saunders Company *becomes* WB Saunders
Brown & Black, Inc. *becomes* Brown & Black

REFERENCES: THE PHYSICAL-DESCRIPTION, SERIES-STATEMENT, AND NOTES GROUPS OF BIBLIOGRAPHIC ELEMENTS

15.22 The physical-description group of elements includes extent of work (such as statement of number of pages in a book), packaging method (pages in the book format), and some other elements particularly relevant to nonprint media. The total number of pages in a book is usually not needed in references for articles.

15.23 The series-statement group of elements includes author name, author role, issue-identification, title, and volume-identification data relevant to identifying the series of which the primarily cited work is a part.

(Stoner GD, ed; Methods and perspectives in cell biology; vol 1).

The notes group of elements includes information appearing on the work that may be useful for readers but cannot be properly placed in a preceding group; an example is an International Standard Book Number (ISBN). Information on availability of a work (seller, address, price) is properly placed in the notes group.

REFERENCES: PUNCTUATION AND TYPOGRAPHY

15.24 Conventional punctuation marks serve in references as delimiters and not for the usual functions defined in Chapter 5. Note, for example, that the period following the abbreviation "eds" for "editors" in one of the

Table 15.2: Punctuation in bibliographic references [fn1]

Mark		Function
Period	.	Closes a group of bibliographic elements. Closes the entire reference.
Comma	,	Separates closely related elements (for example, author names in the authorship group or a secondary-author name) from an author-role indicator like "ed".
Semicolon	;	Separates different elements within a group. Precedes volume-identification data.
Parenthesis marks	( )	Enclose issue-identification data and the series-statement group of elements.
Square brackets	[ ]	Enclose information not carried on the referenced work or added for clarity.
Colon	:	Precedes publisher name. Precedes subordinate title. Precedes extent of work element (such as the inclusive page numbers for journal articles). Follows a connective term (such as the "In:" that connects a chapter title to the title of the book).
En dash (or hyphen)	–	Connects numbers of first and last pages in a range of pages.
Space		Separates a bibliographic group (closed with a period) from a following group. Separates bibliographic elements not separated by punctuation; follows punctuation signs except those linking parts of bibliographic elements and after the colon preceding a "location-extent of work" element.

fn1: This table is based on Table 1, "Types and Uses of Punctuation," in the ANSI standard (14) but does not follow it precisely and omits some details rarely relevant to medical publishing. The en dash (or hyphen) has been added.

examples in the discussion of authorship group in the preceding section is not a period serving as an abbreviation sign; the period serves here to mark the end of the authorship group of elements (see section 15.12). The delimiting functions most often needed in references in the medical literature are summarized in Table 15.2

Note that the example references given in this manual for books, monographs, and similar publications carry a semicolon after the publisher name and preceding (with a space) the date of publication. This punctuation is a minor departure from the original Vancouver style (which used a comma) and is in accord with the ANSI standard; this use of the semicolon preserves the comma for separation of subelements of the same kind in a bibliographic group such as, for example, author names.

Particular kinds of typefaces for different groups of bibliographic elements can serve to distinguish them for readers' convenience. The use, however, of the same typeface for all groups as that of the journal's text (usually a roman or other upright typeface) is more economical of costs in time and effort in copy-marking and typesetting and reduces problems in converting computer typesetting tapes to forms usable in online databases.

EXAMPLE REFERENCES

The remainder of this chapter (sections 15.25 to 15.63) illustrates how references to journal articles, books, newspaper articles, magazine articles, organizational documents, and other kinds of publications are built on the principles (see sections 15.10 to 15.24) incorporated in the Vancouver style from the ANSI standard for bibliographic references (14). Not every possible type of publication is represented by these examples, but the illustrations of how the principles are applied should enable authors and editors to construct references themselves. For the key to example references by type of publication see Table 15.3.

Table 15.3: Key to section numbers of example references for publications of various types

Type of publication	Section number
Journal articles and supplements	
Article with personal author(s)	
6 or fewer authors	15.25
7 or more authors	15.26
Article with corporate (collective) author	15.27

Table 15.3: *(continued)*

Type of publication	Section number
Article with unidentified author	15.28
Part of journal article; personal author	15.29
Journal article accepted but not yet published	15.30
Entire supplement	15.31
Article in supplement	15.32
Journal article with continuous pagination in a journal paginated by issue	15.33
Journal article with discontinuous pagination in a journal paginated by issue	15.34
Books and other monographs	
Personal author; edition; reference to specific pages	15.36
Personal author; total number of pages	15.37
Book with editor	15.38
Chapter with author	15.39
Monograph in a series	15.40
Volume in a multivolume book	15.40
Paper in a published proceedings	15.41
Dissertation or thesis	15.42
Book without named author; compiled by publisher	15.43
Book without named author; issued by organization	15.43
Governmental and organization documents	
Agency publication	
Personal author	15.45
Agency as author	15.46
US Congressional document	
Law	15.47
Hearing report	15.48
Agency report	15.49
Article in a governmental periodical	15.50
Newspaper or magazine articles	
Newspaper article; personal author	15.51
Newspaper article; unnamed author	15.51
Magazine article; personal author	15.52
Manuscripts and other unpublished documents available for scholarly research	
Letter	15.53
Manuscript	15.54
Classic and historic works	
Well-known work	15.55
Particular edition	15.56
Maps	15.57
Nonprint media	
Computer program ("software")	15.59
Videorecording	15.60
Legal documents	
US court report	15.62
US Constitution	15.63

EXAMPLE REFERENCES: JOURNAL ARTICLES AND SUPPLEMENTS

The examples given here for journal articles apply, unless indicated otherwise, only to journals paginated continuously by volume. Some specific examples are given for articles in journals and magazines paginated continuously only in each issue

15.25 JOURNAL ARTICLE WITH 6 OR FEWER AUTHORS

You CH, Lee KY, Chey RY, Menguy R. Electrogastrographic study of patients with unexplained nausea, bloating and vomiting. Gastroenterology. 1980;79:311–4.

Authorship group	
You CH, Lee KY, Chey RY, Menguy R.	Author(s), primary
Title group	
Electrogastrographic study of patients with unexplained nausea, bloating and vomiting.	Title, analytic
Gastroenterology.	Title, collective
Imprint group	
1980	Date of publication (for title, collective)
;79	Volume-identification data
:311–4.	Pagination (location — extent of work)

15.26 JOURNAL ARTICLE WITH 7 OR MORE PERSONAL AUTHORS

Brickner PW, Scanlan BC, Conanan B, et al. Homeless persons and health care. Ann Intern Med. 1986;104:405–9.

Authorship group	
Brickner PW, Scanlan BC, Conanan B, et al.	Author(s), primary
(List all authors when 6 or fewer; when 7 or more, list only the first 3 and add "et al". The article has 7 authors.)	
Title group	
Homeless persons and health care.	Title, analytic
Ann Intern Med.	Title, collective
Imprint group	
1986	Publication date (for title, collective)
;104	Volume-identification data
:405–9.	Pagination (location — extent of work)

15.27 JOURNAL ARTICLE WITH CORPORATE AUTHOR(S)

The Royal Marsden Hospital Bone-Marrow Transplantation Team. Failure of syngeneic bone-marrow graft without preconditioning in post-hepatitis marrow aplasia. Lancet. 1977;2:242–4.

Authorship group	
The Royal Marsden Hospital Bone-Marrow Transplantation Team.	Author(s), primary
Title group	
Failure of syngeneic bone-marrow graft without preconditioning in post-hepatitis marrow aplasia.	Title, analytic
Lancet.	Title, collective
Imprint group	
1977	Date of publication
;2	Volume-identification data
:242–4.	Pagination (location – extent of work)

15.28 JOURNAL ARTICLE WITH UNIDENTIFIED AUTHOR

[Anonymous]. Coffee drinking and cancer of the pancreas [editorial]. Br Med J. 1981;283:628.

Authorship group	
[Anonymous].	Author(s), primary
Title group	
Coffee drinking and cancer of the pancreas	Title, analytic
[editorial].	Information added for clarity
Br Med J.	Title, collective
Imprint group	
1981	Date of publication
;283	Volume-identification data
:628.	Pagination (location – extent of work)

15.29 PART OF JOURNAL ARTICLE: INDIVIDUAL AUTHOR

Overstreet JW. Semen analysis. In: Swerdloff RS. Infertility in the male. Ann Intern Med. 1985;103:907–09.

Authorship group (analytic level)	
Overstreet JW.	Author(s), primary
Title group (analytic level)	
Semen analysis.	Title, analytic

Authorship group (monographic level)	
In:	Connective term
Swerdloff RS.	Author(s), primary
	(first author at mono-
	graphic level)

Title group (monographic level)	
Infertility in the male.	Title, monographic
Title group (collective level)	
Ann Intern Med.	Title, collective
Imprint group	
1985	Date of publication
;103	Volume-identification data
:907–09.	Pagination (location—
	extent of work)

(Illustrates article treated as being at a monographic level when reference is to a part, or analytic level, within it. The article used for this example is a review article derived from a conference presentation. The individual speakers each served as author for a section of the review: Overstreet is author of the section on semen analysis; Swerdloff was moderator of the conference and is first author on the review, designated "moderator".)

15.30 JOURNAL ARTICLE ACCEPTED FOR PUBLICATION
BUT NOT YET PUBLISHED

You CH, Lee KY, Chey RY, Menguy R. Electrogastrographic study of patients with unexplained nausea, bloating and vomiting. Gastroenterology. [In press].

Authorship group	
You CH, Lee KY, Chey RY, Menguy R.	Author(s), primary
Title group	
Electrogastrographic study of patients with unexplained nausea, bloating and vomiting.	Title, analytic
Gastroenterology.	Title, collective
Imprint group	
[In press].	Information substituted for unavailable volume-identification data and pagination

15.31 JOURNAL SUPPLEMENT

Dunn MJ, ed. Proceedings of the Council for High Blood Pressure Research, 1985: Cleveland, Ohio, September 18–20, 1985. Hypertension. 1986;8(6 Pt 2):IIi–III92.

Authorship group	
Dunn MJ	Author(s), primary
, ed.	Author-role indicator

Title group
  Proceedings of the Council for High   Title, monographic
    Blood Pressure Research, 1985
  : Cleveland, Ohio, September 18–20,   Title, subordinate
    1985.
  Hypertension.   Title, collective
Imprint group
  1986   Date of publication
  ;8   Volume-identification
                              data
  (6 Pt 2)   Issue-identification
                              data
  :IIi–II192.   Pagination
                              (location – extent
                              of work)

(Note that the pagination of this supplement uses the roman number "II" to indicate a special sequence for the supplement; the sequence proper includes two sets, "II-i" to "II-xii" and "II-1" to "II-192". This kind of sequence special to a supplement is not recommended style. Recommended pagination is the sequence that continues the pagination of issues adjacent to the supplement and the "Part 1" of the issue carrying the supplement as "Part 2"; see section 1.26.)

15.32   ARTICLE IN JOURNAL SUPPLEMENT

Mastri AR. Neuropathy of diabetic neurogenic bladder. Ann Intern Med. 1980;92(2 Pt 2):316–8.

Authorship group
  Mastri AR.   Author(s), primary
Title group
  Neuropathy of diabetic neurogenic   Title, analytic
    bladder.
  Ann Intern Med.   Title, collective
Imprint group
  1980   Date of publication
  ;92(2 Pt 2)   Volume- and issue-
                              identification data
  :316–8   Pagination (location – extent
                              of work)

15.33   ARTICLE WITH CONTINUOUS PAGINATION
       IN A JOURNAL PAGINATED BY ISSUE

Seaman WB. The case of the pancreatic pseudocyst. Hosp Pract. 1981;16(Sep):24–5.

Authorship group
  Seaman WB.   Author(s), primary

Title group
  The case of the pancreatic   Title, analytic
  pseudocyst.
  Hosp Pract.   Title, collective
Imprint group
  1981   Date of publication
  ;16(Sep)   Volume- and issue-
                              identification data
  :24–5.   Pagination (location –
                              extent of work)

(For abbreviations of names of months, see Table 11.3. The journal in this example is a monthly; for a weekly, place the day of issue after the abbreviation for the month after one space, for example, "(Sep 15)".)

15.34 ARTICLE WITH DISCONTINUOUS PAGINATION
IN A JOURNAL PAGINATED BY ISSUE

Thomas P. Across-the-board diet reform for CAD—is the table tilted?. Med World News. 1986;27(May 26):60–2,67–9,73.

Authorship group
  Thomas P.   Author(s), primary
Title group
  Across-the-board diet reform for   Title, analytic
    CAD—is the table tilted?.
  Med World News.   Title, collective
Imprint group
  1986   Date of publication
  ;27   Volume-identification data
  (May 26)   Issue-identification data
  :60–2,67–9,73.   Pagination (location – extent
                            of work)

(An alternative form for the issue-identification data for this example is "(10)", the issue number, rather than the date of issue; the date of issue is preferred for periodicals with new pagination in each issue because it serves as a signal for this distinction from continous pagination through a volume [see section 1.33] for scholarly journals usually bound in volumes in libraries. Note that the "?" is carried from the original title but that the entire analytic title is closed with a period.)

EXAMPLE REFERENCES: BOOKS AND OTHER MONOGRAPHS

15.35 Bibliographic references to books take the same form, in general, as references to journal articles: author(s); title; imprint data. Variations on this basic form are occasionally needed, for example, for references to particular chapters and to specific pages. Note, however, that bibliographic descriptions that head up book reviews are more useful to readers if they begin with title and supply data such as price not usually given in references (see sections 3.11 to 3.13 and Table 3.1).

15.36 BOOK WITH PERSONAL AUTHOR; EDITION;
REFERENCE TO SPECIFIC PAGES

Eisen HN. Immunology: an introduction to molecular and cellular principles of the immune response. 5th ed. New York: Harper and Row; 1974:215–7.

Authorship group	
Eisen HN.	Author(s), primary
Title group	
Immunology	Title, monographic
: an introduction to molecular and cellular principles of the immune response.	Title, subordinate
Edition group	
5th ed.	Edition statement
Imprint group	
New York	Place of publication
: Harper and Row	Publisher name
; 1974	Date of publication
:215–7.	Location–extent of work [reference to specific pages, pages 215 to 217]

15.37 BOOK WITH PERSONAL AUTHORS; PHYSICAL DESCRIPTION

Rowson KEK, Rees TAL, Mahy BWJ. A dictionary of virology. Oxford: Blackwell; 1981. 230 p.

Authorship group	
Rowson KEK, Rees TAL, Mahy BWJ.	Author(s), primary
Title group	
A dictionary of virology.	Title, monographic
Imprint group	
Oxford	Place of publication
: Blackwell	Publisher name
; 1981.	Date of publication
Physical description group	
230	Extent of work
p.	Packaging method [pages]

15.38 BOOK WITH EDITOR, COMPILER, CHAIRMAN AS AUTHOR;
REFERENCE TO PAGES

Dausset J, Colombani J, eds. Histocompatibility testing 1972. Copenhagen: Munksgaard; 1973:12–8.

Authorship group	
Dausset J, Colombani, J	Author(s), primary
, eds.	Author-role indicator
Title group	
Histocompatibility testing 1972.	Title, monographic
Imprint group	
Copenhagen	Place of publication
: Munksgaard	Publisher name
; 1973	Date of publication
:12–8.	Pagination (location— extent of work)

15.39 CHAPTER IN A BOOK

Weinstein L, Swartz MN. Pathogenic properties of invading microorganisms. In: Sodeman WA Jr, Sodeman WA, eds. Pathologic physiology: mechanisms of disease. Philadelphia: WB Saunders; 1974:457–72.

Authorship group (analytic level)	
Weinstein L, Swartz MN.	Author(s), primary
Title group (analytic level)	
Pathogenic properties of invading microorganisms.	Title, analytic
Authorship group (monographic level)	
In:	Connective term
Sodeman WA Jr, Sodeman WA	Author(s), primary
, eds.	Author-role indicator
Imprint group	
Philadelphia	Place of publication
: WB Saunders	Publisher name
; 1974	Date of publication
:457–72.	Pagination (location— extent of work)

15.40 MONOGRAPH IN A SERIES

Hunninghake GW, Gadek JE, Szapiel SV, et al. The human alveolar macrophage. In: Harris CC, ed. Cultured human cells and tissues in biomedical research. New York: Academic Press; 1980:54–6. (Stoner GD, ed; Methods and perspectives in cell biology; vol 1).

Authorship group (analytic level)	
Hunninghake GW, Gadek JE, Szapiel SV, et al.	Author(s), primary
Title group (analytic level)	
The human alveolar macrophage.	Title, analytic
Authorship group (monographic level)	
In:	Connective term

Harris CC	Author(s), primary
, ed.	Author role indicator
Title group (monographic level)	
Cultured human cell and tissues in biomedical research.	Title, monographic
Imprint group	
New York	Place of publication
: Academic Press	Publisher name
; 1980	Date of publication
:54–6.	Pagination (location – extent of work)
Series statement group	
(Stoner GD	Author(s) primary
, ed	Author role indicator
; Methods and perspectives in cell biology	Title, collective
; vol 1).	Volume-identification data

VOLUME IN A MULTIVOLUME BOOK

Cowie AP, Mackin R. Volume 1: verbs with prepositions and particles. In: Oxford dictionary of current idiomatic English. London: Oxford University Press; 1975.

Authorship group (analytic level)	
Cowie AP, Mackin R.	Author(s), primary
Title group (analytic level)	
Volume 1: verbs with prepositions and particles.	Title, analytic
Title group (monographic level)	
In:	Connective term
Oxford dictionary of current idiomatic English	Title, monographic
Imprint group	
London	Place of publication
: Oxford University Press	Publisher name
; 1975.	Date of publication

15.41 PAPER IN PUBLISHED PROCEEDINGS

DuPont B. Bone marrow transplantation in severe combined immunodeficiency with an unrelated MLC compatible donor. In: White HJ, Smith R, eds. Proceedings of the third annual meeting of the International Society for Experimental Hematology. Houston: International Society for Experimental Hematology; 1974:44–6.

Authorship group	
DuPont B.	Author(s), primary
Title group (analytic level)	

Bone marrow transplantation in severe combined immunodeficiency with an unrelated MLC compatible donor.	Title, analytic
Authorship group (monographic level)	
In:	Connective term
White HJ, Smith R	Author(s), primary
, eds.	Author role indicator
Title group (monographic level)	
Proceedings of the third annual meeting of the International Society for Experimental Hematology.	Title, monographic
Imprint group	
Houston	Place of publication
: International Society for Experimental Hematology	Publisher name
; 1974	Date of publication
:44-6.	Pagination (location — extent of work)

15.42   DISSERTATION OR THESIS

Cairns RB. Infrared spectroscopic studies of solid oxygen [Dissertation]. Berkeley, California: University of California; 1965. 156 p.

Authorship group	
Cairns RB.	Author(s), primary
Title group	
Infrared spectroscopic studies of solid oxygen [Dissertation].	Title, monographic Information added
Imprint group	
Berkeley, California	Place of publication
: University of California	Publisher name
, 1965.	Date of publication
Physical description group	
156	Extent of work
p.	Packaging method (pages)

15.43   BOOK OR MONOGRAPH WITHOUT AUTHOR; COMPILED BY PUBLISHER

Webster's standard American style manual. Springfield, Massachusetts: Merriam-Webster; 1985. 464 p.

Title group	
Webster's standard American style manual.	Title, monographic

Imprint group

Springfield, Massachusetts	Place of publication
: Merriam-Webster	Publisher name
; 1985.	Date of publication

Physical description group

464	Extent of work
p.	Packaging method (pages)

(Widely recognized works at the monographic level without author statements may be so adequately identified with the kind of bibliographic elements illustrated in this example that authorship need not be stated as "[Anonymous]". But note that anonymous articles at the analytic level should carry the authorship element "[Anonymous]"; see section 15.28.)

Monographs compiled and issued by an organization other than a publisher should have the organization given as author; see the next example and sections 15.12, 15.27, 15.44, and 15.46 to 15.50.

BOOK OR MONOGRAPH WITH ORGANIZATION AS AUTHOR

World Health Organization. The SI for the health professions. Geneva: World Health Organization; 1977.

Authorship group

World Health Organization	Author, primary

Title group

The SI for the health professions.	Title, monographic

Imprint group

Geneva	Place of publication
: World Health Organization	Publisher name
; 1977.	Date of publication

EXAMPLE REFERENCES: GOVERNMENTAL AND ORGANIZATIONAL DOCUMENTS

15.44 Documents issued or published by governmental bodies, international organizations such as the World Health Organization, professional societies, and private organizations often present problems in constructing references to them because of uncertainties about authorship and the complexities of report numbers and series designations. A detailed and exhaustive guide through many of these problems is *The Complete Guide to Citing Government Documents* (15), which covers documents of international organizations as well as those of federal, state, local, and regional bodies in the United States. The guide's analysis of bibliographic problems is developed in large part on the principles of the ANSI standard on bibliographic references (14). The examples in sections 15.45 to 15.50 illustrate some of the most frequent types of references.

If the title page does not list personal primary-author(s), the author is, in general, the issuing organizational unit. If the title page carries more than one agency, the unit directly responsible for authorship must be named as author; if the unit is widely known in the readership of the journal, its designation as author is adequate. If the unit is not widely known in the readership, the authorship statement should include, as first author, the name of the highest agency named, for example "US Congress".

> Office of Technology Assessment
> US Congress, Office of Technology Assessment

If the title page of the document carries a personal-author statement, that name (or names) becomes the "author, primary".

The publisher of a federal document is usually either the US Government Printing Office, the National Technical Information Service (NTIS), or the issuing agency. If the US Government Printing Office is named on the title page or the back of the title page, it should be designated the publisher.

15.45 AGENCY PUBLICATION WITH PERSONAL AUTHOR

Ranofsky AL. Surgical operations in short-stay hospitals: United States—1975. Hyattsville, Maryland: National Center for Health Statistics; 1978; DHEW publication no (PHS)78-1785. (Vital and health statistics; series 13; no 34).

Authorship group	
Ranofsky AL.	Author(s), primary
Title group	
Surgical operations in short-stay hospitals	Title, monographic
: United States—1975.	Title, subordinate
Imprint group	
Hyattsville, Maryland	Place of publication
: National Center for Health Statistics	Publisher name
; 1978	Date of publication
DHEW publication no (PHS)78-1785.	Report identifier
Series-statement group	
(Vital and health statistics	Title, collective
series 13	
; no 34).	Issue-identification data

15.46 AGENCY PUBLICATION WITH AGENCY AS AUTHOR

National Center for Health Services Research. Health technology assessment reports, 1984. Rockville, Maryland: National Center for

Health Services Research; 1985; DHHS publication no (PHS) 85-3373. Available from: National Technical Information Service, Springfield, VA 22161.

Authorship group
    National Center for Health Services   Author(s), primary
      Research
Title group
    Health technology assessment reports,   Title, monographic
      1984.
Imprint group
    Rockville, Maryland   Place of publication
    : National Center for Health   Publisher name
      Services Research
    ; 1985   Date of publication
    ; DHHS publication no (PHS)   Report identifier
      85-3373.
Notes group
    Available from: National Technical   Availability
      Information Service, Springfield,
      VA 22161.

15.47   CONGRESSIONAL DOCUMENT: LAW

US House of Representatives, 98th Congress, 1st Session. House resolution 1776, An act to regulate Medicare fees. Washington: US Government Printing Office; 1981.

Authorship group
    US House of Representative, 98th   Author(s), primary
      Congress, 1st Session.
Title group
    House resolution 1776, An act to   Title, monographic
      regulate Medicare fees.
Imprint group
    Washington   Place of publication
    : US Government Printing Office   Publisher name
    ; 1981.   Date of publication

15.48   CONGRESSIONAL DOCUMENT: HEARING REPORT

US House of Representatives, Committee on Energy and Commerce, Subcommittee on Commerce, Transportation, and Tourism. Disapproving the FTC funeral rule, hearing 4 May 1983. Washington: US Government Printing Office; 1983; Serial no 98-18. [Y4.En2/3:98-18].

Authorship group
    US House of Representatives,   Author(s), primary
      Committee on Energy and Commerce,

Subcommittee on Commerce,
Transportation, and Tourism.
Title group
  Disapproving the FTC funeral rule,   Title, monographic
  hearing 4 May 1983.
Imprint group
  Washington   Place of publication
  : Government Printing Office   Publisher name
  ; 1983   Date of publication
  ; Serial no 98-18.   Volume-identification
          number

Notes group
  [Y4.En2/3:98-18].   Acquisition number
          (Superintendent of
          Documents number)

15.49 CONGRESSIONAL DOCUMENT: AGENCY REPORT

US Congress, Office of Technology Assessment. Status of biomedical research and related technology for tropical diseases. Washington: US Government Printing Office; 1985; OTA-H-258.

Authorship group
  US Congress, Office of Technology   Author(s), primary
  Assessment.
Title group
  Status of biomedical research and   Title, monographic
  related technology for tropical
  diseases.
Imprint group
  Washington   Place of publication
  : US Government Printing Office   Publisher name
  ; 1985   Date of publication
  ; OTA-H-258.   Volume-identification
          data

15.50 FEDERAL PERIODICALS: *FEDERAL REGISTER*

US Department of Labor, Occupational Health and Safety Administration. Hazard communication: final rule. Federal Register. 1985 Nov 25;48:53343–4.

Authorship group
  US Department of Labor,   Author(s), primary
  Occupational Health and
  Safety Administration.
Title group
  Hazard communication   Title, analytic
  : final rule.   Title, subordinate
  Federal Register.   Title, collective

Imprint group	
1985 Nov 25	Date of publication
;48	Volume-identification number
:53343-4.	Pagination (location – extent and mode of work)

FEDERAL PERIODICALS: *CONGRESSIONAL RECORD*

Claghorn T. The virtues of chewing tobacco. Congressional Record. 1888 Apr 25;21(Pt 1):435-7.

Authorship group	
Claghorn T.	Author(s), primary
Title group	
The virtues of chewing tobacco.	Title, analytic
Congressional Record.	Title, collective
Imprint group	
1888 Apr 25	Date of publication
;21	Volume-identification data
(Pt 1)	Issue-identification data
:435-7.	Pagination (location – extent and mode of work)

EXAMPLE REFERENCES: NEWSPAPER AND MAGAZINE ARTICLES

15.51 Although newspapers and magazines (in distinction from scholarly journals) may carry volume and issue-number identifiers, the Vancouver style specifies the more useful and readily found date of issue. Titles of publications are given in unabbreviated form.

NEWSPAPER ARTICLE: PERSONAL AUTHOR

Shaffer RA. Advances in chemistry are starting to unlock mysteries of the brain: discoveries could help cure alcoholism and insomnia, explain mental illness. Wall Street Journal. 1977 Aug 12:1(col 1), 10(col 5).

Authorship group	
Shaffer RA.	Author(s), primary
Title group	
Advances in chemistry are starting to unlock mysteries of the brain	Title, analytic
: discoveries could help cure alcoholism and insomnia, explain mental illness.	Title, subordinate
Wall Street Journal.	Title, collective

Imprint group	
1977 Aug 12	Date of publication
:1(col 1), 10(col 5).	Pagination (location — extent and mode of work), column numbers (location — work unit fraction)

NEWSPAPER ARTICLE: ANONYMOUS

[Anonymous]. Dr Milton Birnkrant [Obituary]. The New York Times. 1986 Jun 15;sect 1:30(col 5).

Authorship group	
[Anonymous].	Author(s), primary
Title group	
Dr. Milton Birnkrant	Title, analytic
[Obituary].	Information added
The New York Times.	Title, collective
Imprint group	
1986 Jun 15	Date of publication
;sect 1	Volume-identification data
:30(col 5).	Pagination (location — extent of work); column number (location — work-unit fraction)

15.52 MAGAZINE ARTICLE

Roueché B. Annals of medicine: the Santa Claus culture. The New Yorker. 1971 Sep 4:66–81.

Authorship group	
Roueché B.	Author(s), primary
Title group	
Annals of medicine: the Santa Claus culture.	Title, analytic
Imprint	
1971 Sep 4	Date of publication
:66–81.	Pagination (location — extent of work)

EXAMPLE REFERENCES: MANUSCRIPTS AND OTHER UNPUBLISHED DOCUMENTS AVAILABLE FOR SCHOLARLY RESEARCH

15.53 LETTER

Herrick JB, [and others]. [Letter to Frank R Morton, Secretary, Chicago Medical Society]. Herrick papers. [1923]. Located at: University of Chicago Special Collections, Chicago, Illinois.

Authorship group	
Herrick JB, [and others].	Author(s), primary

Title group
    [Letter to Frank R Morton, Secretary,   Title, monographic
        Chicago Medical Society].   Information added
    Herrick papers.   Title, collective
Imprint group
    [1923]   Date of "publication"
                                 (estimated)
Notes group
    Located at: Connective term
    University of Chicago Special   Availability – name
        Collections
    Chicago, Illinois.   Availability – city

15.54   MANUSCRIPT

[Anonymous]. Ms D c 2-392; Novum organum botanicum. 1 leaf. Located at: University Library, Edinburgh, Scotland.

Authorship group
    [Anonymous].   Author(s), primary
Title group
    Ms D c 2-392   Manuscript identifier
    ; Novum organum botanicum.   Title, monographic
Imprint group
    1   Extent of work
    leaf   Packaging method
Notes group
    Located at: Connective term
    University Library,   Availability – name
    Edinburgh, Scotland.   Availability – city

EXAMPLE REFERENCES: CLASSIC AND HISTORIC WORKS

15.55   References to passages in well-known works available in many editions that do not seek to direct the reader to a particular edition or translation can take simple forms if they will be widely recognized.

    Cymbeline, V, iv, 4.   (title of play by Shakespeare, act, scene, line)
    Ecclesiastes, 5:12   (title of a biblical book, chapter:verse)

15.56   References to particular editions or translations must take the form of a reference to a monograph.

    Freud S. A general introduction to psychoanalysis. Riviere J, tr. Garden City, New York: Garden City; 1943. 412 p.

Authorship group
    Freud S.   Author(s), primary
Title group
    A general introduction to psychoanalysis.   Title, monographic

Edition group
  Riviere J   Author(s), secondary
  , tr.   Author-role indicator
Imprint group
  Garden City, New York   Place of publication
  : Garden City   Publisher name
  ; 1943.   Date of publication
Physical-description group
  412   Extent of work
  p.   Packaging method

(Note that although the title page of this edition does not specify that it is a specific edition, the provision of the edition group of data, in addition to the imprint-group data, makes clear that this is a specific edition, in this case, an edition in translation.)

EXAMPLE REFERENCES: MAPS

15.57 References in the literature of economics, geography, geology, and history to maps may have to be comprehensively detailed, including such information as projection, dimensions, scale. Such references in the medical literature usually need give only enough information to enable the reader to find a cited map.

National Endowment for Ecologic Studies. Density of industry and the incidence of pulmonary malignancies [Statistical map]. San Jose, California: National Endowment for Ecologic Studies; 1978. (Ecologic series; [sheet] EC-7).

Authorship group
  National Endowment for Ecologic   Author, primary
    Studies.
Title group
  Density of industry and the   Title, monographic
    incidence of pulmonary
    malignancies
  [Statistical map].   Information added
Imprint group
  San Jose, California   Place of publication
  : National Endowment for   Publisher name
    Ecologic Studies
  ; 1978.   Date of publication
Series-statement group
  (Ecologic series   Title, collective
  ; [sheet] EC-7).   Sheet number (volume-
                                   identification data)

EXAMPLE REFERENCES: NONPRINT MEDIA

15.58   The kinds of nonprint works most likely to be cited in medical journals are computer programs ("software"), videorecordings, audiorecordings, films (motion pictures), and transparencies (slides). The general form of references is this sequence of bibliographic groups: title group, authorship group, edition group, imprint group, physical-description group, notes group. The authorship group comes second because title data are usually more important than authorship data and many works in nonprint media are essentially anonymous works; the authorship group may be placed first when authorship is more important to the journal's readers than title, which is most likely to be the case when the work is not a commercial product (as with an unmarketed computer program). Most of such works should be treated for bibliographic references as the equivalent of books and other monographs (see section 15.35); occasionally a collective title is needed to represent a work within a titled series of nonprint works.

As with books, bibliographic references to computer programs and other nonprint works such as videorecordings usually need less detail (such as price, technical specifications) than bibliographic headings of reviews of the same kinds of work (see sections 3.11 to 3.13 and Table 3.1).

A medium designator (such as "Videorecording") should usually be included at the end of the title as square-bracketed added information.

For computer programs, "version" is the equivalent of "edition".

15.59   COMPUTER PROGRAM ("SOFTWARE")

Sci-Mate [Computer program]: the manager, the searcher, the editor. Version 2.0. Philadelphia: Institute for Scientific Information; 1985. 5 5.25-inch disks. 3 manuals.

Title group	
Sci-Mate	Title, monographic
[Computer program]	Medium designator
: the manager, the searcher, the editor.	Title(s), subordinate
(No authorship group)	
Edition group	
Version 2.0.	Edition statement
Imprint group	
Philadelphia	Place of publication
: Institute for Scientific Information	Publisher name
; 1985.	Date of publication
Physical-description group	
5 5.25-inch disks.	Extent of work, packaging method

Notes

3 manuals.   Accompanying material

(Note that *Sci-Mate* is treated here as a single work with section subordinate titles, the equivalent of a book with chapters. Alternatively in a reference to one of the three components, *Sci-Mate* could be treated as a separate work, with "Sci-Mate" as a series title.)

15.60 VIDEORECORDING

Understanding chemotherapy [Videorecording]. Westlake, Ohio: Grandview Hospital Audiovisual Communications; [1983]. 1 videocassette; 17.5 minutes; color; 0.5 inch, U-matic. Available from: Grandview Hospital Audiovisual Communications, PO Box 45132, Westlake, OH 44145.

Title group	
Understanding chemotherapy	Title, monographic
[Videorecording].	Medium designator
Imprint group	
Westlake, Ohio	Place of publication
: Grandview Hospital Audiovisual Communications	Publisher name
; [1983].	Date of publication
Physical-description group	
1 videocassette	Extent of work, packaging method
; 17.5 minutes	Extent of work
; color	Medium/packaging, special features
; 0.5 inch, U-matic.	Size
Notes group	
Available from:	Connective phrase
Grandview Hospital Audiovisual Communication, PO Box 45132, Westlake, OH 44145.	Availability — name, address

EXAMPLE REFERENCES: LEGAL DOCUMENTS

15.61 Citations of, and references to, documents in the literature of law are governed by a large and complex set of rules, sequences, and abbreviations described in great detail in *A Uniform System of Citation* (USC) (16). This system is used not only in the strictly legal literature but in some medical journals and books closely related to it (for example, *Journal of Legal Medicine* published by the American College of Legal Medicine). Although most readers of medical journals may personally find references built on the USC system virtually incomprehensible because of unfamiliarity with its conventions, the references will be adequate for locating referenced documents in some large general and law libraries. This is the best reason for not converting references from the USC style to the Vancouver style.

Medical journals wishing to make legal references more comprehensible to medical readers should modify them by giving full terms rather than abbreviations and punctuating them in accord with the principles of the ANSI standard (14), summarized in Table 15.2. The examples immediately below are based on examples in the ANSI standard. The full terms represented by the USC abbreviations can be found in *A Uniform System of Citation* (16). The examples represent both the USC style and versions recommended here.

Whether or not legal references in medical papers are converted as suggested in the paragraph above, the citations should be in the Vancouver style, reference numbers within parenthesis marks at appropriate points in text, tables, or figure legends, and not in the style of citations specified in the USC system.

15.62 FEDERAL COURT REPORT (US SUPREME COURT) IN A CIVIL ACTION

[USC style] Speiser v. Randall, 357 U.S. 513(1958).
Speiser versus Randall. US Supreme Court. 357:513. 1958.

Title group	
Speiser versus Randall.	Title, monographic (case name)
US Supreme Court.	Title, collective
Imprint group	
357	Volume-identification data
:513.	Location – extent of work (beginning pagination)
Notes group	
1958.	Date of decision

15.63 SECTION OF AN ARTICLE IN THE US CONSTITUTION

[USC style] U.S. Const. art. I, § 9.
US Constitution. Article I, section 9.

Title group	
US Constitution	Title, monographic
Imprint group	
Article I	Volume-identification data
, Section 9.	Location

REFERENCES

1. Huth EJ. Critical argument: the basic structure of papers. In: Huth EJ. How to write and publish papers in the medical sciences. Philadelphia: ISI Press; 1982:47–9.

2. CBE Style Manual Committee. CBE style manual. 5th ed. Bethesda, Maryland: Council of Biology Editors; 1983:1–2.
3. Bibliographic forms. In: The Chicago manual of style. 13th ed. Chicago: University of Chicago Press; 1982:437–83.
4. CBE Style Manual Committee. References. In: CBE style manual. 5th ed. Bethesda, Maryland: Council of Biology Editors; 1983:47–65.
5. Dodd JS, ed. The ACS style guide: a manual for authors and editors. Washington: American Chemical Society; 1986:106–7.
6. American Psychological Association. Publication manual of the American Psychological Association. 3rd ed. Washington: American Psychological Association; 1983:107–33.
7. Notes and documentation of sources. In: Webster's standard American style manual. Springfield, Massachusetts: Merriam-Webster; 1985:179–212.
8. Haas E. Uniform requirements for manuscripts submitted to biomedical journals. CBE Views. 1980;3:12–5.
9. [Huth EJ]. Uniform requirements for manuscripts. Ann Intern Med. 1979;90:120.
10. International Steering Committee of Medical Editors. Uniform requirements for manuscripts submitted to biomedical journals. Ann Intern Med. 1979;90:95–9.
11. International Steering Committee of Medical Editors. Uniform requirements for manuscripts submitted to biomedical journals. Br Med J. 1978;1:1334–6.
12. International Committee of Medical Journal Editors. Uniform requirements for manuscripts submitted to biomedical journals. Ann Intern Med. 1982;96:766–71.
13. International Committee of Medical Journal Editors. Uniform requirements for manuscripts submitted to biomedical journals. Br Med J. 1982;284:1766–70.
14. Subcommittee 4 on Bibliographic References, American National Standards Committee on Library Work, Documentation, and Related Publishing Practices, Z39. American national standard for bibliographic references. New York: American National Standards Institute; 1977; ANSI Z39.29-1977. [The activities of ANSI Z39 are now carried out by the National Information Standards Organization (NISO).]
15. Garner DL, Smith DH. The complete guide to citing government documents: a manual for writers & librarians. Bethesda, Maryland: Congressional Information Service; 1984.
16. [Anonymous]. A uniform system of citation. 13th ed. Cambridge, Massachusetts: Harvard Law Review Association; 1981.

Chapter 16

Scientific Style in Medical Sciences

The recommendations in this chapter include some conventions established by formal agreement in various disciplines and other conventions established informally by widespread use. Some of its sections discuss in detail some aspects of nomenclature set forth only briefly in Chapter 10. This manual cannot accommodate full descriptions of the rationales and rules for the formal conventions summarized here and a complete bibliography of the documents that prescribe them. This chapter does little more than illustrate recommended usage, and for only some fraction of potential questions of style. Authors highly experienced in the scientific fields represented here are likely to know the conventions illustrated, so the aim in this chapter is to help editors not familiar with these conventions as well as manuscript editors with little or no experience in science. The references direct authors needing more detailed guidance on style to the more detailed documents on which some of these recommendations are based. Editors of journals in these fields will, of course, build larger collections of style conventions for their needs than what this chapter holds.

ANATOMY, EMBRYOLOGY, AND HISTOLOGY

See section 10.8.

BACTERIOLOGY

16.1   Bacteriologic organisms are classified into taxonomic ranks; see Table 16.1. The names of organisms in the ranks from kingdom down to subspecies are governed by official international conventions; names in infrasubspecific ranks do not have official standing in nomenclature but

Table 16.1: Main taxonomic ranks in bacteriology

Rank	Nomenclatural standing	Synonym	Example name
Kingdom	Official		*Procaryotae*
Division	Official		*Firmicutes*
Class	Official		*Archaeobacteria*
Order	Official		*Spirochaetales*
Family	Official		*Legionellaceae*
Genus	Official		*Brucella*
Species	Official		*Flavobacterium meningosepticum*
Subspecies	Official		*Campylobacter fetus* subspecies *venerealis*
Infrasubspecific ranks			
Biovar	Not official	Biotype	
Serovar	Not official	Serotype	
Pathovar	Not official	Pathotype	
Morphovar	Not official	Morphotype	

must, of course, be presented accurately. Authoritative sources for the form and spelling of bacterial names include *Bergey's Manual of Systematic Bacteriology* (1), *Approved Lists of Bacterial Names* (2), and *Catalogue of Bacteria, Phages and rDNA Vectors* (3). The standard medical dictionaries (4–7) are convenient sources for the most common names. For a general introduction to bacteriologic nomenclature, see the chapter "Bacterial Nomenclature" by Peter H A Sneath in reference 1. Many details of taxonomic nomenclature are clearly defined and explained in *A Dictionary of Microbial Taxonomy* (8). For style in mycology, see sections 16.50 and 16.51; in parasitology, section 16.57; in virology, sections 16.63 to 16.65.

16.2   Designated suffixes for stem terms indicate the rank of a name for the ranks order through subtribe (see Table 16.2).

BACTERIAL GENUS, SPECIES, AND SUBSPECIES NAMES

16.3   A genus name is a single name, capitalized and printed in italic (slanted)

Table 16.2: Suffixes indicating bacterial taxonomic ranks

Rank	Suffix
Order	*-ales*
Suborder	*-ineae*
Family	*-aceae*
Subfamily	*-oideae*
Tribe	*-eae*
Subtribe	*-inae*

type. It refers to all species and subspecies within the genus and should be used as a noun only in this sense; it should not be used as a short substitute for the name of a species known or unknown. It may be used adjectivally in a taxonomic context, as in modifying the word "species" but a common, or vernacular, form of a genus name is preferred in other contexts; see section 16.9.

> . . . cultured several species of *Pseudomonas* from . . .
> . . . cultured several *Pseudomonas* species from . . .
> . . . classified the genus *Pseudomonas*.
>
> INCORRECT   . . . cultured *Pseudomonas* from the wound.
> CORRECT   . . . cultured a *Pseudomonas* species from . . .

If a genus name appears within text set in an italic (slanted) typeface (for example, in an italicized title), set the name in a roman (upright) typeface.

> . . . his classic work, *A New Taxonomy for* Salmonella *and Other Genera*, first suggested that . . .

16.4   The name of a species is a binomen (two-component name) consisting of the name of its genus and the specific epithet (epithet for the species). The genus name is capitalized (see section 16.3) and the specific epithet is not capitalized even when the species name appears in a context ordinarily calling for capitalization, as in a title; both components must be in an italic (slanted) typeface. Do not use the specific epithet by itself.

> . . . methods for culturing *Staphylococcus aureus* were . . .
> *Staphylococcus aureus* and Wound Infections [article title]
>
> INCORRECT   . . . cultured *coli* from the wound.
> CORRECT   . . . cultured *Escherichia coli* from the wound.

When a species name is in text that must be set in an italic (slanted) typeface, as in a title, set the name in a roman (upright) typeface.

> *Theodor Escherich and* Escherichia coli [book title]

16.5   Subspecies names follow the rules for species names (section 16.4), but the designation "subspecies" between the specific epithet and the subspecific epithet is not set in an italic (slanted) typeface. Do not omit the specific epithet.

> . . . infections with *Campylobacter fetus* subspecies *venerealis*.
>
> INCORRECT   . . . infections with *Campylobacter venerealis*.
> CORRECT   . . . infections with *C. fetus* subspecies *venerealis*.

16.6   Designations for strains and infrasubspecific categories are not governed by official nomenclatural rules and use various alphanumeric terms added to species names. These designations must be in a roman (upright) typeface; a type-culture number is separated from the type-culture abbrevia-

Table 16.3: Abbreviations for names of some culture collections [fn1]

Abbreviation	Name of culture collection
AMRC	FAO-WHO International Reference Centre for Animal Mycoplasmas
ATCC	American Type Culture Collection
CBS	Centraalbureau voor Schimmelcultures
CCEB	Culture Collection of Entomophagous Bacteria
CDC	Centers for Disease Control
CIP	Collection of the Institut Pasteur
DSM	Deutsche Sammlung von Mikroorganismen
IAM	Institute of Applied Microbiology, University of Tokyo
ICPB	International Collection of Phytopathogenic Bacteria
IFO	Institute for Fermentation [Osaka, Japan]
IMRU	Institute of Microbiology, Rutgers—The State University
INA	Institute for New Antibiotics
IPV	Istituto di Pathologia Vegetale
KCC	Kaken Chemical Company
LSU	Louisiana State University
LMD	Laboratorium voor Microbiologie
NCDO	National Collection of Dairy Organisms
NCIB	National Collection of Industrial Bacteria
NCPPB	National Collection of Plant Pathogenic Bacteria
NCTC	National Collection of Type Cultures
NIAID	National Institute of Allergy and Infectious Diseases
NIHJ	National Institute of Health [Japan]
NRC	National Research Council
NRL	Neisseria Reference Laboratory
NRRL	Northern Utilization Research and Development Division
PDDCC	Culture Collection of Plant Diseases Division
TC	Thaxter Collection
TPH	Microbiological Culture Collection, Public Health Laboratory [Toronto]
UMH	University of Missouri Herbarium

fn1: Complete addresses for these collections can be found on pages 29 and 30 of reference 1. Abbreviations for additional institutions can be found on pages xviii and xix of reference 3.

tion (Table 16.3) by a space, but the other types of designations (as for a serovar) are closed up.

> *Escherichia coli* O6:K15:H16 [serovar of an enteropathogenic *E. coli*]
> *Escherichia* coli ATCC 27325 [American Type Culture Collection strain 27325]

The term "strain" should not be used with the species name but can be used with the strain designation in a context indicating in another way the species to which it refers.

> INCORRECT   *Escherichia coli* strain ATCC 27325
> CORRECT   ... from the possibilities among *Pseudomonas* species, we selected the strain ATCC 14718.

16.7   The names of bacterial taxa above genus (kingdom, classes, orders, and families; see Tables 16.1 and 16.2) should also be capitalized and in an italic (slanted) typeface.

> *Spirochaetales* [order]   *Leptospiraceae* [family]

These names are plurals and encompass all bacteria in the taxon; they must not be applied to some bacteria within the taxon.

> INCORRECT   . . . *Leptospiraceae* have been isolated from . . .
> CORRECT   . . . members of the family *Leptospiraceae* have been . . .

BACTERIOLOGIC ABBREVIATIONS AND COMMON NAMES

16.8   The genus name in a species binomen may be abbreviated after the first mention in the text of the full name if a species in a single genus is a subject of the paper. Care must be taken, however, not to use the same abbreviation within a paper for different genera such as "*S aureus*" and "*S pyogenes*" for *Staphylococcus aureus* and *Streptococcus pyogenes;* suitable abbreviations here might be "*S aureus*" and "*Str pyogenes*". There are no official abbreviations for genus names, and abbreviated forms of species binomens should be stated within parenthesis marks at the first mention of the binomen in the text. Do not abbreviate taxonomic names in titles; do not abbreviate genus names when they stand by themselves. Widely used abbreviations for *species* (singular), *species* (plural), and *subspecies* (singular) are, respectively, "sp", "spp", and "subsp". In general these abbreviations and those for genus names in binomens should not be used unless the binomens are used frequently in a paper or space must be saved, as in a table.

16.9   Common, or vernacular, names are frequently used for some genera and species. There are no official rules for their formation; editors unfamiliar with such names and their acceptability as idiomatic forms should confirm their spelling and acceptability in a standard medical dictionary (4–7). The plural forms of common generic names may be used to refer informally to some unspecified species within a genus. Such names are not capitalized unless they are used in a title or at the beginning of a sentence or table row-heading; they must appear in a roman (upright) typeface, not in an italic (slanted) typeface.

Genus name or binomen	Singular	Plural
Streptococcus pneumoniae	the pneumococcus	pneumococci
Neisseria gonorrhoeae	the gonococcus	gonococci
Salmonella	a salmonella	salmonellas
Pseudomonas	a pseudomonad	pseudomonads

The plural forms of common names of species may be used to describe many individual organisms of a species seen in a particular circumstance, such as, for example, in a microscopic view of a stained sputum specimen.

Examination of the smear showed many pneumococci.

16.10 Adjectival forms of genus names are frequently used non-taxonomically to modify nouns such as *abscess, infection, pneumonia*. These forms are usually derived by adding "-al" or "-ic" to the stem of the genus name, but an unchanged genus name is sometimes used adjectivally. Such adjectives should not be in an italic (slanted) typeface; this rule holds even if the adjective has the same form as its noun equivalent because the adjective in noun form is not being used taxonomically in such a context.

> ... a pseudomonal pneumonia ...   ... a streptococcal pneumonia ...
> ... a staphylococcal abscess ...   ... a salmonella dysentery ...

Adjectival forms should not be used if ambiguous implications might arise from such usage.

> INCORRECT   ... a pneumocystic pneumonia ... [implies a "cystic" type of pneumonia]
> CORRECT   ... a pneumocystis pneumonia ...

A taxonomic species or genus name should not be used adjectivally in a nontaxonomic sense, as in "*Pneumocystis carini* pneumonia" or "*Staphylococcus* abscess".

BACTERIAL GENETICS

16.11 Genotypes are designated by 3-letter symbols in a lowercase italic (slanted) typeface.

> *ara   his   lac*

Symbol elements attached to the basic 3-letter symbol add various specific designations.

> Capital letters (italic typeface) for related loci
>
> *araB   lacZ*
>
> Italic (slanted) lowercase letters *p, t,* and *o* for, respectively, promoter, terminator, and operator sites
>
> *lacZp   lacZp   lacZo*
>
> Superscript (roman typeface) plus sign for wild-type genes
>
> *ara*⁺   *his*⁺   *lac*⁺
>
> Serial isolation numbers (allele numbers) in an italic typeface
>
> *arab   araC2*

Symbols specifying genetic characteristics of a strain are spaced after the species name.

Escherichia coli hisB lacC

16.12 Phenotypes are symbolized by similar conventions but the letters must be in a roman (upright) typeface with the initial letter capitalized.

AraA   His⁺   LacC

Phenotype symbols following the strain name must be in roman (upright) characters.

Escherichia coli lacA His⁺

16.13 Plasmids are symbolized by various alphanumeric combinations; the symbols should be enclosed by parenthesis marks and placed immediately after the species name, designation of strain, or genotype without spacing.

Escherichia coli(pEH421)   *E. coli* K-11(pEH421)   *E. coli lacB*(pEH421)

Additional details on style for bacterial genetics, including phenotypic symbols for drug resistance and sensitivity, can be found in the section "Genetics" of *ASM Style Manual for Journals and Books* (9). The originating document for this system is a paper (10) by Demerec, Adelberg, Clark, and Hartman.

CARDIOLOGY

ELECTROCARDIOGRAPHIC RECORDINGS

16.14 Electrocardiographic leads (the combinations of positions for the electrodes from which tracings are recorded) are designated by alphabetic and numeric characters (11).

The standard leads from electrodes on the limbs ("limb leads") are designated with roman numerals.

lead I   [electrodes on the right and left arms]
lead II   [electrodes on the right arm and left leg]
lead III   [electrodes on the left arm and left leg]

In the unipolar lead system, 1 electrode ("central terminal") is represented by combined potentials from the 3 limbs and the other electrode is on 1 of the limbs. The letter "V" stands for the central terminal and the letter "R" or "L" or "F" for the single-limb lead.

VR   VL   VF

In a variant of the unipolar lead system, the augmented unipolar lead system, the central lead is designated by "aV" and a capital (or small capital) letter R, L, or F (for, respectively, the right-arm lead, the left-arm lead, and the left-"foot" lead).

lead aVR   lead aVL   lead aVF

The chest leads are designated with the capital letter V (for the central terminal) and a number for the position of the chest electrode; the number 1 stands for the first electrode position, which is just to the right of the lower sternum, and the last number, 6, for the last electrode on the left side of the precordium.

lead V1   lead V2   [and so on to]   lead V6

Leads proceeding rightward from the V1 position are designated similarly with an added capital (or small-capital) letter "R".

V3R   V4R   [and so on]

Leads taken at the same vertical line but over a higher intercostal space are designated by adding a roman number for the space.

V3III   [third intercostal space, same vertical line as V3]

Esophageal leads are designated with a capital letter V (for the central terminal), a capital (or small capital) letter E (for "esophageal"), and the distance from the nares (in centimeters, implied) to the esophageal electrode.

lead VE28   lead VE31

Such modifiers as "R" and "L" may be styled as subscript small-capital letters (subscript or on-line) as in "V_R" and "V_L" but such styling is no more effective for clear meaning than capital-letter modifiers and makes unjustified work for typists, manuscript editors, and compositors.

16.15   Designations for electrocardiographic waves (deflections from the baseline), wave complexes, segments, and wave intervals were standardized in 1943 by a committee of the American Heart Association (12) and affirmed by the Criteria Committee of the New York Heart Association (11). Waves are designated with capital letters P, Q, R, S, T, and U. Wave complexes are represented by unspaced wave letters; if distinctions must be made between minor and major waves, the lesser wave is indicated by a lowercase letter. Prime signs are used to indicate waves after their usual position.

P wave   T wave   U wave   QRS complex   rS   rR'

A segment of tracing between 2 waves is designated by the capital letters for the waves at the beginning and the end of the segment separated by a hyphen. The hyphen symbolizes the distance on the tracing between the 2 waves, which are not immediately adjacent as are the waves indicated in "QRS complex". The same convention is used to indicate the time interval between 2 waves.

> S-T segment P-R interval Q-T interval prolongation

GRADING OF SEVERITY OF CLINICAL CARDIOVASCULAR MANIFESTATIONS

16.16 The severity of retinal hypertensive vascular changes (and the other accompanying retinal changes) in the ocular fundus (13) is indicated by a roman number from I to IV spaced after the word "grade"; a "grade IV" change is the most severe.

The loudness of cardiac and vascular murmurs is indicated by an arabic number in the range 1–6, 6 representing the loudest; the use of the scale of 1–6 is sometimes indicated by the convention, loudness of the heard murmur/the scale number for the loudest possible murmur, as in "grade 2/6".

The severity of cardiac disease ("status") and the prognosis in a patient are indicated in the nomenclatural system of the New York Heart Association (11) by a number in the range 1–4 for each component, with the 2 numbers connected by a period; 1 represents the mildest state and the best prognosis, 4 the worst.

> Cardiac status and prognosis: 3.2

CARDIOLOGIC SYMBOLS AND ABBREVIATIONS

16.17 Symbols and abbreviations for the variables measured in cardiovascular research and clinical function tests should be styled in accord with the international conventions for symbolization of quantities (see sections 11.1, 14.1, and 14.2). Single-letter symbols for quantities must be in an italic (slanted) typeface; superscript or subscript letters that are not themselves quantities and that modify the symbol to which they are attached should be in a roman (upright) typeface.

> area under left ventricular dye curve ($mg \cdot s \cdot L^{-1}$): A_{LV}
> right-to-left shunt ($L \cdot min^{-1}$): $\dot{Q}_{R-L}$

The 6 kinds of quantities that represent most of the variables measured in cardiovascular investigations can be represented by 6 already widely used symbols that hold to the international convention of single-letter symbols printed in an italic (slanted) typeface.

pressure	P	flow [volume/unit time]	$\dot{Q}$ OR $\dot{V}$
volume	V	saturation	S
velocity	v	work	W

In one system of this kind (14) a superscript symbol indicates anatomic structure and a subscript, condition or time.

left ventricular end-diastolic pressure: P_{ed}^{lv} [lv = left ventricle, ed = end-diastolic]

If abbreviation groups must be used to represent quantities (an undesirable practice), the letters should be in a roman (upright) typeface, to avoid any possible confusion between a single represented quantity and multiplication of two or more quantities. A convention that can indicate unequivocally that a multiletter group represents a single quantity is placement of the group within parenthesis marks.

pulmonary vascular resistance (dyne·s·cm⁻⁵):   PVR   or   (PVR)

pulmonary vascular resistance (dyne·s·cm^{-5}):   PVR   or   (PVR)

time-tension index (mmHg·s·min^{-1}):   TTI   or   (TTI)

Authors should be asked, however, to convert such upright-letter abbreviations to the slanted (italic) single-letter symbols and upright-letter modifiers that are in accord with international conventions.

pulmonary vascular resistance: R_{vr}

UNITS OF MEASUREMENT IN CARDIOLOGY

16.18 Cardiologic measurements may be reported by authors in the earlier and still widely-used metric units or in SI units. European usage, in general, is favoring SI units but conversion to SI units is beginning in North America. Individual journals will have to come to decisions on whether to require reporting in SI units. Blood pressure will probably continue to be reported in the unit mmHg for a relatively long period because of the ubiquitous use of sphygmomanometers with scales thus marked. See Table 16.4 for SI units for the main variables of importance in cardiology.

Note that in the preceding paragraph and in Table 16.4 the "mm" and "Hg" in the unit symbol "mmHg" for "millimeters of mercury" are unspaced. This style is in accord with international recommended practice (15) and with the style for the symbol for degree Celsius, °C (see section 13.16 and Appendix A).

Table 16.4: SI and older metric units for cardiovascular variables

Quantity	SI unit	Older metric unit
Blood pressure	kPa [kilopascal]	mmHg [fn1]
Vascular resistance	kPa·s·L^{-1}	mmHg·min·L^{-1} [fn2]
Flow: cardiac output	L·min^{-1}·kg^{-1}	
Oxygen consumption	L·min^{-1}	
Viscosity	Pa·s	

fn1: To convert mmHg to kPa, multiply the value in mmHg by 0.133.
fn2: To convert mmHg·min·L^{-1} to kPa·s·L^{-1}, multiply the value in mmHg·min·L^{-1} by 8.0.

THE RENIN-ANGIOTENSIN SYSTEM

For designations of components of the renin-angiotensin system, see section 16.34.

CHEMISTRY, INCLUDING BIOCHEMISTRY

16.19 The sections under this heading describe only the style conventions needed most frequently in journals of the medical sciences and clinical medicine. Additional details can be found in the style manuals of the American Chemical Society (16) and the Council of Biology Editors (17). The authoritative recommendations for biochemistry are those issued by the International Union of Biochemistry (IUB) from time to time in separate documents and in a compendium of these documents (18); the Union has issued a separate document on enzyme nomenclature (19) [fn1].

CHEMICAL SYMBOLS AND ABBREVIATIONS

16.20 Symbols for chemical elements whether standing alone or in formulas have initial capitals and must be in roman type (see Table 16.5); the number of atoms of an element in a formula is indicated by a subscript number to the right of the symbol.

$$H \quad H_2 \quad H_2O \quad H_2SO_4 \quad NaOH \quad Na_2SO_4 \quad C_4H_6HgO_4$$

Chemical symbols may be used in text for reference to gases and chemicals that are subjects of investigation or experiment or are agents or reagents in chemical methods or diagnostic test but should not be used mixed with words or alone, in general, to refer to elements.

... studied N_2 in expired air ...   ... toxic effects of CCl_4 ...
... percent of hydrogen in the body ...   ... atmospheric O_3 ...
NOT   ... a Na chloride solution ...   ... percent of H in the body ...

Concentrations of elements or compounds (molarity, mol/L) are

---

fn1: A new edition of the IUB compendium has been scheduled for publication in 1986. It will include the documents in the 1978 edition (18) (stereochemistry, natural products and related compounds, biochemical equilibria, citation of bibliographic references, conformation of polypeptide chains, synthetic polypeptides, peptide hormones, multiple forms of enzymes, nucleic acids and related topics, lipids, steroids, quinones, carotenoids, folic acid, corrinoids, carbohydrates, cyclitols, phosphorus, vitamin B-6); modifications to documents in the 1978 edition (isotopically-modified compounds, abbreviations and symbols for chemical names of interest in biochemistry, human immunoglobulins, α-amino acids, modifications of natural peptides, one-letter notation for amino-acid sequences, tocopherols); and documents issued since 1978. Inquiries should be sent to The Biochemical Society, 7 Warwick Court, London WC1R 5DP, United Kingdom.

Table 16.5: Symbols for chemical elements and for isotopes with medical applications

Symbol	Element	Symbol	Element	Symbol	Element
Ac	actinium	Gd	gadolinium	Pr	praeseodymium
Ag	silver	Ge	germanium	Pt	platinum
Al	aluminum (aluminium)	H	hydrogen	Pu	plutonium
		Ha	hafnium	Ra	radium
Am	americium	He	helium	^{226}Ra	
^{241}Am		Hg	mercury	Rb	rubidium
Ar	argon	^{197}Hg		Re	rhenium
As	arsenic	^{203}Hg		Rf	rutherfordium
At	astatine	Ho	holmium	Rh	rhodium
Au	gold	I	iodine	Rn	radon
^{198}Au		^{123}I		^{222}Rn	
B	boron	^{125}I		Ru	ruthenium
Ba	barium	^{131}I		^{106}Ru	
Be	beryllium	In	indium	S	sulfur
Bi	bismuth	^{111}In		^{35}S	
Bk	berkelium	^{113m}In		Sc	scandium
Br	bromine	K	potassium	Se	selenium
C	carbon	^{42}K		^{75}Se	
^{14}C		Kr	krypton	Si	silicon
Ca	calcium	^{85}Kr		Sm	samarium
^{47}Ca		La	lanthanum	Sn	tin
Cd	cadmium	Li	lithium	Sr	strontium
Ce	cerium	Lr	lawrencium	^{85}Sr	
Cf	californium	Lu	lutetium	^{87m}Sr	
Cl	chlorine	Md	mendelevium	^{90}Sr	
Cm	curium	Mg	magnesium	Ta	tantalum
Co	cobalt	Mn	manganese	Tb	terbium
^{57}Co		Mo	molybdenum	Tc	technetium
^{60}Co		N	nitrogen	^{99m}Tc	
Cr	chromium	Na	sodium	Te	tellurium
^{51}Cr		^{24}Na		Th	thorium
Cs	cesium	Nb	niobium	Ti	titanium
^{137}Cs		Nd	neodymium	Tl	thallium
Cu	copper	Ne	neon	^{201}Tl	
^{64}Cu		Ni	nickel	Tm	thulium
Dy	dysprosium	No	nobelium	U	uranium
Er	erbium	Np	neptunium	V	vanadium
Es	einsteinium	O	oxygen	W	tungsten
Eu	europium	Os	osmium	Xe	xenon
F	fluorine	P	phosphorus	^{133}Xe	
^{18}F		^{32}P		Y	yttrium
Fe	iron	Pa	protactinium	Yb	ytterbium
^{59}Fe		Pb	lead	^{169}Yb	
Fm	fermium	^{210}Pb		Zn	zinc
Fr	francium	Pd	palladium	Zr	zirconium
Ga	gallium	Pm	promethium		
^{67}Ga		Po	polonium		

indicated in equations by symbols within square brackets (see section 5.32) rather than by chemical names.

[Na⁺] [NaCl]   NOT   [sodium ion] [sodium chloride]

Do not use this symbolism in narrative text but write out the equivalent as a term.

NOT   . . . and measured [NaCl] in . . .
BUT   . . . and measured the concentration of NaCl in . . .

16.21 Nuclides are indicated by left superscripts and subscripts adjacent to the symbol for an element.

- Left superscript: Mass number

   ^{198}Au ^{14}C ^{67}Ga

- Left subscript number: Atomic number

   $_{79}$Au $_{6}$C $_{31}$Ga

Right superscripts and subscripts serve other functions.

- Right superscript: Ionic charge, oxidation number, or state of electronic excitation

   Ca^{2+} $Cl_6H_2Pt^{IV}$ NO^*

- Right subscript: Number of atoms of the element or radical thus modified in the molecule or in the radical demarcated by parenthesis marks.

   N_2 H_2SO_4 C_2H_5OH $(CH_3)_2CHCH_2CH(NH_2)COOH$

Isotopic labeling is indicated by the number and symbol within square brackets immediately before the name of the compound; if the labeled position is known, it is indicated before the superscript by the appropriate italicized prefix (see section 16.26) or arabic number.

[^{15}N]alanine   [1-^{14}C]acetic acid   [^{32}P]AMP

In text an isotope can be identified by attaching the mass number by a hyphen to the name of the element written out.

iodine-131   phosphorus-32

For the style of names of radioactive pharmaceuticals, see section 10.4.

An oxidation number (roman numerals) specified only for an element and not within a formula should be on the line and within parenthesis marks.

lead(IV)   Cr(III)

16.22 An abbreviation for a long chemical name used frequently in an article may be acceptable if it is well known among the journal's readers or is explained within parenthesis marks immediately after the first mention of the name in text. Such abbreviations range from those widely accepted in all of the medical sciences (such as "DNA" for deoxyribonucleic acid) to coinages by authors for particular articles; use of the second type should be discouraged for names not excessively long. The editor of a journal should compile a list of such abbreviations likely to be well known among its readers.

DNA	deoxyribonucleic acid
DHPG	9-(1,3-dihydroxy-2-propoxymethyl) guanine
EEDQ	N-ethoxycarbonyl-2-ethoxy-1,2-dihydroquinoline
NADH	reduced nicotinamide-adenine dinucleotide

Abbreviations for chemical names should, in general, not be used in titles (see section 2.2). Such abbreviations can be used in abstracts if, as in text, they are explained at first mention

CHEMICAL DIMENSIONS AND STRUCTURE

16.23 Chemical concentrations in solutions generally should be reported as moles per litre (mol/L or mol·L^{-1}), millimoles per litre (mmol/L or mmol·L^{-1}), or micromoles per litre (μmol/L or μmol·L^{-1}); the choice is determined by the magnitude of values to be reported for a particular measurement; see the table for clinical chemistry determinations in Appendix A. Values for measurements of osmotic pressure should, for clinical purposes, be reported in terms of the osmole as osmolality with the unit, mol/kg (kilogram of fluid measured), rather than as freezing point depression.

16.24 The term *molecular weight* should be replaced (20) by the term *relative molecular mass* (symbol, M_r), a dimensionless number representing the ratio of the mass of the element or compound measured to one-twelfth the mass of the pure nuclide carbon-12. The dalton (symbol, Da), a mass equal to one-twelfth of the mass of the pure nuclide carbon-12, is not recognized internationally as an appropriate unit for relative molecular mass ("molecular weight") but is conveniently used to express the mass of a very small biological entity with complex chemical composition such as a ribosome.

16.25 The names of some organic compounds begin with multiplying prefixes derived from Latin or Greek. The Latin prefixes run in the sequence di, tri, tetra, penta, and so on; the Greek prefixes are bis, tris, tetrakis, and so on. These prefixes are closed up with the stem word and are set in a roman (upright) typeface; names thus formed follow the conventional rules for capitalization at the beginning of sentences and in titles (see sections 7.1 and 7.2). The same rules apply to the 2 structural prefixes cyclo and iso.

dihydroxyaluminum aminoacetate
tris(hydroxymethyl)nitromethane
Tris(hydroxymethyl)nitromethane was the bactericide used . . .
cyclopropane   isopropyl alcohol   tetraethyl pyrophosphate

16.26   The names of many organic compounds begin with prefixed locants and descriptors that indicate structural characteristics. Locants and descriptors can be numerals, letters, or short prefix-terms; they are prefixed, and attached by a hyphen, to the stem name. Successive prefixes of this type and of like meaning are linked by commas unspaced; those of unlike meaning are hyphenated. Capitalization at the beginning of sentences and in titles is applied to the stem name, not the prefix. The letters of the stem name determine the position of the name in an alphabetically sequenced index. Numeric and small-capital prefixes must be in a roman (upright) typeface; other prefixes must be in an italic (slanted) typeface or in greek letters as appropriate for a particular convention.

N,N,N',N'-tetraethylphthalamide   2,2,3,3-tetrafluoro-1-propanol
trans-cisoid-trans-perhydrophenanthrene   D-1,2,4-butanetriol
trans-cisoid-trans-Perhydrophenanthrene was suspected of being . . .

See Table 16.6 for a summary of locants and descriptors and their typographic conventions.

Table 16.6:   Locants and descriptors in chemical names [fn1]

Typeface	Locant or descriptor	Example
Italic (slanted)	Chemical-element symbol locant	*N,N'*-dimethylurea
	Greek-letter locant	β-sitosterol
	Positional descriptor: *cis-, m-, o-, p-, sec-, tert-, trans-*	*cis*-dichloroethene *p*-bromoaniline *tert*-butyl bromide
	Stereoisomer descriptor: (*R*)-, (*S*)-, (*Z*)-, (*E*)-, *cis-, trans-, cisoid-, rel-, d-, l-, s-, meso-, sn-, endo-, exo-, syn-, sym-, anti-, amphi-, erythro-, threo-, altro-, ribo-, xylo-, vic-, gem-, M-, P-*	*d*-amphetamine 13-*cis*-retinoic acid *meso*-tartaric acid
Roman (upright)	Number locant	2-hexanone 5-iodo-2-thiouracil
	Small-capital letter locant	L-methionine

fn1:   This table is based in part on Table VIII in reference 16, which gives a much larger number of examples.

16.27   Optical rotation (not configuration) is indicated by a plus sign $(+)$ or minus sign $(-)$ within parenthesis marks and connected to the stem name by a hyphen.

$(-)$-tartaric acid $(+)$-glucose

ENZYMES

16.28   *Enzyme Nomenclature: 1984* (19) is the current authority in which to confirm the correctness of enzyme-classification code numbers (EC numbers), recommended enzyme names, and systematic enzyme names

Table 16.7:   Symbols for enzyme kinetics [fn1]

Symbol	Meaning
$[A]$	concentration of substrate A
$[A]_{0.5}$	value of $[A]$ at which $v = 0.5\ V$
$[B]$	concentration of substrate B
$[E]_0$	stoichiometric concentration of active centers
h (or n_H)	Hill coefficient
$[I]$	concentration of inhibitor I
k	rate constant of any order n
$\tilde{k}$	pH-independent value of k
k^{app}	apparent value of k
k_A, k_B	specificity constants for A, B
k_{cat}	catalytic constant
k_i, k_{-i}	forward and reverse rate constants, respectively, for ith step
K_i	inhibition constant (inhibition type unspecified)
K_{iA}	inhibition constant for A
K_{ic}	competitive inhibition constant
k_{ij}	rate constant for step from E_i to E_j
K_{iu}	uncompetitive inhibition constant
K_m	Michaelis constant (or Michaelis concentration)
K_{mA}	Michaelis constant for A
K_{sA}	value of K_s for substrate A
k_0	catalytic constant
$[Q]$	concentration of activator Q time
t	time
v	rate (or velocity) of reaction
V (or V_{max})	limiting rate (or maximum rate, or maximum velocity)
v_A	rate of consumption of A
v_{max}	true maximum value of v
v_0	initial rate of reaction
$[Y]$	concentration of product Y
$[Z]$	concentration of product Z
ε_a	degree of activation
ε_i	degree of inhibition
τ	relaxation time

fn1: Based on Table 1 in reference 21.

The proper use of names for an enzyme depends on the topic of the paper and the readership of the journal, but all journals should give the EC number at the first mention of an enzyme in the text (if a number has been assigned).

> ... and in our studies of inhibition of alcohol dehydrogenase (EC 1.1.1.1) by ...

16.29 A committee of the International Union of Biochemistry has recommended symbols and terms (21) for enzyme kinetics. The symbols are individual and combined roman (upright), italic (slanted) capital and lowercase, and lowercase greek letters in various combinations (see Table 16.7). These symbols are in accord with the international conventions for symbols of quantities and their modifiers (see sections 11.1 and 14.1). The symbols are characteristically combined in equations.

$$v = k_A [E]_0 [A]$$

POLYPEPTIDES AND POLYNUCLEOTIDES

16.30 The amino acid residues in polypeptides are represented (22) by 3-letter symbols (usually the first 3 letters [the first capitalized] of the common

Table 16.8: Symbols for amino acids

Common name	3-Letter symbol	1-Letter symbol [fn1]
alanine	Ala	A
arginine	Arg	R
asparagine	Asn	N
aspartic acid	Asp	D
cysteine	Cys	C
glutamine	Gln	Q
glutamic acid	Glu	E
glycine	Gly	G
histidine	His	H
isoleucine	Ile	I
leucine	Leu	L
lysine	Lys	K
methionine	Met	M
phenylalanine	Phe	F
proline	Pro	P
serine	Ser	S
threonine	Thr	T
tryptophan	Trp	W
tyrosine	Tyr	Y
valine	Val	V
unspecified amino acid	Xaa	X

fn1: The 1-letter symbols are to be used only for summary presentation of large amounts of data, comparisons of long sequences, and computer handling of data; see reference 20 for further details.

name of the amino acid). A known sequence is indicated by hyphens (representing peptide bonds) between the symbols; known residues in an unknown sequence are represented by a sequence within parenthesis marks with the amino acid symbols separated by commas.

Asp-His-Pro   (Asp,His,Pro)

For 3-letter symbols for amino acids, see Table 16.8

16.31   Sequences of nucleotides in polynucleotides and in codons are represented by strings of single capital-letter symbols standing for individual nucleotides and by other economical devices. A recently published recommendation deals with additional single-letter symbols to represent incompletely specified bases (see Table 16.9) (23); it also allows for discontinuance of the use of hyphens connecting nucleotide symbols to represent the -OPO$_2$H-O- group (phosphodiester linkage). The lowercase letter p can be used at the left end of a sequence to represent a terminal 5'-phosphate and at the right for a terminal 3'-phosphate.

pG-A-C-C-T-T-A-G-C-A-A-T-Gp   pGACCTTAGCAATp
or 5'-GACCTTAGCAAT-3'

For a concise summary of the earlier recommendations, see reference 17.

IMMUNOGLOBULINS

16.32   Classes of immunoglobulins are represented by the symbol for immunoglobulin, Ig, and a capital letter (unspaced) for the class.

Table 16.9: Symbols for specified or incompletely specified nucleotides in nucleic acid sequences

Symbol	Meaning	Origin of designation
G	G	Guanine
A	A	Adenine
T	T	Thymine
C	C	Cytosine
R	G or A	pu**R**ine
Y	T or C	p**Y**rimidine
M	A or C	a**M**ino
K	G or T	**K**eto
S	G or C	**S**trong interaction (3 H bonds)
W	A or T	**W**eak interaction (2 H bonds)
H	A or C or T	not-G, **H** follows G in the alphabet
B	G or T or C	not-A, **B** follows A
V	G or C or A	not-T (not-U), **V** follows U
D	G or A or T	not-C, **D** follows C
N	G or A or T or C	a**N**y

IgG IgA IgM IgD IgE

Subclasses are indicated by a number attached to the class symbol; potential subclasses are indicated by a parenthetic alphabetic code representing a city or initials of a patient.

IgG2 IgM3 IgE(Ph)

The two major groups of polypeptide chains in immunoglobulin molecules are the light (L) and heavy (H) chains. The heavy chains are designated by lowercase greek letters that correspond to the roman capital letter of the class, for example, μ ("mu") corresponding to the M of IgM: "μ-chain". The light chains are designated as κ (kappa) and λ (lambda). The 2 well-defined regions of the polypeptide chains are designated "the V region" (the variable region) and "the C region" (the constant region). The symbols "V_L" and "C_L" represent the variable and constant regions of the light chains, and "V_H" and "C_H" the variable and constant regions of heavy chains. Subdivisions within a variable region associated with a light chain of a given type are designated "subgroups" and are identified with roman numerals. With the established symbolic system, an immunoglobulin molecule can be represented as a formula.

$$[(V_{\kappa I}C_{\kappa})(V_{\gamma}C\gamma_{I})]_2$$ [an IgG1 molecule with κ light chains of subgroup I]

A clear summary of the characteristics of immunoglobulins and the conventions for their nomenclature and symbolization has been published by DS Rowe (24). Two subsequent memoranda on immunoglobulins have been published (25,26), the second extending the rules of immunoglobulins of animal [non-human] origin.

INTERFERONS

16.33 Interferons and their genes can be represented by symbols based on a standard nomenclature (27, 28). The three defined interferon types correspond to the type of inducer and the cell type producing the interferon: types α (alpha), β (beta), and γ (gamma). The alpha type is induced in leukocytes and lymphoblastoid lines, the beta type is induced in cells in solid tissues, the gamma type is induced in T cells; other greek letters may be assigned in the future to new species of interferon genes and their corresponding protein products. An interferon is represented by the symbol IFN to which is attached by a hyphen the lowercase greek letter representing its type; to the greek letter may be attached a subscripted or unsubscripted arabic number or a capital letter (with the greek letter unhyphenated) to indicate a non-allelic variant. The symbol IFN may be prefixed with a symbol to indicate the animal species from which the interferon has been derived, for example, "Hu" to represent "human",

"Mu" to represent "murine". The genes corresponding to the three main types of interferons are represented by corresponding symbols in an italic (slanted) typeface.

IFN-α   IFN-β   IFN-γ   HuIFN-α²   HuIFNαA
IFN-α   *IFN*-β

Natural and undefined interferons should be simply designated by the prefix for species of origin, the IFN symbol, and a parenthetic suffix indicating producing cell and inducer: for example, HuIFN(Namalwa/Sendai). This sytem is being modified by geneticists to bring it into accord with their conventions for gene symbols (see section 16.37).

THE RENIN-ANGIOTENSIN SYSTEM

16.34   Conventions for nomenclature and symbolization of the renin-angiotensin system have been established by the Nomenclature Committee of the International Society of Hypertension (29). The numbering

Table 16.10:   Nomenclature and symbols for the renin-angiotensin system [fn1]

Common name	Systematic name	Abbreviation
angiotensinogen	renin substrate	
- - - - - - - - - - -	renin substrate-(1–14)tetra-decapeptide	TDP renin substrate [fn2]
angiotensin I	angiotensin-(1–10)decapeptide	ANG I [fn3] ANG-(1–10)
ox ("beef") ANG	[Val⁵]angiotensin-(1–10) decapeptide	[Val⁵]ANG I [Val⁵]ANG-(1–10)
angiotensin II	angiotensin-(1–8)octapeptide	ANG II ANG-(1–8)
angiotensin III	angiotensin-(2–8)heptapeptide	ANG III ANG-(2–8)
saralasin	[Sar¹,Val⁵,Ala⁸]angiotensin-(1–8)octapeptide	[Sar¹,Val⁵,Ala⁸]ANG II [fn4] [Sar¹,Val⁵,Ala⁸]ANG-(1–8)
- - - - - - - - - - -	[Pro⁸ᵃ]angiotensin-(1–8)nona-peptide	[Pro⁸ᵃ]ANG II (extension at C-terminal with proline residue)
converting enzyme	(EC 3.4.15.1)	CE
renin-angiotensin system		RAS

fn1: This table has been adapted from the table in reference 29.
fn2: The amino-acid sequence and its numbering for TDP.

    1   2   3   4   5   6   7   8   9   10 11 12 13 14
    Asp-Arg-Val-Tyr-Ile-His-Pro-Phe-His-Leu-Leu-Val-Tyr-Ser

fn3: The amino-acid sequence and its numbering for ANG I.

    1   2   3   4   5   6   7   8   9   10
    Asp-Arg-Val-Tyr-Ile-His-Pro-Phe-His-Leu

fn4: Sar is the symbol for sarcosine (*N*-methylglycine).

of peptides follows that established for the 2 reference compounds, human renin substrate-(1–14) tetradecapeptide and human angiotensin-(1–10) decapeptide. The systematic names and the abbreviations for components are prefixed to indicate amino acid substitutions and their position; the amino acid sequence-numbering is suffixed to the systematic root name or abbreviation.

[Val^5]ANG-(1–8)   [Tyr^{4a}]ANG II

See Table 16.10 for common (trivial) and systematic names, abbreviations, and the peptide amino-acid sequences; the amino acid symbols are those in Table 16.8

ENDOCRINOLOGY

16.35 Abbreviations for polypeptide hormones are widely recognized in the medical sciences but they should be defined within parenthesis marks at their first mention in text and in an abstract; they should not be used in titles. Lowercase prefixes designate species. See Table 16.11 for abbreviations and prefixes.

Common names for some steroids may be used without being defined by the systematic nomenclature for steroids (see Table 16.12). Common names for other steroids are acceptable if defined by systematic nomenclature at first mention in text and accompanied by any necessary explanation of letter abbreviations.

A committee of the American Thyroid Association has recommended nomenclature, symbols, and abbreviations relevant to tests for thyroid hormones in serum (30); see Table 16.13 but note the departure in the table from some of the recommendations as explained in a footnote.

GENETICS

Nomenclature and symbolization for human genetics and genetic disorders now comprise a staggering number of symbols and terms. The two basic reference works for verification of symbols and terms are the successive catalogs issued by the meetings of the International Workshop on Human Gene Mapping (31) and the McKusick catalog of phenotypes (32) representing disorders determined in man by mechanisms of mendelian inheritance.

SYMBOLIZATION OF CHROMOSOMES

16.36 The well-established and comprehensive system for symbolizing normal and abnormal human chromosomes (33) uses linear assemblies of lower-

Table 16.11: Abbreviations and prefixes for polypeptide hormones [fn1]

Hormone	Abbreviation
ACTH-releasing hormone	CRH
adrenocorticotropin	ACTH
arginine vasopressin	AVP
calcitonin	CT
follicle-stimulating hormone	FSH
FSH- and LH-releasing hormone	GnRH
GH-inhibiting hormone (somatostatin)	SRIH
GH-releasing hormone	GHRH
growth hormone (somatotropin)	GH
bovine GH	bGH
human GH	hGH
ovine GH	oGH
porcine GH	pGH
rat GH	rGH
human chorionic gonadotropin	hCG
insulin-like growth factor I	IGF-I
insulin-like growth factor II	IGF-II
luteinizing hormone	LH
lysine vasopressin	LVP
melanocyte-stimulating hormone	MSH
oxytocin	OT
parathyroid hormone	PTH
proopiomelancortin	POMC
prolactin	PRL
somatomedin-C	Sm-C
thyroid-stimulating autoantibodies	TSab
thyrotropin	TSH
thyroxine	T4 [fn2]
3,5,3′-triiodothyronine	T3 [fn2]
3,3′,5′-triiodothyronine	rT3 [fn2]
TSH-releasing hormone	TRH

fn1: The species prefix for "human" (see example under "growth hormone") need not be used to designate a human hormone unless ambiguity might result from incomplete designation.

fn2: These abbreviations have often carried subscripted numbers rather than on-line numbers. The on-line style is to be preferred; it reserves subscripted numbers for their general use in chemical formulas (see section 16.21) and saves some work for typists and compositors.

Table 16.12: Common names for steroids that need not be defined in most journals by systematic nomenclature

aldosterone	cortisol	estriol
androsterone	cortisone	estrone
androstenedione	dehydroepiandrosterone	etiocholanolone
cholesterol	deoxycorticosterone	progesterone
corticosterone	17β-estradiol	testosterone

Table 16.13: Abbreviations relevant to tests for thyroid hormones in serum [fn1]

Test	Abbreviation
Iodine concentration	
Total iodine	TI
Protein-bound iodine	PBI
Iodide	I⁻
Extractable iodine	EI
Nonextractable iodine	NEI
Butanol-extractable iodine	BEI
Butanol-nonextractable iodine	BNEI
Thyroxine iodine (chromatographic)	T4I(C)
Hormone concentration	
Thyroxine (chromatographic)	T4(C)
Thyroxine (displacement)	T4(D)
Thyroxine (radioimmunoassay)	T4(RIA)
Triiodothyronine (displacement)	T3(D)
Triiodothyronine (radioimmunoassay)	T3(RIA)
Free thyroxine	FT4
Free triiodothyronine	FT3
Inverse of unoccupied thyroxine-binding sites	
Percent free thyroxine	%FT4
Percent free triiodothyronine	%FT3
Resin triiodothyronine uptake	RT3U
Resin thyroxine uptake	RT4U
Erythrocyte triiodothyronine uptake	ET3U
Indirect indicators of free hormone concentration	
Thyroxine-resin T_3 index	T4-RT3 index
Thyroxine-resin T_4 index	T4-RT4 index
Thyroxine-binding proteins	
Thyroxine-binding globulin capacity	TBG_{cap}
Thyroxine-binding prealbumin capacity	$TBPA_{cap}$
Thyroxine-binding globulin concentration	TBG
Thyroxine-binding prealbumin concentration	TBPA

fn1: See footnote 2 to Table 16.11 on placing modifying numbers on-line instead of sub-scripted.

case and capital letters, arabic and roman numerals, and specific punctuation and signs (all in a roman [upright] typeface); see Table 16.14 for these symbols. The sequence of symbols is specified: total number of chromosomes including the sex chromosomes, comma, the sex chromosome constitution, comma, chromosomal aberrations (with specified conventions for letters, numbers, signs, and punctuation).

46,XY,+18,−21   [46 chromosomes, XY sex chromosomes, an extra chromosome 18, a missing chromosome 21]

46,XY,t(Bp−;Dq+)   [a balanced reciprocal translocation between the short arm of a B- and the long arm of a D-group chromosome]

47,XY,+21,var(21)(p13,Q12),var(21=2)(p13,Q54)mat   [male with 47 chro-

Table 16.14: Symbols (including abbreviated terms) for representing human chromosomes and their aberrations

Symbol or abbreviation	Meaning
→ (arrow)	from-to
* (asterisk)	multiplication sign
: (colon)	break (in detailed descriptions)
:: (double colon)	break and re-union (in detailed descriptions)
= (equal sign)	sum of
− (minus sign)	loss of
( ) (parenthesis marks)	surround structurally altered chromosome
+ (plus sign)	gain of
? (question mark)	questionable identification of chromosome or chromosome structure
; (semicolon)	separates chromosomes and chromosome regions in structural rearrangements involving more than one chromosome
/ (slant line)	separates cell lines in describing mosaics or chimeras
= (double underline)	distinguishes homologous chromosomes
AI	first meiotic anaphase
AII	second meiotic anaphase
ace	acentric fragment
b	break
cen	centromere
chi	chimera
cs	chromosome
ct	chromatid
cx	complex
del	deletion
der	derivative chromosome
dia	diakinesis
dic	dicentric
dip	diplotene
dir	direct
dis	distal
dit	dictyate
dmin	double minute
dup	duplication
e	exchange
end	endoreduplication
f	fragment
fem	female
g	gap
h	secondary constriction
i	isochromosome
ins	insertion
inv	inversion
lep	leptotene
MI	first meiotic metaphase
MII	second meiotic metaphase
mal	male
mar	marker chromosome

Table 16.14: (*continued*)

Symbol or abbreviation	Meaning
mat	maternal origin
med	median
min	minute
mn	modal number
mos	mosaic
oom	oogonial metaphase
p	short arm of chromosome
PI	first meiotic prophase
pac	pachytene
pat	paternal origin
pcc	premature chromosome condensation
Ph[1]	Philadelphia chromosome [fn1]
prx	proximal
psu	pseudo
pvz	pulverization
q	long arm of chromosome
qr	quadriradial
r	ring chromosome
rcp	reciprocal
rea	rearrangement
rec	recombinant chromosome
rob	robertsonian translocation
s	satellite
sce	sister chromatid exchange
sdl	side-line, sub-line
sl	stem line
spm	spermatogonial metaphase
t	translocation
tan	tandem translocation
ter	terminal (end of chromosome)
tr	triradial
tri	tricentric
var	variable chromosome region
xma	chiasma, chiasmata
zyg	zygotene

fn1: The symbol Ph[1] is in the recommendation; a recent recommendation (34) calls for omitting the superscript number 1, Ph by itself to be the form.

mosomes and trisomy 21; one chromosome 21 has very small satellites of pale intensity after Q-banding; the two remaining chromosomes 21 are identical, with very large and intensely fluorescent satellites, and both are of maternal origin]

The system includes conventions for human meiotic chromosomes.

SYMBOLIZATION OF GENES

16.37 Comprehensive conventions for human gene nomenclature and symbolization were established in 1979 (35).

Gene loci are designated by symbolic groups of 3 to 5 (occasionally 6) capital letters (and in some groups arabic numerals) set in an italic (slanted) typeface (underlined in typescript); lowercase letters are still allowed in blood-group symbols. Hyphens, greek letters, and roman numerals are not allowed; hyphens are allowed in *HLA* designations.

> *BR   CFAG   HLA-DR1A   PPY   RAF1   TUBBP1*

Allele characters are separated from the initial gene symbol by an asterisk without spacing. The allele character is also in an italic (slanted) typeface. Genotype symbols follow the same conventions and are separated by a slant line. Various linkage relationships are variously indicated by semicolons, spaces, and dashes separating allele pairs.

> *ADA*1   ADA*2   HBB*6V   AMY1*A/AMY1*B*
> *ENO1*1/ENO1*2; PGM2*1/PGM2*2*

Phenotype symbols follow the same conventions but must be in a roman (upright) typeface; a space rather than an asterisk separates gene and allele characters.

> *ADA*1/ADA*1* [genotype]   ADA 1 [phenotype]

The recommendations for symbols for genes coding for enzymes, other proteins, hemoglobins, cell surface markers, and inherited clinical syndromes follow the same conventions.

> *G6PD*A/G6PD*B* [genotype]   G6PD AB [phenotype]
> Cystic fibrosis: *CF* [gene symbol]   *R* [allele symbol]
>   *CF*N/CF*R* [heterozygote genotype]

Reference 31 is the authoritative source in which to confirm gene symbols; note, however, that it applies (with underlining) the convention of italic (slanted) characters for gene symbols in most of its text but not in its tables.

Conventions for oncogenes have developed along somewhat different lines, being prefixed with upright (roman) letters, but they are being converted among geneticists to the conventions described above (31,35). The prefixes capital letter N, lowercase letter c, and lowercase letter v refer, respectively, to "nuclear", "cellular", and "viral".

> N-*myc*   *NMYC*   *Raf-1   Raf1*   v-*ros*

Similar changes are being applied to symbols for interferon genes; also see section 16.33

> *IFN*-α   *IFNA*

A valuable reference source in which to verify oncogene symbols is the catalog issued by the American Type Culture Collection (36), *Catalogue of Recombinant DNA Collections.*

CELL LINES

16.38   A cell line representing a human genetic mutation may have to be specified by a number assigned by the cell repository (37) maintaining the line, for example, GM1234Z, in which GM is the code for the repository, 1234 is the assigned number, and Z indicates that the cell is stored frozen.

CLINICAL GENETIC SYNDROMES

16.39   If an established descriptive and noneponymic term for a disease, disorder, or other kind of clinical genetic syndrome is available and is in good standing in an authoritative catalog (32), use it in preference to an eponymic term. Eponymic terms that must be used should be in the nonpossessive form (see section 10.10). Syndrome names in the nonpossessive form are idiomatically preceded by "the".

> metatropic dwarfism, type II   *not*   Kniest disease
> Krabbe disease   *not*   Krabbe's disease
> . . . described a new case of Krabbe disease in a girl.
> . . . described a new case of the Keutel syndrome with onset. . .

HUMAN PEDIGREES

16.40   Successive generations in a pedigree should be designated (38) by roman numbers beginning with I for the oldest generation. Members of a generation should be numbered with arabic numbers beginning with 1 for the most senior (at the leftmost end in a linear pedigree diagram) and proceeding to the right. Individual members are then designated by combined generation roman number and individual arabic number.

> The 5th child in a sibship that is the 3rd generation in the pedigree: III5

Individuals can be identified unambiguously by the initial letters of their names coupled to numerals representing date of birth: "EJH19230515".

HEMATOLOGY

HEMOGLOBIN

16.41   The term *hemoglobin* can be represented by the symbol Hb. The various normal and abnormal human hemoglobins are identified by the capital letters A, C through Q, and S, the major and minor human adult hemoglobins being designated A and A_2.

> Hb A   hemoglobin A_2 hemoglobin F ["fetal"]   Hb S

Subsequently identified hemoglobins have been named for the laboratory, hospital, or locality in which they were found.

> Hb Hammersmith   Hb Torino   Hb Presbyterian

Some authors have subscripted these modifying names, but this practice is proscribed by the generally accepted recommendations (39,40) on nomenclature of hemoglobins.

The 4 polypeptide chains of the normal human hemoglobin (Hb, A, Hb_2, Hb F) are designated by the greek letters α (alpha), β (beta), γ (gamma), and δ (delta). The paired chains are designated by formulas of the chemical type.

$$\alpha_2\beta_2 \text{ [Hb A]} \qquad \alpha_2\delta_2 \text{ [Hb A}_2]$$

Hemoglobin F has mixed gamma chains which may be designated with following superscripts for the identifying amino acid and its position in the chain or by a preceding single-letter superscript standing for the amino acid.

$$\alpha_2\gamma_2^{136Gly} \ (^G\gamma) \qquad \alpha_2\gamma_2^{136Ala} \ (^A\gamma)$$

Two embryonic chains are designated by ε (epsilon) and ζ (zeta).

$$\alpha_2\varepsilon_2 \text{ [Hb Gower 2]}$$

Notations for an amino acid substitution in an abnormal hemoglobin indicate, in order, the chain and the numbered position in it, the helix position within parenthesis marks (letters NA, A, B, C, CE, E, EF, F, FG, G, GH, H, HC with attached arabic numbers), the amino acid replaced, a right-pointing arrow, and the amino acid substituted.

$$\alpha86(F7)Leu \rightarrow Arg \text{ [Hb Moabit]}$$

Such notation can be used as an entire superscript to a chain designation in a chain formula

$$a_2\beta_2^{(86Lys \rightarrow Asn,Asp)} \text{ [Hb Providence]}$$

16.42 The thalassemias are notated with the greek letters for the globin chains preceding "thalassemia" to indicate which chain (or chains) is characteristically synthesized at a lower than normal rate. Lehman and Carrell (41) have proposed a symbolization for the α-thalassemias that reflects which of the 4 potentially responsible genes are in fact responsible for the particular thalassemia.

1α-thalassemia $\quad -\alpha/\alpha\alpha \qquad 4\alpha$-thalassemia $\quad - -/- -$
2α-thalassemia $\quad -\alpha/-\alpha$ (trans) *or* $- -/\alpha\alpha$ (cis)

BLOOD GROUPS

16.43 The human blood groups have been designated by largely non-systematic alphabetic and numeric symbols (capital and lowercase letters on the line and superscripted, numeric subscripts) and names.

A   AB   A$_s$ D^u Levay   Le^b hr^H A$_{hel}$

Phenotypes have been represented with roman (upright) letters and genotypes with italic (slanted) letters.

A$_2$B   *A$_2$B*   MNs   *Ms/Ns*

Efforts are being made to systematize symbolization for blood groups (42,43) but until a new system is clearly established, editors unfamiliar with customary and recently proposed symbols may have to consult current textbooks in hematology for verification of styles for symbols.

COAGULATION FACTORS

16.44   Coagulation factors are designated by the term "factor" and a roman number (44–46). The activated form of a factor is indicated by adding "a" to the roman numeral. The designations for factor VIII and von Willebrand factor can be further modified (47) with a colon and an alphabetic symbol: "C" for coagulant activity, "Ag" for antigenic activities. "VWF" designates *von Willebrand factor*.

factor II   factor VIIa   VIII:Ag   VIII:C   VWF:Ag

The factors also have widely used names, and factor abnormalities are associated with a number of disorders (see Table 16.15).

A system for a genetic nomenclature for human blood coagulation (48) recommends use of the factor designations with roman (upright) characters for symbolized phenotypes and italic (slanted) characters for inferred genotypes.

F.XIIaa$^+$ [symbolized phenotype]   *XIIaa$^+$/aa$^+$*

HEMATOLOGIC UNITS OF MEASUREMENTS

16.45   Most hematologic measurements should be reported in SI units. The volume of reference for cell counts is the litre (L) rather than the decilitre ("100 ml"). The unit for the erythrocyte sedimentation rate remains the mm/h. The American National Metric Council recommends that for the near future hemoglobin be reported in the United States in the mass-concentration unit, g/L, rather than in the substance-concentration unit, mmol/L; for a discussion of this question and for a table of SI units in hematology with conversion factors and significant digits, see Table A.8 in Appendix A.

HEMATOLOGIC MALIGNANT DISEASES

For nomenclature of hematologic malignant diseases, see sections 16.54 and 16.55.

Table 16.15: Coagulation factors, synonyms, and associated disorders

Factor	Synonym	Associated disorder
factor I	fibrinogen	afibrinogenemia hypofibrinogenemia dysfibrinogenemia
factor II	prothrombin	hypoprothrombinemia
factor III	thromboplastin	
factor IV	calcium	
factor V	proacclerin labile factor accelerator globulin (AcG)	parahemophilia, Owren disease
factor VI	accelerin	
factor VII	proconvertin serum prothrombin conversion accelerator (SPCA) stable factor autoprothrombin I	hypoproconvertinemia
factor VIII	antihemophilic factor (AHF) antihemophilic globulin (AHG) thromboplastinogen platelet cofactor I plasma thromboplastic factor A antihemophilic factor A	hemophilia A and von Willebrand disease
factor IX	plasma thromboplastin compo- nent (PTC) Christmas factor platelet cofactor II autoprothrombin II plasma thromboplastic factor B antihemophilic factor B	hemophilia B, Christmas disease
factor X	Stuart-Prower factor Stuart factor	Stuart deficiency, heredi- tary factor X deficiency
factor XI	plasma thromboplastin antece- dent (PTA)	plasma thromboplastin antecedent deficiency, Rosenthal syndrome
factor XII	Hageman factor	(Hageman trait)
factor XIII	fibrin-stabilizing factor (FSF)	factor XIII deficiency
Fletcher factor	prekallikrein	Fletcher factor deficiency
Fitzgerald		Fitzgerald factor deficiency
Passovoy factor		Passovoy factor deficiency

IMMUNOLOGY

For nomenclature and symbolization of immunoglobulins, see section 16.32.

THE COMPLEMENT SYSTEMS

16.46 Complement components in the classical complement system are designated (49) by the capital letter C and an attached arabic number from 1 to 9. Note that the sequence representing the reaction sequence is not in numeric order, a concession to prior usage. The subcomponents of C1 are designated by suffixed lowercase letters q, r, and s.

C1 (C1q C1r C1s)   C4   C2   C3   C5   C6   C7   C8   C9

Intermediate complexes are designated with prefixed capital letters, E for *erythrocyte* and A for *antibody*, attached to the C for *complement* followed by the arabic numbers for the components that have interacted. Where component activity is lost from a complex, the corresponding numbers are omitted.

EAC1423   [the complex produced by interaction of the 1st four components of complement]

EA43   [loss of C1 and C2 activity from EAC1423]

A bar over component numbers indicates acquired enzymatic or other biologic activity. The bar replaces the previously used lowercase letter a that had designated acquired activity.

$C\overline{42}$ *for*   C(42)a

16.47 For the alternative activating pathway of complement (50) the 5 proteins are symbolized by the capital letters B, D, P, H, and I; C3 retains its symbolization in the classical system (49). The lesser protein fragment produced during a reaction is symbolized by the lowercase letter a, the larger fragment by the lowercase letter b. Complexes between proteins are symbolized by linking the symbols for the 2 proteins with an unspaced comma. Loss by a protein of a defined activity is indicated by the lowercase letter i.

C3   B   Ba   Bb   C3b,Bb   Bbi

HISTOCOMPATIBILITY LEUKOCYTE ANTIGENS

16.48 Symbolization for the histocompatibility complex (histocompatibility leukocyte antigens) uses a notation (51–54) with capital letters, lowercase letter w, and arabic numbers.

HLA designates the region or system
Capital letters A, B, C, and so on designate the locus
Lowercase letter w designates provisional assignment of specificity
Numbers 1, 2, 3, and so on indicate specificity of each locus

To the original designation of locus D (51) have been added the specificities DP, DQ, and DR. Broad specificities may be indicated within parenthesis marks after a narrow specificity.

HLA-A1   HLA-Aw24(9)   HLA-Bw21   HLA-Bw56(w22)   HLA-DRw10

Genetic symbols for loci, alleles, and genotypes should follow the conventions established in human genetics (see section 16.37) and be printed in an italic (slanted) typeface (underlined in typescripts).

CELL-TYPE ABBREVIATIONS

16.49   Various alphabetic and alphanumeric designations are applied to lymphocytes and antibodies used to detect them. These should be in a roman (upright) typeface. The designations by capital letters T (for *thymic*) and B (for *bursal*) should not be attached to the cell term by a hyphen unless the letter and term are used together as an adjective (see section 9.16).

T lymphocyte   T-cell leukemia   OKT3   HNK-1

MYCOLOGY

16.50   Taxonomic names of yeasts and other fungi of importance in clinical medicine and the medical sciences are styled, in general, by the same conventions that apply to bacteriologic names (see sections 10.5 and 16.3). Genus names and species names (binomens) must be in italic (slanted) typeface when they are in text set in a roman (upright) typeface; when these names must appear in text set in an italic (slanted) typeface, as in a book title mentioned in text, they are set in a roman (upright) typeface. The species epithet (second component in a species name) is never capitalized and must not be used by itself.

Candida   *Candida albicans*   *Rhizopus nigricans*
. . . in the classic monograph A Study of Candida *in South America*, he . . .

Authoritative sources for the names of yeasts and other medically important fungi are the standard medical dictionaries (4–7) and the American Type Culture Collection catalog of fungi (55).

16.51   The names of the diseases caused by infection with fungi are formed, in general, by adding the suffixes -osis or -iasis to a stem drawn from the genus name of the causative fungus. An exception is the term *mycetoma* applied to chronic infection with, or a non-neoplastic tumor caused by, a mycelial fungus. "Candidiasis" and "candidosis" are alternatively acceptable terms for candidal infection (56).

ONCOLOGY

ONCOLOGIC NOMENCLATURE

16.52 Most terms for benign and malignant tumors can be verified in one of the standard medical dictionaries (4–7). In general, histologically descriptive terms should be preferred to eponymic terms (see section 10.9). The 2 main authoritative sources for classification and nomenclature of tumors by their histologic characteristics are the fascicles of *Atlas of Tumor Pathology* published by the Armed Forces Institute of Pathology (57) and publications (58,59) of the World Health Organization (*International Histological Classification of Tumors* and *ICD-O: International Classification of Diseases for Oncology*).

TUMOR STAGING

16.53 Accurate case-record keeping in oncology needs precise description of the characteristics of the patient's disease; accurate comparison of cases and reliable deductions from case series call for uniformity in criteria for case description. A system widely used in the United States for some cancers is the TNM system of the American Joint Committee on Cancer (AJCC) (60); T stands for *tumor*, N for *nodes*, M for *metastasis*. An alphanumeric set of codes (see Table 16.16) determine the capital-letter and numeric symbols to be used to describe a particular case; the TMN

Table 16.16: Symbols in the TMN system for classification and staging of cancer [fn1]

Symbol	Meaning
	CHRONOLOGY OF CLASSIFICATION
c	Clinical-diagnostic
p	Postsurgical treatment-pathologic
s	Surgical-evaluative
r	Retreatment
a	Autopsy
	TUMOR
TX	Primary tumor cannot be assessed
T0	No evidence of primary tumor
Tis	Carcinoma *in situ*
T1, T2, T3, T4	Tumor size or involvement

Table 16.16: (*continued*)

Symbol	Meaning
	METASTASIS
MX	Presence of distant metastasis cannot be assessed
M0	No evidence of distant metastasis
M1	Distant metastasis present (sites of metastasis: BRA, brain; EYE, eye; HEP, hepatic; LYM, lymph nodes; MAR, bone marrow; OSS, osseous; OTH, other; PLE, pleural; PUL, pulmonary; SKI, skin)
	HISTOPATHOLOGY: GRADE
GX	Grade cannot be assessed
G1	Well differentiated
G2	Moderately well differentiated
G3, G4	Poorly to very poorly differentiated
	HISTOPATHOLOGY: LYMPHATIC INVASION
LX	Lymphatic invasion cannot be assessed
L0	No evidence of lymphatic invasion
L1	Invasion of superficial lymphatics
L2	Invasion of deep lymphatics
	HISTOPATHOLOGY: VENOUS INVASION
VX	Venous invasion cannot be assessed
V0	Veins do not contain tumor
V1	Efferent veins contain tumor
V2	Distant veins contain tumor
	RESIDUAL TUMOR
R0	No residual tumor
R1	Microscopic residual tumor
R2	Macroscopic residual tumor
	HOST PERFORMANCE SCALE [fn2]
H0	Normal activity
H1	Symptomatic; ambulatory; cares for self
H2	Ambulatory more than 50% of time; occasionally needs help
H3	Ambulatory less than 50% of time; needs nursing care
H4	Bedridden; may need hospitalization

fn1: Adapted from pages 6–8 in reference 60; TNM stands for "*t*umor", "*n*ode", and "*m*etastasis".

fn2: Other scales of physical state and performance summarized in reference 60 are the Karnofsky Scale: Criteria of Performance Status (PS), which uses 11 categories (0, 10, 20, and so on to 100), and the Eastern Cooperative Oncology Group Scale (ECOG), which has grades 0–4.

symbols may be preceded by a lowercase letter that indicates the chronology of the classification.

cT2,N0,M1LYM   aT3,N2,M1BRA

Such classifications may appear in descriptions of individual cases and in specifications for stages of cancer (see section 16.54).

16.54   In addition to the case-characterization for cancer by the criteria and symbols in the TMN system, there are notations for the staging of cases of some specific diseases that use other symbolic systems. In general the stage of a case is specified by a roman number to which may be added alphabetic modifiers; see Table 16.17 for stage notation for Hodgkin disease.

stage IVB [for uterine cancer with spread to distant organs]
stage I_E [for Hodgkin disease; single extralymphatic site involved]

Note that "stage" is not capitalized in running text.

. . . treated the 16 patients in stage $III_{E+S}B$ with . . .

Special additional notations to be used within the TMN system have been developed for specific malignancies such as the notation developed

Table 16.17:   Staging symbols for Hodgkin disease [fn1]

Stage category	Symbol
DISEASE EXTENT	
Single lymph-node region	I
A single extralymphatic organ or site	I_E
Two or more lymph node regions on the same side of the diaphragm	II
An extralymphatic organ or site and of one or more lymph node regions on the same side of the diaphragm	II_E
Lymph node regions on both sides of the diaphragm	III
Stage III with an extralymphatic organ or site	III_E
Stage III and the spleen	III_S
Stage III with E and S	III_{E+S}
SYSTEMIC SYMPTOMS	
No systemic symptoms (such as weight loss, fever, night sweats, pruritus)	A
Systemic symptoms	B

fn1: Various staging classifications have been in use, with somewhat differing criteria, but the symbols illustrated here are representative of those used in the several systems; the same, or similar, stagings have also been applied to non-Hodgkin lymphomas.

by the American Thoracic Society (61) to designate regional nodal stations in staging primary lung cancer.

SPECIAL ONCOLOGIC CLASSIFICATIONS

16.55 Some hematologic malignant diseases have been classified into subcategories specified by cellular criteria based on electron microscopy and immunologic methods (62); the categories are symbolized for shorthand representation in text. Examples are the FAB (French-American-British Cooperative Group) classifications of acute leukemias (63–65) symbolized by an alphanumeric notation, for example, L3 for a specific type of lymphoblastic leukemia.

A convention (66) has been developed for designating antibodies used in immunologic characterization of hematologic malignancies by cluster differentiation (in cell culture). The designation takes the form CD#[cell designation, designation of protein or glycoprotein or glycolipid or carbohydrate or unknown type and relative molecular mass] "designation of particular monoclonal antibody"; # is the arbitrary number officially specified for the cluster; *cell designation* is the symbolic notation for the most typical cell lineage or cell type from which the relative molecular mass ("molecular weight") was established; the chemical designation is p for *protein*, gp for *glycoprotein*, gl for *glycolipid*, CHO for *carbohydrate*, u for *unknown*; relative molecular mass ("molecular weight") is expressed in kilodaltons; *designation of particular monoclonal antibody* is the author's own notation.

CD10[nT-nB,p100]"J5"

CANCER CHEMOTHERAPY: ABBREVIATIONS

16.56 Some cancer chemotherapies are multidrug regimens and cannot be designated by a simple or short compound term. These regimens may be reasonably designated in text by an abbreviation derived in some way from the drug names; the abbreviation must be explained at its first mention in the text and abstract. Such abbreviations can be used in titles (although the general rule for titles excludes abbreviations and full drug names should be used when possible; see section 2.2); the title should make clear that the abbreviation refers to a chemotherapeutic program.

NOT MACOP-B for the Treatment of . . .
BUT MACOP-B Chemotherapy for the Treatment of . . .
[*m*ethotrexate with leucovorin rescue, doxorubicin ("*A*driamycin"), *c*yclophosphamide, vincristine ("*O*ncovin"), *p*rednisone, *b*leomycin]

ONCOGENE SYMBOLIZATION

For the system of symbolization for oncogenes, see section 16.37.

PARASITOLOGY AND MEDICAL ENTOMOLOGY

16.57   The scientific (taxonomic) names of protozoa, worms, and insects are capitalized at the taxonomic levels of genus and above. In species names (binomens; see section 10.5), the genus name is capitalized but the species epithet is not, even in titles. Genus and species names (and names of lower taxa) must be in an italic (slanted) typeface; if they must appear within text or a title set in an italic (slanted) typeface, they can be set in a roman (upright) typeface. Names of taxa above genus must be in a roman (upright) typeface. In running text the genus name of a binomen may be abbreviated (capital letter) after its first mention but only if confusion as to genus names will not result.

> *Amnicola*   [a genus of freshwater snails]
> Nematoda   [a phylum of worms]
> Muscidae   [a family of flies]
> *Solenopsis*   [a genus of ants]
>
> . . . and anaphylaxis due to stings by *Solenopsis* species, including *S richteri*, *S geminata*, and *S invicta* has been . . .
>
> . . . infested with larvae of *Musca domestica vicina* in two wounds of the . . . [reference to a subspecies of *Musca domestica*]
>
> . . . wrote his classic monograph, *The Ecology of* Musca domestica *in Brazil*, while he was ill with . . .

Many organisms of importance in parasitology and other fields of clinical medicine have common names. These names and the names of diseases derived from them are acceptable for nontaxonomic use.

> . . . saw many amebas in the stool preparation. [reference to individual organisms of an unspecified species in one of the genera of the order Amoebida]
>
> . . . the differential diagnosis of diarrheas includes amebiasis.

The taxonomic names of protozoa can be verified in *Catalogue of Protists—Algae and Protozoa* (67). Names for zoologic taxonomic ranks down to the rank Family can be verified in *Synopsis and Classification of Living Organisms* (68).

PHARMACOLOGY

For drug names, see section 10.3. Chemical names should be in the styles recommended in sections 16.21 and 16.25 to 16.28 for chemistry and biochemistry.

16.58   Style for pharmacokinetic symbols and equations has been recommended by the Committee for Pharmacokinetic Nomenclature of the American College of Clinical Pharmacology in their *Manual of Symbols, Equations & Definitions* (69). The symbols are various combinations of capital, lowercase, and greek letters. Subscripted variables are specific qualifiers for sites of measurement, organs and elimination routes, and routes of administration; superscripts are for other kinds of qualifiers such as *steady-state*. For examples of the main variables (quantities) and their modifiers, see Table 16.18.

Note that the single-letter symbols for quantities are presented in Table 16.18 in an italic (slanted) typeface to bring their style into accord

Table 16.18: Representative symbols and modifiers for pharmacokinetics [fn1]

Symbol	Term symbolized
A	Amount of drug in the body at any time t
A^{ss}	Amount of drug in the body at steady-state
(AUC)	Area under concentration-time curve during any dosing interval (τ)
C	Drug concentration in plasma at any time t
C_{ur}	Drug concentration in urine at any time t
C	Maximum (peak) steady-state dose concentration in plasma during dosing interval
$(CL)_{CR}$	Creatinine clearance
K_m	Michaelis-Menten constant
τ	Dosing interval (time)
V_{ur}	Urine volume excreted

Symbol modifiers

Sites of measurement		Organs and elimination routes		Routes of administration	
p	plasma	H	hepatic	iv	intravenous
b	blood	R	renal	po	peroral
u	unbound species	NR	nonrenal	sc	subcutaneous
sal	saliva	e	excreted into	im	intramuscular
ur	urine		urine	sl	sublingual
t	tissue	m	metabolized	pr	rectal
				ip	intraperitoneal
				top	topical
				oral	oral

fn1: These representative symbols and the modifiers are derived from *Manual of Symbols, Equations & Definitions in Pharmacokinetics* (69) prepared by the Committee for Pharmacokinetic Nomenclature of the American College of Clinical Pharmacology. The style here differs slightly from that in the recommendations of the manual to bring the symbols into accord with the recommendations of the International Union for Biochemistry; see section 16.29. The main symbols (for quantities) are in an italic (slanted) typeface if they are single-letter symbols and in a roman (upright) typeface and enclosed by parenthesis marks if they are multiletter symbols; modifiers are in a roman (upright) typeface or a greek letter.

with international usage for symbolization of quantities (see sections 11.1, 14.1, and 14.2) and the style specified by the International Union of Biochemistry for enzyme kinetics (see section 16.29 and Table 16.7); double-letter and triple-letter symbols have been kept in roman (upright) type and enclosed by parenthesis marks as recommended in section 16.17 to distinguish them from single-letter italicized symbols. Subscript and superscript modifiers are in a roman (upright) typeface.

Drug doses and drug concentrations are still most widely stated in mass units, but shifts are likely to be made in the not-too-distant future to molar units (70; also see Appendix A).

PSYCHIATRY

16.59 Articles on psychiatric and psychologic topics may specify psychiatric diagnoses with classification numbers from the system described in *Diagnostic and Statistical Manual of Mental Disorders* (71), widely known as "DSM-III".

> 292.11 cannabis delusional disorder
>
> . . . met the criteria for antisocial personality disorder (DSM-III 301.70) in both examinations while hospitalized.

Another widely used numeric classification of psychiatric disorders is that in *The International Classification of Diseases, 9th Revision, Clinical Modification* (ICD-9-CM) (72), which is also used for diagnoses in relation to payments for services.

A useful reference for definitions, street names of abused drugs and chemicals, and abbreviations is *Psychiatric Glossary* (73).

PULMONARY MEDICINE

SYMBOLS FOR QUANTITIES

16.60 Symbols for quantities measured in respiratory physiology and pulmonary medicine and the units in which they are expressed have differed in the United States and other parts of the world, particularly Europe. The general rules stated below and the symbols presented in Table 16.19 represent an attempt to bring usages into convergence, if not an immediate unity, and to simplify for authors and typists the preparing of typescripts. These recommendations are derived from related recommendations in three authoritative sources (74–76) and internationally accepted principles for symbolization (see sections 8.4, 11.1, 14.1, 14.2, 16.17, and 16.29).

Single-letter symbols (preferred) for quantities should be in an italic (slanted) typeface; see the general rules in section 8.4. Such symbols are marked in a typescript for an italic typeface by single-underlining.

Table 16.19: Symbols for measurements in respiratory physiology and pulmonary medicine

Symbol	Definition	Symbol	Definition
	RESPIRATORY MECHANICS: MAIN SYMBOLS		
C	compliance, concentration	t	time
E	elastance	$\dot{V}$	volume
f	frequency	$\dot{V}$	flow of gas
G	conductance	$\ddot{V}$	acceleration of volume
I	inertance	W	work
P	pressure	$\dot{W}$	power
R	resistance	Z	impedance
sG	specific conductance		
	RESPIRATORY MECHANICS: MODIFIERS		
A	alveolar	ia	intercostal or accessory muscles
ab	abdomen		
am	ambient	L	transpulmonary, lung, pulmonary
ao	airway opening		
aw	airway	lam	laminar
B	barometric	m	mouth
bs	body surface	max	maximum
ca	convective acceleration	mus	muscle
di	diaphragm	pl	pleural
ds	downstream	rc	rib cage
dyn	dynamic	rel	relaxed, relaxation
E	expiratory	rs	respiratory system
el	elastic	st	static
es	esophageal	T	tidal
fr	frictional or flow resistive	ti	tissue
		tm	transmural
ga	gastric	tur	turbulence
I	inspiratory	us	upstream
		w	chest wall
	RESPIRATORY MECHANICS: SUBDIVISIONS OF LUNG VOLUME		
(CC)	closing capacity	(IRV)	inspiratory reserve volume
(CV)	closing volume	(RV)	residual volume
(ERV)	expiratory reserve volume	(TLC)	total lung capacity
(FRC)	functional residual capacity	(VC)	vital capacity
(IC)	inspiratory capacity	V_T	tidal volume
	RESPIRATORY MECHANICS: MEASUREMENTS ON FORCED RESPIRATORY MANEUVERS		
(EPP)	equal pressure points	$(FET)_x$	time required to expire forcibly percent of (VC), x from (TLC)
$(FEF)_{x-y}$	mean forced expiratory flow between 2 designated volume points in $(FVC) = (V_x - V_y)/t$	$(FEV)_t$	forced expiratory volume in time interval t

Table 16.19: *(continued)*

Symbol	Definition	Symbol	Definition
(FVC)	forced vital capacity		ventilation
(IVPF)	isovolume pressure-flow	(PEF)	peak expiratory flow
(MEFV)	maximum expiratory flow-volume [curve]	(PEFV)	partial expiratory flow-volume [curve]
(MFSR)	maximum flow static recoil [curve]	$\dot{V}max_{xx}$	maximum expiratory flow at xx% of (VC)
(MIFV)	maximum inspiratory flow-volume [curve]	$\dot{V}max_{xx,(TLC)}$	
(MVV)	maximum voluntary		maximum expiratory flow at xx% of (TLC)

RESPIRATORY MECHANICS: EXAMPLES OF COMBINATIONS

C_L	lung compliance	$sGaw$	specific airway conductance
$Cst,_L$	static lung compliance	Wdi	diaphragmatic power
P_A	alveolar pressure	$W_{I,el,L}$	elastic work performed on the lung during inspiration
Pao	pressure at airway opening		
$P_{E,m,max_{xx,(TLC)}}$	maximum expiratory mouth pressure at xx% of (TLC)		

ALVEOLAR GAS EXCHANGE AND PULMONARY CIRCULATION: MAIN SYMBOLS

C	concentration (in a liquid)	Q	volume of liquid
(Cap)	capacity	$\dot{Q}$	flow of blood, perfusion
D	diffusing capacity	R	gas-exchange ratio
f	respiratory frequency	S	saturation
F	fraction	V	volume of gas
G	conductance	β	slope of dissociation curve
P	pressure, total or partial	θ	reaction rate

ALVEOLAR GAS EXCHANGE AND PULMONARY CIRCULATION: MODIFIERS

a	arterial	pc	pulmonary capillary
A	alveolar	pc′	pulmonary end capillary
B	barometric	pv	pulmonary venous
c	capillary	pw	pulmonary wedge
DS	dead space	s	shunt
e	effective	t	time
E	expired	T	total
I	inspired	ti	tissue
la	left atrial	v	venous
m	membrane	$\bar{v}$	mixed venous
p	plasma	va	venous admixture
pa	pulmonary arterial	0	zero initial value

ALVEOLAR GAS EXCHANGE AND PULMONARY CIRCULATION: SPECIAL GAS-PHASE SYMBOLS

ATPD	ambient temperature and pressure, dry	ATPS	ambient temperature and pressure, saturated

Table 16.19: (*continued*)

Symbol	Definition	Symbol	Definition
BTPS	body temperature, ambient pressure, saturated with water vapor	STPD	standard temperature and pressure, dry

ALVEOLAR GAS EXCHANGE AND PULMONARY CIRCULATION: EXAMPLES OF COMBINATIONS

Symbol	Definition	Symbol	Definition
$C\bar{v}_{O_2}$	concentration of O_2 in mixed venous blood	Q_T	cardiac output
O_2 (Cap)	O_2 capacity	Sa_{O_2}	saturation of hemoglobin with O_2 in arterial blood
Pa_{O_2}	partial pressure of O_2 in arterial blood	$\dot{V}_A/\dot{Q}$	ventilation-perfusion ratio
		$\dot{V}_E$	expired minute ventilation
$PA_{O_2}\text{-}Pa_{O_2}$	alveolar-arterial difference in partial pressure of O_2	$V\max_{O_2}$	maximum O_2 consumption
P_{O_2}	partial pressure of O_2		

CONTROL OF BREATHING

Symbol	Definition	Symbol	Definition
T_E	expiratory time	T_T	total respiratory cycle time
T_I	inspiratory time		

Table 16.20: Units of measurement in respiratory physiology and pulmonary medicine

Measurement	Unit	
	Customary Metric	SI
Flow, ventilatory and capacity (V and others)	$L \cdot min^{-1}$, $L \cdot s^{-1}$	$L \cdot min^{-1}$, $L \cdot s^{-1}$, $m^3 \cdot s^{-1}$
Flow, blood ($\dot{Q}$)	$L \cdot min^{-1}$	$L \cdot min^{-1}$
Capacity and volume, static	L	L
Compliance (C)	$L \cdot cmH_2O^{-1}$	$L \cdot kPa^{-1}$
Conductance (G)	$L \cdot s^{-1} \cdot cmH_2O^{-1}$	$L \cdot s^{-1} \cdot kPa^{-1}$
Diffusing capacity (D)	$ml \cdot min^{-1} \cdot mmHg^{-1}$	$mmol \cdot min^{-1} \cdot kPa^{-1}$
Gas exchange (V)	$ml \cdot min^{-1}$	$mmol \cdot min^{-1}$
Pressure (P)	mmHg, cmH_2O	kPa
Reaction rate of CO with oxyhemo-globin (r)	$mlCO \cdot min^{-1} \cdot mmHg^{-1} \cdot ml^{-1}$	$mmol \cdot min^{-1} \cdot kPa^{-1} \cdot L^{-1}$
Resistance (R)	$cmH_2O \cdot L^{-1} \cdot s$	$kPa \cdot L^{-1} \cdot s$
Time (t)	s	s

Multiple-letter abbreviations (not preferred) should be in a roman typeface and grouped within parenthesis marks to indicate that the group of letters must be regarded as a single quantity.

Modifying symbols suffixed to the symbols for quantities should be either small-capital letters or lowercase letters, in a roman (upright)

typeface, and on the line (with a small number of minor exceptions). Small-capital letters are marked in typescript by double-underlining; alternatively a subscripted capital letter can be used in typing.

Modifying symbols are separated, unspaced, with commas.

A dash over a symbol (an overbar) indicates a mean value; a single dot, a time derivative; two dots, the second time derivative.

A percent sign preceding a symbol indicates percentage of predicted normal value; a following percent sign, a ratio expressed as a percentage.

UNITS FOR RESPIRATORY PHYSIOLOGY

16.61 SI units for measurements in respiratory physiology and pulmonary medicine are generally used in Europe and will be increasingly used in the United States. See Table 16.20 for customary metric units and SI units.

RADIOLOGY

16.62 SI units for units of importance in radiology are already in wide use in radiology journals and should be used in other journals. See Table 16.21 for symbols for quantities and for customary metric units and SI units; this table is based on recommendations in references 77–79.

VIROLOGY

VIRUS NOMENCLATURE

16.63 The authority for the names of viruses is the International Committee on Taxonomy of Viruses (ICTV), whose reports (80) establish taxonomic names and list acceptable common (vernacular) names.

All names (families, groups, genera, species) approved by the ICTV should be in an italic (slanted) typeface (REF Mathews, personal communication). Family, group, and genus names are capitalized. Nomenclature for species has not been systematic for the most part, and the present equivalents of bacterial species names (see section 16.3) are mostly English common (vernacular) names, which are not systematically capitalized and should not be in an italic (slanted) typeface. Most of the common names are written solid; those incorporating the name of a disease are written as compound terms.

> *Retroviridae* [family]   *Coronavirus* [genus]   coxsackievirus
> herpesvirus   measles virus   varicella-zoster virus
> Newcastle disease virus   echovirus   vaccinia virus

16.64 The group of retroviruses associated with the acquired immunodeficiency syndrome (AIDS) has been named by a subcommittee of the ICTV (81) "human immunodeficiency viruses", abbreviated HIV. To the abbrevia-

Table 16.21: Symbols and units in radiology

Quantity	Symbol for quantity	SI unit	SI unit: special name and symbol		Customary metric unit: name and symbol	
			name	symbol	name	symbol
Activity	A	s^{-1}	becquerel	Bq	curie	Ci
Absorbed dose	D	$J \cdot kg^{-1}$	gray	Gy	rad	rad
Absorbed dose rate	$\dot{D}$	$J \cdot kg^{-1} \cdot s^{-1}$		$Gy \cdot s^{-1}$	rad per second	$rad \cdot s^{-1}$
Average energy per ion pair	W	J			electron volt	eV
Dose equivalent	H	$J \cdot kg^{-1}$	sievert	Sv	rem	rem
Dose equivalent rate	$\dot{H}$	$J \cdot kg^{-1} \cdot s^{-1}$		$Sv \cdot s^{-1}$	rem per second	$rem \cdot s^{-1}$
Electric current	I	A			ampere	A
Electric potential difference	U, V	$W \cdot A^{-1}$	volt	V	volt	V
Exposure	X	$C \cdot kg^{-1}$			roentgen	R
Exposure rate	$\dot{X}$	$C \cdot kg^{-1} \cdot s^{-1}$			roentgen per second	$R \cdot s^{-1}$
Fluence	Φ	m^{-2}			1 per centimetre squared	cm^{-2}
Kerma	K	$J \cdot kg^{-1}$	gray	Gy	rad	rad
Kerma rate	$\dot{K}$	$J \cdot kg^{-1} \cdot s^{-1}$		$Gy \cdot s^{-1}$	rad per second	$rad \cdot s^{-1}$
Lineal energy	y	$J \cdot m^{-1}$			kiloelectronvolt per micrometre	$keV \cdot \mu m^{-1}$
Linear energy	L	(same units as for "Linear energy" above)				
Mass attenuation coefficient	μ/ρ	$m^2 \cdot kg^{-1}$			centimetre squared per gram	$cm^2 \cdot g^{-1}$
Mass energy transfer coefficient	μ_{tr}/ρ	(same units as for "Mass attenuation coefficient")				
Mass energy absorption coefficient	μ_{en}/ρ	(same units as for "Mass attenuation coefficient")				
Mass stopping power	S/ρ	$J \cdot m^2 \cdot kg^{-1}$			MeV centimetre squared per gram	$MeV \cdot cm^2 \cdot g^{-1}$
Power	P	$J \cdot s^{-1}$	watt	W	watt	W
Pressure	p	$N \cdot m^{-2}$	pascal	Pa	torr	torr
Specific	z	$J \cdot kg^{-1}$	gray	Gy	rad	rad

tion can be added within parenthesis marks an abbreviated designation for a specific isolate including an abbreviation for the laboratory and a number for the place of isolate in a sequence of isolates: "for example, the 42nd isolate at the University of Chicago could be described as HIV(CHI-42)" (81). The preceding abbreviated designations for this group of viruses have included "HTLV-III" (human T-cell lymphotropic virus type III), "LAV" (lymphadenopathy-associated virus), "ARV" (AIDS-associated retrovirus), and "IDAV" (immunodeficiency-associated virus).

Several staging classifications have been proposed (82–84) for the syndrome (AIDS) associated with HIV infection. These code the stages by various alphanumeric combinations.

> group II   group IVC-2   group IVE   category 1   category 4B
> WR5   WR4K   WR3CNS

HEPATITIS VIRUSES

16.65 The nomenclature and symbolization for infection with the agent associated with hepatitis formerly known as "δ-agent" ("delta-agent") (85) should follow the patterns for hepatitis B virus.

> HDV   hepatitis D virus   HDAg   hepatitis D antigen
> viral hepatitis, type D

See Table 16.22 for the well-established abbreviations for hepatitis viruses and their antigens and antibodies.

Table 16.22: Abbreviations for viral hepatitis, the viruses, and the viral antigens and antibodies

Abbreviation	Term
HA	hepatitis A
HAV	hepatitis A virus
HAAg	antigen associated with hepatitis A virus (HAV)
anti-HA	antibody to HAAg
HB	hepatitis B
HBV	hepatitis B virus
HBsAg	surface antigen of hepatitis B virus (HBV)
HBcAg	core antigen of hepatitis B virus (HBV)
HBeAg	"e" antigen associated HBV infection
anti-HBs	antibody to HBsAg
anti-HBc	antibody to HBcAg
anti-HBe	antibody to HBeAg
non-A, non-B	presumed viral agent not producing HA or HB

REFERENCES

1. Krieg NR, Holt JG, eds. Bergey's manual of systematic bacteriology: volume 1. Baltimore: Williams & Wilkins; 1984. Volume 2 is to become available in the second half of 1986.
2. Skerman VBD, McGowan V, Sneath PHA. Approved lists of bacterial names. Int J Syst Bacteriol. 1980;30:225–40.
3. Gherna R, Nierman W, Pienta P. American Type Culture Collection catalogue of bacteria, phages and rDNA vectors. Rockville, Maryland: American Type Culture Collection; 1985. Published every four years.
4. Critchley M, ed. Butterworths medical dictionary. 2nd ed. London: Butterworths; 1978
5. Friel JP, ed. Dorland's illustrated medical dictionary. 26th ed.
6. Landau SI, ed. International dictionary of medicine and biology. New York: John Wiley; 1986.
7. Illustrated Stedman's medical dictionary. 24th ed. Baltimore: Williams & Wilkins; 1982.
8. Cowan ST; Hill LR, ed. A dictionary of microbial taxonomy. Cambridge: Cambridge University Press; 1978.
9. American Society for Microbiology. ASM style manual for journals and books. Washington: American Society for Microbiology; 1985:31–6.
10. Demerec M, Adelberg EA, Clark AJ, Hartman PE. A proposal for a uniform nomenclature in bacterial genetics. Genetics. 1966;54:61–76.
11. The Criteria Committee of the New York Heart Association. Nomenclature and criteria for diagnosis of diseases of the heart and great vessels. 8th ed. Boston: Little, Brown; 1979.
12. American Heart Association. The standardization of electrocardiographic nomenclature: report of a committee of the American Heart Association. JAMA. 1943;121:1347–51.
13. Keith NM, Wagener HP, Barker NW. Some different types of essential hypertension: their cause and prognosis. Am J Med Sci. 1939;197:332–43.
14. Werf TVD. Cardiovascular pathophysiology. Oxford: Oxford University Press;1980:viii.
15. World Health Organization. The SI for the health professions. Geneva: World Health Organization: 1977.
16. Dodd JS, ed. The ACS style guide. Washington: American Chemical Society; 1986.
17. CBE Style Manual Committee. CBE style manual: a guide for authors, editors, and publishers in the biological sciences. 5th ed. Bethesda, Maryland: Council of Biology Editors; 1983:214–26.
18. International Union of Biochemistry. Biochemical nomenclature and related documents. London: The Biochemical Society; 1978.
19. Nomenclature Committee of the International Union of Biochemistry on the Nomenclature and Classification of Enzyme-Catalyzed Reactions. Enzyme nomenclature: 1984. Orlando, Florida: Academic Press; 1984.
20. Committee of Editors of Biochemical Journals. Recommendations to editors of biochemical journals: circular no 338. Liege, Belgium: Committee of Editors of Biochemical Journals; 1984.
21. Nomenclature Committee of the International Union of Biochemistry. Symbolism and terminology in enzyme kinetics. Eur J Biochem. 1982;128:281–91.
22. IUPAC-IUB Joint Commission on Biochemical Nomenclature. Nomenclature and symbolism for amino acids and peptides. Eur J Biochem. 1984;138:9–37.

23. Nomenclature Committee of the International Union of Biochemistry. Nomenclature for incompletely specified bases in nucleic acid sequences. Eur J Biochem. 1985;150:1-5.
24. Rowe DS. Nomenclature of immunoglobulins. Nature. 1970: 228:509-511.
25. World Health Organization. Nomenclature of human immunoglobulins. Bull WHO. 1973;48:373.
26. World Health Organization. Proposed rules for the designation of immunoglobulins of animal origin. Bull WHO. 1978;56:815-7.
27. Stewart WE II, Blalock JE, Burke DC, et al. Interferon nomenclature. J Immunol. 1980;125:2353. Letter.
28. Interferon Nomenclature Committee. Interferon nomenclature. J Gen Virol. 1984;65:669-70.
29. Nomenclature Committee of the International Society of Hypertension. Nomenclature of the renin-angiotensin system: report of the Nomenclature Committee of the International Society of Hypertension. Hypertension. 1979;1:654-6.
30. Solomon DH, Benotti J, DeGroot LJ, et al. A nomenclature for tests of thyroid hormones in serum: report of a committee of the American Thyroid Association. J Clin Endocrinol Metab. 1972;34:884-90.
31. Eighth International Workshop on Human Gene Mapping. Human gene mapping 8: Helsinki Conference (1985), Eighth international workshop on human gene mapping. Cytogenet Cell Genet. 1985;40(1-4):1-823). Simultaneously published in: Birth Defects: Original Article Series, Vol 21(4). White Plains, New York: March of Dimes Birth Defects Foundation; 1985.
32. McKusick VA. Mendelian inheritance in man: catalogs of autosomal dominant, autosomal recessive, and X-linked phenotypes. 6th ed. Baltimore: Johns Hopkins University Press; 1983.
33. Standing Committee on Human Cytogenetic Nomenclature. An international system for human cytogenetic nomenclature (1978) ISCN (1978): report of the Standing Committee on Human Cytogenetic Nomenclature. Cyotgenet Cell Genet. 1978;21:309-409.
34. Sandberg AA, Hecht BK, Hecht F. Nomenclature: the Philadelphia chromosome or Ph without superscript. Cancer Genet Cytogenet. 1985;14:1.
35. Shows TB, Alper CA, Bootsma D, et al. International system for human gene nomenclature (1979), ISGN (1979). Cytogenet Cell Genet. 1979;25:96-116.
36. American Type Culture Collection. Catalogue of recombinant DNA collections. Rockville, Maryland: American Type Culture Collection; 1986.
37. National Institutes of Health. 1985 catalog of cell lines: NIGMS human genetic mutant cell repository sponsored by the National Institute of General Medical Sciences, NIA aging cell repository sponsored by the National Institute on Aging. Bethesda, Maryland: National Institutes of Health; 1985; NIH publication no 85-2011.
38. Chicago Conference. Chicago Conference: standardization in human cytogenetics. In: Birth defects original article series. New York: National Foundation-March of Dimes; 1966. (Vol 1(2)).
39. Tenth International Congress of Haematology. Nomenclature of hemoglobins. Br Med J. 1964;2:1258.
40. International Society of Haematology. Recommendations by the International Society of Haematology on the nomenclature of abnormal haemoglobins. Br J Haematol. 1965;11:121-2.
41. Lehmann H, Carrell RW. Nomenclature of the α-thalassemias. Lancet. 1984;1:552-3.
42. Allen FHJr, Anstee DJ, Bird GWG, et al. ISBT working party on terminology for red cell surface antigens. Vox Sang. 1983;42:164-5.

43. Lewis M, Allen FHJr, Anstee DJ, et al. ISBT working party on terminology for red blood cell surface antigens: Munich report. Vox Sang. 1985;49:171–5.
44. International Committee on Nomenclature of Blood Clotting Factors. Nomenclature of blood clotting factors: four factors, their characterization and international number. JAMA. 1959;170:325–8.
45. International Committeee on Blood Clotting Factors. New blood clotting factors: transactions of the conference held under the auspices of the International Committee on Blood Clotting Factors, Montreux, Switzerland, August 24–26, 1959. Thromb Diath Haemorrh. 1940;4[Suppl]260–78.
46. International Committee for the Nomenclature of Blood Clotting Factors. The nomenclature of blood clotting factors. JAMA. 1962;180:733–5.
47. Marder VJ, Mannucci PM, Firkin BG, Hoyer LW, Meyer D. Standard nomenclature for factor VIII and von Willebrand factor: a recommendation by the International Committee on Thrombosis and Haemostasis. Thromb Haemost. 1985;54:871–2.
48. International Committee of Haemostasis and Thrombosis. I A Genetic nomenclature for human blood coagulation. Thromb Diath Haemorrh. 1973;30:1–11.
49. World Health Organization. Nomenclature of complement. Bull WHO 1968;39:935–8.
50. World Health Organization. Nomenclature of the alternative activating pathway of complement. Bull WHO. 1981;59:489–91.
51. World Health Organization. Nomenclature for factors of the HLA system. Bull WHO. 1975;52:261–5.
52. World Health Organization. Nomenclature for factors of the HLA system, 1977. Bull WHO. 1978;56:461–5.
53. World Health Organization. Nomenclature for factors of the HLA system, 1980. Bull WHO. 1980;58:945–8.
54. World Health Organization. Nomenclature for factors of the HLA system. Bull WHO. 1985;63:399–405.
55. American Type Culture Collection. Catalog of fungi/yeasts. 16th ed. Rockville, Maryland: American Type Culture Collection; 1984.
56. McGinnis MR, Ajello L, Schell WA. Mycotic diseases: a proposed nomenclature. Int J Dermatol. 1985:24:9–15.
57. [Various authors]. Atlas of tumor pathology. Washington: Armed Forces Institute of Pathology. Issued in fascicles.
58. Sobin LH. The international histological classification of tumours. Bull WHO. 1981;59:813–9.
59. World Health Organization. ICD-O: international histological classification of diseases for oncology. 1st ed. Geneva: World Health Organization, 1976.
60. American Joint Committee on Cancer; Beahrs OH, Myers MH, eds. Manual for staging of cancer. 2nd ed. Philadelphia: JB Lippincott; 1983.
61. Committee on Lung Cancer, American Thoracic Society. Clinical staging of primary lung cancer. Clinical staging of primary lung cancer. Am Rev Resp Dis. 1983; 127:659–64.
62. Foon KA, Todd RF. Immunologic classification of leukemia and lymphoma. Blood. 1986;68:1–31.
63. French-American-British (FAB) Co-operative Group: Bennett J, Catovsky D, Daniel M-T, et al. Proposals for the classification of acute leukemia. Br J Haematol. 1976;33:451–8.
64. Bennett JM, Catovsky D, Daniel MT, et al. Criteria for the diagnosis of acute leukemia of megakaryocytic lineage (M7): a report of the French-American-British Cooperative Group. Ann Intern Med. 1985;103:460–2.

65. Bennett JM, Catovsky D, Daniel MT, et al. Proposed revised criteria for the classification of acute myeloid leukemia: a report of the French-American-British Cooperative Group. Ann Intern Med. 1985;103:620–5.
66. Bernard A, Boumsell L, Dausset J, Milstein C, Schlossman SF, eds. Leucocyte typing: human leucocyte differentiation antigens detected by monoclonal antibodies: specification – classification – nomenclature. Berlin: Springer; 1984.
67. American Type Culture Collection. Catalogue of protists – algae/protozoa. 16th ed. Rockville, Maryland: American Type Culture Collection; 1985.
68. Parker SP, ed. Synopsis and classification of living organisms. New York: McGraw-Hill; 1982.
69. Committee for Pharmacokinetic Nomenclature. Manual of symbols, equations & definitions in pharmacokinetics. J Clin Pharmacol. 1982;22(7; supplement):1S–23S.
70. Ratcliffe JG, Worth HGJ. Recommended units for reporting drug concentrations in biological units. Lancet. 1986;1:202–3.
71. American Psychiatric Association. Diagnostic and statistical manual of mental disorders. 3rd ed. Washington: American Psychiatric Association; 1980.
72. Commission on Professional and Hospital Activities. The international classification of diseases, 9th revision, clinical modification. Ann Arbor, Michigan: Commission on Professional and Hospital Activities; 1978.
73. American Psychiatric Association. The American Psychiatric Association's psychiatric glossary. 5th ed. Washington: American Psychiatric Association; 1984.
74. CBE Style Manual Committee. CBE style manual. 5th ed. Bethesda, Maryland: Council of Biology Editors; 1983:207–10.
75. ACCP-ATS Joint Committee on Pulmonary Nomenclature. Pulmonary terms and symbols: a report of the ACCP-ATS Joint Committee on Pulmonary Nomenclature. Chest. 1975;67:583–93.
76. Macklem PT. Symbols and abbreviations. In: Fishman AP, ed. The respiratory system. Bethesda, Maryland: American Physiological Society; 1985:ix–xi. (Handbook of Physiology, vol 1, sec 3).
77. National Council on Radiation Protection and Measurements. SI units in radiation protection and measurements. Bethesda, Maryland: National Council on Radiation Protection and Measurements; 1985. (NRCP report no 82).
78. International Commission on Radiation Units and Measurements. Radiation quantities and units. Washington: International Commission on Radiation Units and Measurements; 1980. (ICRU report 33).
79. International Electrotechnical Commission. Medical radiology – terminology. Geneva: Bureau Central de la Commission Electrotechnique Internationale; 1984. (Publication 788).
80. Matthews REF. Classification and nomenclature of viruses: third report of the International Committee on Taxonomy of Viruses. Basel: S Karger; 1979.
81. Coffin J, Haase A, Levy JA, et al. Human immunodeficiency viruses. Science. 1986;232:697.
82. Centers for Disease Control. Classification system for human T-lymphotropic virus type III/lymphadenopathy-associated virus infections. MMWR. 1986;35:334–9.
83. Haverkos HW, Gottlieb MS, Killen JY, Edelman R. Classification of HTLY-III/LAV-related diseases. J Infect Dis. 1985;152:1095.
84. Redfield RR, Wright DC, Tramont EC. The Walter Reed staging classification for HTLV-III/LAV infection. N Engl J Med. 1986;314:131–2.
85. Jacobson IM, Dienstag JL. The delta hepatitis agent: "viral hepatitis, type D". Gastroenterology. 1984;86:1614–7.

Chapter 17

Prose Style

How a fabric strikes us is determined by its parts and how they are put together: its threads and their roughness and colors; the tightness of the weave; the patterns. So it is with prose style. Each and every element of a piece of prose and how they are put together create a style that may be lean, clear, accurate, and strong, or stuffed, unclear, inaccurate, and flabby. This chapter does not review all of the details of vocabulary, grammatical rules, and syntax for expository prose in English; some of the many good guides are described briefly in Appendix C. This chapter takes up only some problems and defects that occur widely in medical prose.

Editors must take care not to confuse defects in prose style with authors' legitimate preferences. Wrong words, inaccurate statement, and windy writing should be cleaned up, but authors must be allowed to have their styles when meaning is accurately and efficiently conveyed to the reader.

ABBREVIATION

17.1 A blight spreading through medical prose is the myriad of abbreviations coined *ad hoc* to substitute for the formal names of diseases, variables, procedures, syndromes, tests, therapies. Some examples are "CAD" ("coronary artery disease"), "COLD" (chronic obstructive lung disease), "LVEDP" (left-ventricular end-diastolic pressure), "NANBH" (non-A, non-B hepatitis), "IVP" (intravenous pyelography). Such coinages tend to pass into acceptance for formal medical prose, but authors should usually be expected to replace such abbreviations with full and formal terms. Enforcing this requirement is aided by a journal's publishing in its information-for-authors page (see section 1.23) a list of acceptable abbreviations. Abbreviations should not be used in titles of papers (see section 2.2); occasionally exceptions may have to be made for widely-known abbreviations for long names of therapies or chemicals. Abbreviations acceptable in the journal but not widely recognized outside of its field should be explained parenthetically in the abstract and at their first mention in the text of a paper (see sections 2.8 and 11.2).

Excessive use of abbreviations can often be avoided by deleting those needed as modifiers.

> NOT . . . included 75 control subjects and 57 SLE patients.
> BUT . . . included 75 control subjects and 57 patients.
> [in a paper concerned only with systemic lupus erythematosus (SLE)]

Similarly, the context of a sentence may make clear the term to which a short substitute for it refers.

> [In a paper about only one enzyme, propanediol-phosphate dehydrogenase]
> . . . and no evidence of the enzyme was found in the other subjects.
> [In a paper about only the acquired immunodeficiency syndrome (AIDS)]
> . . . and the other patients had no evidence of the syndrome.

Formal symbolic representation of many quantities measured in function tests may be available in place of such coinages as "LVEDP" (see sections 14.2 and 16.17). Authors should be encouraged to use symbols for quantities rather than multiletter abbreviations, and journal editors have a responsibility to develop consensus in their fields for appropriate formal symbols.

VOCABULARY

17.2 Clear and accurate statement in scientific prose calls for choice of the right word at every point. Editors should consider authors' choices and improve them whenever a change will lead to a gain in clarity and accuracy. They must take care, however, in making such changes lest an acceptable idiom be distorted; this risk is greatest for editors, notably manuscript editors (*subeditors* in British usage) not familiar with the idiom of the discipline represented by the journal.

ABSTRACT NOUNS SUBSTITUTING FOR ACTIVE VERBS

17.3 Much scientific prose takes too much time for its message and tires its readers. Its central fault lies in the heavy use of abstract nouns that have taken the place of the active verbs from which they were derived. This fault is often quickly identified by spotting "-tion" nouns and gerunds (verbal nouns) ending in "ing", either likely to be followed by "of".

> . . . and the findings have led to increased *understanding of* the likely modes of *transmission* as well as the *identification of* persons at risk for infection.

Such a passage can be revised to more direct and concise statement by rewriting it to convert the abstract nouns to verbs.

> . . . and from the findings we *understand* better how the infection is *transmitted* and how to *identify* persons at risk.

Among the most frequent of the "-tion" nouns in clinical medicine are those that represent processes in the body, organs, tissues, or cells.

excretion by the kidney of	the kidney excretes
migration of xxxxxx through the	xxxxxx migrates through the

Prose revised to correct this fault will hold more readers. Note, however, that such revision may change the tone from impersonal to personal voice. The tone of a paper should not obviously shift throughout its text; a paper should be thus revised throughout or not at all.

CONFUSED AND MISUSED WORDS

17.4   Many pairs or small groups of words have, or appear to have, closely related meanings. The right choice is needed for accurate statement.

a; the   A full discussion of these sometimes-confused articles might run for pages. The most frequent fault in their use in medical prose is failure to select the right one for the specificity needed. The article *a* implies that the noun it precedes represents an item with more than one representative of its class; the article *the* implies that the phrase "*the* (noun)" refers to a unique item of its class.

. . . is not a treatment for . . .	[there are other treatments]
. . . is not the treatment for . . .	[there is only one proper treatment among possible treatments]

> NOT   We present a case of an immunocompetent patient who . . .
> BUT   We present the case of an immunocompetent patient who . . . [The patient did not have more than one "case", only that presented.]

accuracy; precision   *Accuracy* is the degree to which the value of a measurement is correct; *precision* is the degree of refinement to which something is measured, or to which a measured value is reported. *Precision* and *precise* applied to statements in prose indicate qualities of definiteness, terseness, and specificity.

affect; effect   As nouns, *affect* means the feeling apparent to an observer that accompanies an emotional state and *effect*, the result of the action of a causal agent. As a verb, *to affect* means "to produce a change" and implies the lack of intent; *to effect*, "to cause to bring about a change" and an intent to do so.

> His mood affected the whole family.
> His work finally effected a change in staff attitudes.

after; following   Although *follow* (and its participles *following* and *followed*) can be used as an intransitive verb ("to come after, passively"), the priorities of its definitions in dictionaries reflect its preferred use as a transitive (active) verb. Avoid the use of *following* as a preposition and prefer *after*.

> He carefully followed the procedures used by his chief. ["copied the procedures" by intent]
> NOT   He fainted following the operation.
> BUT   He fainted after the operation.

alternate; alternative   *Alternate* indicates successive but different items of the same class; *alternative* indicates choices or options and implies they are mutually exclusive.

> The alternate treatments, applied at intervals of 2 weeks, were radiation and chemotherapy.
>
> The alternative treatments were radiation and chemotherapy; he chose radiation. [OR: The possible treatment was radiation or chemotherapy.]

anatomy; structure   Reserve *anatomy* for the discipline that is concerned with the study of structure.

> NOT   At autopsy the anatomy of the third ventricle was abnormal.
> BUT   At autopsy the third ventricle was structurally abnormal.

Also see *morphology; structure.*

and/or; and . . . , or . . . , or both   Do not use the lazy legalism *and/or.*

> NOT   . . . that nonenzymatic glycosylation of fibrinogen and/or fibrin results in . . .
> BUT   . . . that nonenzymatic glycosylation of fibrinogen and of fibrin results in . . . [the two *of*s link "fibrinogen" and "fibrin" independently to "glycosylation"; either one or both together can be "glycosylated"]

Such a solution often avoids the longer structure of *and . . . , or . . . , or both.*

ante-; anti-   Serving as prefixes, *ante-* means "preceding" and *anti-* means "being against".

> antepartum = before birth
> antiemetic = having an effect against emesis
> [Note that as a Latin phrase rather than as an adjective, *ante partum* is not run together: "She was treated ante partum with iron and a high-protein diet".]

assure; ensure; insure   See *insure; ensure; assure.*

average; typical   Reserve *average* as a synomym for the statistical term *mean*. Use *typical* for *characteristic, natural, regular.*

> NOT   His was an average case of appendicitis.
> BUT   His was a typical case of appendicitis.

believe; think; feel   *Believe* means "actively accept as true"; *think* means "applying mental activity and power" in considering a question without necessarily being sure of the answer. *Feel* can be akin to *believe* and mean "have an inward conviction", with the conviction's not necessarily being held by anyone else as with a belief or supported by external evidence that would convince others.

> We believe that radiation is the better treatment for . . .
> ["We have examined the evidence and conclude that radiation . . ."]
>
> We think that radiation is the better treatment for . . .
> ["There may be some room for disagreement but after pondering the question, we decided that radiation . . ."]
>
> We feel that radiation is the better treatment for . . .
> [Others may disagree but we have the inward conviction that . . .]

bi-; semi-   Prefixes: *bi-* means "two", "occurring every two units of time", or "affecting two elements"; *semi-* means "half" or "partly", "occurring at the first point and half point of a unit of time".

> bigeminy   twinned or paired beats or pulses
> biped   two-legged
> bimonthly   every two months
> biaural   affecting both ears
> semicircular forming a half-circle
> semimonthly   twice a month

Note that some general dictionaries do not draw this distinction, but that which is best for its judgments on usage, *The American Heritage Dictionary* (1), calls the use of *bi-* as a prefix to designate occurrences twice in a period "nonstandard". The clear distinction should be preserved.

biopsy   See *perform.*

case; patient   Reserve *case* for "an instance or episode of disease, disorder, or dysfunction"; use *patient* to refer to the person affected by disease, disorder, or dysfunction.

> NOT   Case 1 was treated for 5 months with . . .
> BUT   In Case 1, the patient was treated for 5 months with . . .

In the first example, *case* is dehumanizing jargon (also see section 17.5).

climatic; climactic   *Climatic* means "having to do with climate"; *climactic,* "having the character of a climax". Do not confuse either with *climacteric,* the endocrine evolution that immediately precedes the end of a woman's reproductive period of life.

comparable; similar   Reserve *comparable* to mean "having characteristics suitable for a comparison"; avoid using it to mean "similar".

> Despite their differences, the two methods yielded data with precisions that made them comparable. [data useful for comparison]
>
> NOT   The two study groups were comparable in age, sex distribution, and mean weights.
>
> BUT   The two study groups were similar in age, sex distribution, and mean weights.

compared to; compared with   *Compared to* means "judged against a standard or reference"; *compared with* means "used in an examination for similarity or difference".

> Compared to Osler, Smith was a cretin.
>
> Chemotherapy was compared with radiation in the study and found to yield a much higher mortality rate.

comprise; compose   Reserve *comprise* for the meaning of the French verb from which it was derived, "to include". A whole entity "comprises" its parts. Parts of a whole "compose" the whole; remember that the "composer" puts together "notes" (parts) to "compose" a musical work as a whole entity.

> The university comprises 6 health-science schools and 10 colleges.
>
> The medical school and 10 colleges compose the university.

council; counsel   A *council* is an administrative, advisory, deliberative, or legislative group of persons. As a noun, *counsel* refers to a lawyer managing a case or representing a client and as a verb, to the giving of advice.

criterion; standard   Reserve *criterion* to mean "a characteristic applied in coming to a judgment"; use *standard* to mean "the specific characteristic or value assigned to a criterion for applying it in judgments".

> The main criterion for improvement was gain in body weight.
>
> The standard for adequate improvement was a weight gain of 1.0 kg in the treatment period.

customary   See *traditional; customary; conventional.*

data; datum   Do not forget that *data* is the plural form of *datum.*

If *datum* is needed as the singular noun but seems unidiomatic, substitute an acceptable singular noun, such as *value, figure, finding*.

NOT   The data is adequate evidence for the conclusion.
BUT   The data are adequate evidence for the conclusion.

demonstrate, exhibit; show   *Demonstrate* and *exhibit* often serve as pompous substitutes for *show*. These three verbs are transitive (active) and thus imply that their subjects are the agents for the action they state, but *show* is less obtrusive. As inanimate things "data" cannot initiate the action of "showing"; the usual use of *show* with an inanimate subject like *data* is simply an elliptical construction accepted as an idiom in scientific prose.

USUAL FORM   The data show that the drug was more effective than the placebo.
MEANING   [We interpret] the data [to] show that the drug was more effective than the placebo.

determine; assess, examine, measure   Reserve *determine* for "fixing conclusively, deciding definitely, settling a question"; avoid using *determine* for simply "carrying out a measurement", "ascertaining the value of a quantity" where conclusive fixing of a value is not involved. More specific choices for the various acts of laboratory measurement are available: *measure, weigh, titrate*. The same point applies to the noun equivalents *determination, measurement, titration*.

ACCEPTABLE   We determined the value of the dissociation constant at . . .
NOT ACCEPTABLE   We determined the serum chloride values of the 16 patients with the method of . . .
ACCEPTABLE   We measured serum chloride with the method of . . .

discreet; discrete   A homophone pair: *discreet*, an adjective that indicates careful behavior in conduct and speech; *discrete*, an adjective that indicates a separate entity.

dosage; dose   *Dosage* is "an amount of medicine to be taken or given in a period of time, or a total amount"; *dose* is "the amount taken or given at one time"; the sum of doses may be *dosage* or *total dose*.

effect; affect   See *affect; effect*.

employ; use   Reserve *employ* for its narrower and original meaning, "putting to work, or engaging the help or services of, a person"; prefer the simpler and broader *use* for "applying a device, tool, method, or some other inanimate item to a task".

PRETENTIOUS   We employed the method of Smith for serum chloride.
SIMPLER   We used the method of Smith for serum chloride.

ensure; insure; assure   See *insure; ensure; assure.*

etiology; cause   Reserve *etiology* for its meaning, "the study of the causes of disease". Do not use *etiology* as a pompous synonym for *cause*; use *cause* when cause is meant.

evaluate; assess, examine, measure, study   Reserve *evaluate* for the meaning "to examine before assigning a value"; do not use it as a stuffy and imprecise substitute for such verbs as *assess, examine, measure, study.*

NOT   We evaluated the patient's pulmonary function with . . .
BUT   We measured the patient's pulmonary function with . . .

exhibit; show   See *demonstrate, exhibit; show.*

feel   See *believe; think; feel*

fewer; less   *Fewer* is correct for "a smaller number of"; *less* means "a smaller amount" of something not measured in individual units.

UNACCEPTABLE   Less persons get infected today with the poliomyelitis virus.
CORRECT   Fewer persons get infected today with the poliomyelitis virus.
We see less paralysis now in typical cases.

following; after   See *after; following.*

homogenous; homogeneous   Reserve *homogenous* as the adjectival form of *homogeny*, in biology, "correspondence of organs or parts having a descent from an origin in common"; the alternative adjectival form is *homogenetic.* Use *homogeneous* for "uniform throughout in structure or composition".

hypothecate; hypothesize   Do not use *hypothecate* for "to form a hypothesis"; it properly has a specific and narrow meaning like "to mortgage".

hypothesis; theory   See *theory; hypothesis.*

imply; infer   See *infer; imply.*

important; significant   See the entry for *significant.*

incidence; prevalence   Reserve *incidence* for "number of cases of a disease, complication, injury occurring (newly appearing) per specified number of persons or patients (the denominator, typically 100, 1000, or 1 million) in a specified period of time, typically 1 year"; the period must be specified. *Prevalence* is "the number of cases existing at a point in time (or in a short specified period needed for ascertainment) per specified number of persons or patients".

NOT   The incidence of wound disruptions was 10%.
BUT   The incidence of wound disruptions was 10% [10 per 100 patients] in the first 6 postoperative months.

The incidence of HIV infections stabilized at 4.5 cases per 100 000 persons in one year [4.5 cases/(100 000 persons)·(1 year)].
The peak prevalence of HIV infection was 1 case per 100 000 inhabitants.

individual; person   Reserve *individual* for contrast specifically with a group and avoid its unnecessary use as a synonym for *person*.

NOT   We found ten individuals with signs suggesting HIV infection.
BUT   We found ten persons with signs suggesting HIV infection.

Social groups tend to behave collectively as if they have a low IQ; their individuals tend to have higher IQs.

Also see *people; persons.*

infective; infectious   Use *infectious* to describe an organism or virus that can readily cause an infection or to describe a disease from which an "infectious agent" can be readily transmitted to another person or animal and cause an infection. Use *infective* to describe a disease that represents an infection but that is highly unlikely to be the source of infection for another person or animal.

We identified 10 species in the genus that are likely to be infectious in the right environmental circumstances.
Gonorrhea was the infectious disease seen most frequently in clinics of VA hospitals.
Our study of 254 cases of infective endocarditis convinced us . . .
[Bacterial endocarditis is highly unlikely to be the source of infection for another person; it is caused by bacterial infection.]

infer; imply   These are not synomyms. *Infer* means "draw a conclusion from specified or unspecified evidence". *Imply* means "suggest a conclusion".

We inferred from the epidemiologic data that HIV was the causative virus.
He implied in his discussion that HIV could be the causative virus.

infested with; infected with   To *infest* and *infestation* refer to parasitic coexistence of small organisms, usually macroscopic, on humans or animals, usually without their causing a disease but only a nuisance; *to infect* and *infection* refer to external or internal coexistence of viruses or microorganisms with humans or animals, usually with production of a disease. Invasion of the body by a microorganism without its producing a disease is termed *colonization*.

> During his week in the USSR, he became infested with lice.
> While he was in that humid climate, his skin became infected with *Staphylococcus aureus*.

insure; ensure; assure   In American English these three verbs all mean "to provide protection (financial, contractual, operational) against a risk". But *assure* is also used to mean "relieve a person of concern or anxiety about a feared event or consequence". For references to financial protection of life or property, *insure* is now generally preferred among the three in American usage. *Ensure* also has the special mean of "make certain of".

localize; locate   *Localize* means "confine, or be confined, to a location"; *locate* means "place something at at particular site" or "find a particular site".

manuscript; paper   A manuscript (or typescript) is the particular record on sheets of paper of the text, tables, references, or any other content of the intellectual work referred to in scholarly settings as "a paper". The "paper" is the ideational content, and the "paper" is carried on the manuscript. A "paper" (the intellectual work in words and numbers) can be sent to an editor but it is sent in the form of a manuscript.

> NOT   His manuscript lacks any real evidence for his conclusion.
> BUT   His paper lacks any real evidence . . .
> NOT   The editor has rejected my manuscript.
> BUT   The editor both rejected my paper and lost the manuscript.

media; medium   *Media* is a plural noun; *medium*, singular. Do not use *media* loosely as a singular noun in the sloppy style of public-relations and advertising experts.

> In an attempt to culture a bacterium, we tried 10 media.
> The best medium for postgraduate education is an on-the-spot clinic.

metastasis; metastatic lesion   *Metastasis* refers in its strict sense to the process by which a disease process, particularly a malignant neoplasm, spreads from its original site to another. Hence a neoplastic lesion or localized disease, for example, an abscess that is the result of metastasis, can be described, respectively, as a *metastatic lesion* and a *metastatic abscess*. In jargon a metastatic tumor is often referred to as "a metastasis", which is undesirable usage. "Metastases" should be avoided as a term for *metastatic tumors* or *metastatic lesions*.

method; technique   See *technique; method; technic.*

morphology; structure   *Morphology* means the study of structure; do not use it as a synonym for *structure.*

> NOT Endoscopy showed abnormal morphology at the lower end of the esophagus.
> BUT Endoscopy showed a mucosal abnormality of unknown type.

mucous; mucus   *Mucous* is an adjective meaning "of a type producing mucus"; do not use it for *mucus,* a noun meaning "a viscous mixture secreted by glands in certain epithelial membranes".

> . . . mucous membrane of the nose . . .
> Bloody mucus drained from his nose for 10 days.

nutrition; nutritional   As an adjective, use *nutrition* with terms for organizations, services, functions. Use *nutritional* as the adjective to modify terms having to do with adequate or inadequate nutrition (diet).

nutrition assessment	nutritional deficiencies
nutrition counseling	nutritional health
nutrition department	nutritional requirements
nutrition research	nutritional status

on, at, in   These prepositions are often used idiomatically in the jargon of clinical medicine. In some of these idioms, the preposition can be properly changed to that preferred in standard English.

> NOT For 2 months we always had at least ten cases of AIDS on the private service.
> BUT . . . in the private service.
> NOT On admission the patient had a fever of 39.0 °C.
> BUT At admission the patient . . .

paper, report; study, trial   *Paper* (journal article) and *report* (published account) are sometimes used incorrectly for the *study* or *trial* reported.

> NOT This report (17) is the first that attempts to measure the . . .
> BUT This study (17) was the first that attempted to measure the . . .
> OR   The paper by Jones (17) first reported attempts to measure . . .

Also see *manuscript; paper* above in this section.

parameter; index, indicator, variable   Reserve *parameter* for its specific meaning in mathematics, "a variable in an equation to which various values or an arbitrary constant can be assigned, a variable that determines or restricts the value defined by the equation as a whole". Do not use *parameter* loosely as a jargon substitute for *index, indicator,* or *variable* (dependent variable).

> NOT   We measured 10 parameters of hematologic status.
> BUT   To the 2nd parameter, q, in equation 9.2, we assigned the value . . .

pathology; abnormality, disease, disorder, lesion   Reserve *pathology* for "the study of disease and its processes"; do not use *pathology* as a synonym for a structural or functional abnormality. The same rule applies to *pathophysiology* as a substitute for *abnormal function.*

> NOT   Endoscopy revealed gastric pathology 10 cm beyond the . . .
> BUT   Endoscopy showed a gastric lesion 10 cm beyond . . .
> NOT   In his description of the patient's pathophysiology . . .
> BUT   In his description of the patient's abnormalities . . .

people; persons   Reserve *people* to refer to a body or large group of persons who have characteristics in common, such as nationality, language, needs; do not use *people* as a simple collective substitute for *persons* unless those persons have some true commonality other than the event described.

> NOT   We estimated that no more than 150 people became infected.
> BUT   We estimated that no more than 150 persons became infected.
>
> Schistosomiasis is the leading disease among the people of . . .
> Persons ["individuals"] who become infected with HIV usually first show . . .
>
> The people [groups of persons] most likely to become infected with HIV include homosexuals and drug addicts.

This distinction is rarely followed in demotic and news-media speech: "You shudda seen da funny people we met at da party".

perform   For the jargon verb *perform* substitute when possible a simpler and more precise verb.

> NOT   As a result, we performed a biopsy through . . .
> BUT   As a result we biopsied the . . .
> NOT   We performed a statistical analysis with the data from . . .
> BUT   We statistically analyzed the data from . . .

Note that the use of *biopsy* as a verb was long taboo; *biopsy* is now widely accepted both as a transitive verb meaning "obtain a tissue specimen and examine it histologically" and a noun meaning "a tissue specimen obtained by the act of biopsy". Note, however, that as a verb *biopsy* is coming to mean only the act of obtaining a specimen.

precision; accuracy   See *accuracy; precision.*

prior to; before   Avoid using *prior to* as a pompous substitute for *before*. This phrase may be properly used to indicate an act necessarily antecedent to (having to be carried out before) a second act but this use is proper only infrequently.

> NOT   Prior to admission, the patient vomited blood twice.
> BUT   The patient vomited blood twice before admission.

> ACCEPTABLE   Assessment of cardiac status must be done prior to any major operation.

proven; proved   The antique past participle *proven* should be used only for its specific and narrow meaning in Scots law. There is no sound reason why the past participle of *prove* (transitive or intransitive form) used adjectivally should differ from the past participial forms of other verbs used similarly.

> NOT   These drugs have proven to be effective in legionellosis.
> BUT   These drugs have proved to be effective in legionellosis.

report   See *paper, report; study, trial*.

require; need   Reserve *require* for use as an active verb that represents the act of setting a requirement or pressing for fullfillment of a need. Do not use *require* as an intransitive verb for passively having a need.

> NOT   The patient became unresponsive and required intubation.
> BUT   The patient became unresponsive and needed intubation.

roentgenograph   See *X ray; roentgen ray; radiograph; roentgen-ograph*.

semi-; bi-   See *bi-; semi-*.

significant; great; important; influential; major; valuable   Reserve *significant* for its statistical meaning, "meeting a value set *a priori* for the test of a statistical hypothesis, such as a P value for a test of a null hypothesis". Alternatively, specify the statistical meaning of *significant* with the phrase *statistically significant*. In non-quantitative contexts, *significant* can be used to mean "indicating" or "signifying" some notable point, but some other modifier such as *important* or *major* or *striking* may be more precise.

> NOT   Medicare costs had a significant effect on the deficit. [What was "signified"?]
> BUT   Medicare costs greatly increased the deficit.

since; because   Prefer *because* to *since* to express a causal relation; reserve *since* to express a sequence without a causal relation.

NOT   Since he broke his leg, we had to delay further studies.
BUT   Because he broke his leg, we had to delay further studies.

He has not been seen since his visit to the clinic in May.

similar; comparable   See *comparable; similar.*

small; few   *Small* refers to size of an entity; *few* refers to the number of items of the same kind.

NOT   Although the published data are small, it appears that . . .
BUT   Although the published data are few, it appears that . . .
OR   Although the body of published data is small, it appears . . .

Also see *fewer; less.*

study   See *paper, report; study, trial.*

technique; method; technic   Reserve *technique* for "the degree of skill, adroitness, or facility with which a procedure, method, or act is carried out". Prefer *method* for the procedure itself. *Technic* is an infrequently used synonym for *technology.*

NOT   . . . titration by the technique of Smith (37) and . . .
BUT   Their superior technique with the method of Smith (37) . . .

Medicine's contemporary technic is costly.

that; which   See *which; that.*

that; who   Do not use *that* to refer to a particular person; *that* can be used to refer to a kind of person.

NOT   We are sure it was Osler that designed the laboratory.
BUT   We are sure it was Osler who designed the laboratory.
OR   We are sure it was an architect that designed the laboratory.

the; a   See *a; the.*

theory; hypothesis   Reserve *theory* for "a broad, integrated, and general concept having substantial support from scientific evidence and useful in predicting a wide range of phenomena"; do not use *theory* trivially for *hypothesis*, "a reasoned conjecture suitable for experimental testing of its validity".

NOT   Our theory was that the malformation was caused by aspirin.
BUT   We hypothesized that the malformation was caused by aspirin.

think; believe; feel   See *believe; think; feel.*

traditional; customary; conventional   Use *traditional* only to indicate an association with a tradition (a practice with historically long use and esteem in a society or group). *Customary* implies having the character of a habit or usual procedure. *Conventional* implies having wide and general acceptance at the time.

> The graduating class repeated the traditional oath.
> The dean gave the customary, but mercifully short, address.
> We compared the new drug with conventional therapies.

utilize; use   Reserve *utilize* for its specific and only rarely needed meaning, "give utility to" or "put to use"; avoid it as a pretentious substitute for *use*. The argument that *use* means "use up" has no merit; other more specific verbs such as *consume, exploit, exhaust* are available.

> NOT   We utilized endoscopy as the method of last resort.
> BUT   We used endoscopy as the method of last resort.

varying, various, variety of; differing, different   Reserve *varying* as an adjective to indicate an entity that changes; a single entity that changes from time to time is *varying* while separate and unlike entities *differ*. *Variety of* is often simply a longer way of saying *various*, but note that *variety* can mean a specific entity in a group with various members, such as a variety of a flower or of a bacterial species (see section 10.5).

> The patient had varying degrees of leg edema.
>
> The patients had differing degrees of leg edema at the end of the study.
>
> Each patient in the group had varying degrees of leg edema throughout the study.

versus; compared with, and, or   Reserve *versus* for its meaning "against, in conflict with".

> NOT   We studied streptomycin versus penicillin in the treatment of . . .
> BUT   We compared streptomycin with penicillin for the treatment of . . .

Note, however, that *versus* is well and properly established in the term *graft-versus-host disease*.

volume; book   *Volume* is frequently and pompously misused to refer to a book. Reserve *volume* for its narrow bibliographic meaning, "a subtitled part of a single work issued in parts called *volumes*". See, as an example, reference 7 at the end of this chapter.

> NOT   Smith has written the best available volume on pneumoconiosis.
> BUT   Smith has written the best book now available on . . .

which; that   Reserve the use of *that* for the relative pronoun opening a restrictive clause, a clause needed for the sense of the sentence. *Which* is a relative pronoun that opens a nonrestrictive clause, a clause that can be omitted from a sentence without loss of the central meaning, a clause that is in essence an "aside".

> This is the procedure that almost all surgeons prefer.
> This procedure, which Cushing developed, is good but difficult.

In speech and less formal writing the "that" is often omitted and simply implied when its effect of emphasis is not needed.

> This is the procedure almost all surgeons prefer.

X ray; roentgen ray; radiograph, roentgenograph   Prefer *roentgen ray* to *X ray*. Do not use *X ray* to refer to the image produced by roentgen rays; use *radiograph; roentgenograph* and *roentgenography* are becoming terms regarded as antique and too narrow in view of the various imaging methods now widely used in radiology.

This section comments on many, but not all, of the words that frequently turn up confused and misused in medical prose. Some of the dictionaries and guides to usage described in Appendix C can help the writer and the editor who strive for precision in style. Especially helpful are *The Penguin Dictionary of Confusibles* (2) and the "Usage Notes" that conclude many definitions in *The American Heritage Dictionary of the English Language* (1).

DEHUMANIZING TERMS

17.5   Persons working steadily in care of the ill and injured tend to protect themselves from its emotional strain by using jargon that objectifies patients and verbally converts them from persons into things. An example is the use of *case* for *patient*, also discussed above in section 17.4.

> NOT   The patients presented here do not represent a clinical entity.
> BUT   These cases do not represent a clinical entity.
>
> NOT   She had been well regulated for nearly 2 years.
> BUT   Her insulin dosage had been well regulated for nearly 2 years.

Another class of dehumanizing terms is the diagnostic label: "diabetics" for *diabetic patients*, "schizophrenic" for a patient with schizophrenia, "alcoholics" for persons with alcoholism. Such terms are such a constant part of informal communication in medicine and its related fields that they tend to creep into the formal writing of even generally careful writers. Editors have an ethical duty to maintain in their journals a tone of caring and concern for the ill and injured that is in keeping with their profession's publicly professed commitment. Dehumanizing terms should be revised to keep the person in the patient.

17.6   Closely related to the kinds of dehumanizing terms pointed out in section 17.5 are the terms *female* and *male* used where *woman* and *man* or *girl* and *boy* would be more accurate. *Female* and *male* may be acceptable, however, in papers reporting patient or study-subject groups that include persons in wide age-ranges, such as childhood through adult life.

EMPTY WORDS AND PHRASES

17.7 Many words and phrases with which we pad out our speech to let us hold our thoughts together are waste words in formal prose and should be cut, or at least trimmed, to keep statement lean and strong. Empty phrases are easier to spot than unneeded epithets (see section 17.8); many empty phrases can be replaced by single words.

Empty phrase	Substitute
a majority of	most
a number of	many
accounted for by the fact that	because
along the lines of	like
an innumerable number of	innumerable
an order of magnitude	ten times
are of the same opinion	agree
as a consequence of	because
at the present moment	now
at this point in time	now
by means of	by, with
caused injuries to	injured
completely filled	filled
definitely proved	proved
despite the fact that	although
due to the fact that	because
during the course of	during, while
during the time that	while
fewer in number	fewer
for the purpose of	for, to
for the reason that	because
from the standpoint of	according to
give rise to	cause
goes under the name of	is called
has the capability of	can, is able to
having regard to	about
if conditions are such that	if
in all cases	always, invariably
in a position to	can, may
in a satisfactory manner	satisfactorily
in an adequate manner	satisfactorily
in case	if
in close proximity to	near
in connection with	about, concerning
in (my, our) opinion it is not an unjustifiable assumption that	(I, we) think

Empty phrase	Substitute
in order to	to
in the event that	if
in view of the fact that	because
it has been reported by Jones	Jones reported
it is believed that	[omit]
it is clear that	clearly
it is often the case that	often
it is possible that the cause is	the cause may be
it is worth pointing out that	note that
it may, however, be noted that	but
it would appear that	apparently
lacked the ability to	could not
large in size	large
large numbers of	many
on account of	because
on behalf of	for
on the basis of	because, by, from
on the grounds that	because
original source	source
owing to the fact that	because
past history	history
prior to [in time]	before
red in color	red
referred to as	called
results so far achieved	results so far
round in shape	round
smaller in size	smaller
subsequent to	after
take into consideration	consider
the question as to whether	whether
through the use of	by, with
was of the opinion that	believed
with a view to	to
with reference to	about [or omit]
with regard to	about, concerning [or omit]
with the result that	so that

17.8 A closely related fault is the unneeded or imprecise modifier (epithet). Many adjectives, notably those for number or severity, add little or no meaning and can be deleted; others can be replaced by a more precise modifier.

> NOT The metastatic bone lesions were very painful.
> BUT . . . were painful.
> OR . . . were excruciatingly painful.
> OR The pain . . . was unbearable.
>
> NOT The patient was lying supine in bed.
> BUT The patient was lying in bed.
>
> NOT Careful hemodynamic monitoring is needed if one is to prevent . . .

BUT   Hemodynamic monitoring is needed if one is to prevent . . .
[Would the author recommend "sloppy" or "negligent" monitoring?]

Follow the rule of Herbert Read (3): ". . . omit all epithets that may be assumed, and . . . admit only those which definitely further action, interest or meaning". Many careful writers would use *that* in place of Read's *which* in this passage; he may have wished to avoid juxtaposing 2 "th-" words, "those" and "that".

ENGLISH: AMERICAN OR BRITISH

17.9   American and British English differ in many minor ways in spelling (see sections 9.1 to 9.7) and vocabulary (for example: *gasoline* and *petrol*; *two weeks* and *fortnight*; *while* and *whilst*). Their medical vocabularies also differ in small ways: some terms for aspects of practice (for example: *office* or *clinic, consulting room* or *surgery*; *operating room, theatre*) and a few terms for disease (such as *chronic obstructive lung disease* and *chronic bronchitis*). In general, a journal should use the spelling and vocabulary of its main readership, including users of its text in an online database. Terms unfamiliar to database searchers can lead to the missing of papers relevant to their searches (also see section 9.4).

Editors must be careful, however, not to change terms in the medical and scientific vocabulary without the consent of authors. A compromise solution is giving the journal's preferred term within square brackets (see section 5.31) immediately after the first mentions in the abstract and the paper's text of the term that needs to be thus clarified.

ETHNIC TERMS

17.10   Do not use ethnic terms where they serve only to perpetuate or create unscientific, unnecessary, and sometimes derogatory associations.

NOT   A 22-year-old black man with sickle cell anemia came to the emergency room with . . .
BUT   A 22-year-old man with sickle cell anemia came to . . .
[Sickle cell anemia may be seen almost exclusively in "black" persons but its occurrence is associated with a particular genotype, not with being "black".]

In describing a new observation, an ethnic modifier may be justified, however, by the possibility that later observations will provide firmer evidence of a causal association of a disease or syndrome with a particular cultural, economic, or ethnic group. In many instances of reporting the cases of groups of patients ("case series"), the ethnic identifiers are meaningless without accompanying data on the ethnic makeup of the population from which they were sampled.

Any ethnic identifiers should be as precise as possible; justified identification of an American Indian, for example, might specify the tribe.

NOT   A 22-year-old American Indian came to the . . .
BUT   A 22-year-old man of the Cherokee tribe . . .

Do not use pseudoprecise ethnic terms. "Caucasian" (4) and "Afro-American" carry no more scientific precision than *white* and *black*, "oriental" no more than *Asian*.

Do not use an ethnic term widely regarded as derogatory by the group to which it applies.

For a thorough discussion of ethnic stereotyping and a list of terms with comments, see "Guidelines for Fair Representation of Minority Groups" in *Guidelines for Bias-Free Publishing* (5).

FOREIGN-LANGUAGE WORDS AND PHRASES

17.11   Some authors cannot resist affecting the posture of a "cultured man" by dropping foreign-language words and phrases into their English text. They forget that most readers of English-language journals know only English (and their own language if they are not anglophones). Such discourtesy should be cleaned up by substituting an equivalent English word or phrase if one is available.

For	Substitute
entre nous	between us
pari passu	together, at the same time
vis-à-vis	about, with regard to
weltschmerz	deep and broad pessimism, painful boredom

For recommendations on replacing abbreviations widely used in scholarly writing for Latin phrases, see section 11.2.

IDIOM: ERRORS OF NON-ANGLOPHONE AUTHORS

17.12   English can be a difficult language in which to write with clear and accurate but fluid style, even for writers born into English. For writers born into another language, English is filled with treacherous details. Two main types of errors in idioms are likely to turn up in generally good English prose written by non-anglophone authors: literal translations of words with a different meaning in English and use of unidiomatic prepositions, most often with verbs.

Erroneous literal translations may be baffling to the editor who does not know the original language. In French *actuel*, for example, means "present" and "current" and thus would be translated erroneously as "actual"; *journal* in French means "newspaper", "magazine", or "journal" but in English, "scholarly magazine" or "diary". The solution for the editor facing an unidiomatic or apparently erroneous word or phrase is to find the apparent cognate in a translating dictionary of the native language of the author and to convert the translated term to the apparently best English idiom.

Prepositions unidiomatic in English may represent the correct idiom in the language of origin. For example, "the natural history of diabetic nephropathy associated to diabetes type II" should read ". . . associated with . . ." but the "to" came from the proper idiom in Spanish. Two English dictionaries will be particularly helpful to non-anglophones in selecting the right prepositions, particularly those associated with verbs. *Chambers 20th Century Dictionary* (6) specifies in the entries for single-word verbs the various idiomatic verb forms that include prepositions as the second element. The *Oxford Dictionary of Current Idiomatic English: Volume 1: Verbs with Prepositions & Particles* (7) is even more thorough in its presentation of such verbs; it has, for example, no fewer than 36 separate entries for the various verb + preposition forms of *hold*.

JARGON AND SLANG

17.13   *Jargon* is the vocabulary and syntax idiomatic for a vocational or cultural group. Medicine has a jargon that seems unidiomatic to manuscript editors (British English, *subeditors*) without medical training but is acceptable usage for physicians and surgeons, even in formal prose.

> The patient left the operating room in good condition. [The surgeon means that at the end of the operation, the patient's blood pressure, pulse rate, respiratory rate, and other indicators showed no evidence of undesirable immediate consequences of the operation. The manuscript editor, not trained in surgery or any other field of medicine, imagines a picture of the patient getting down from the operating table, mopping the floor clean, tidying up in other ways, and walking out the door. In fact the surgeon has made a statement that is idiomatic and clear to other surgeons and would be acceptable in a formal case report.]

The type of idiom in this example is condensation; 3 other types often seen in medical jargon are inflation, euphemism, and the forming of verbs from nouns.

Inflation is the replacing of short, plain, and direct words and phrases with ones that are longer, fancier, and less direct.

outpatient clinic	ambulatory-care facility
medicine and nursing	health-care professions
use of new treatments	utilization of recently introduced therapeutic modalities
spit out blood	expectorated a hemorrhagic production
bled	hemorrhaged

Such words and phrases can usually be deflated but care must be taken not to distort the intended meaning.

Euphemism is the shift to a word or term that softens the reality of the original.

| He died. | He expired. |
| death or disability | adverse outcomes |

A constant tendency in medical jargon is the forming of verbs from nouns.

diagnosis	We diagnosed
intubation	He was intubated
endoscope	I endoscoped
catheter	She catheterized

Some verbs of this kind are acceptable in medical idiom but some are slang.

The editors of a journal should compile its own list of idioms that are acceptable, and even needed, in medical formal prose to be published and which clearly are not. Judgments on what is acceptable may be difficult. The standard medical dictionaries (see Appendix C) are safe guides; they tend to admit only those terms that are in wide use in medical journals and books

17.14 *Slang* in medicine is the informal jargon that is not acceptable in formal medical prose. This is the jargon that usually is confined to hospital-dining room talk and other private conversations among medical students, house officers, physicians, and nurses. The slang is a mixture of short forms of formal terms, thoughtless epithets, neologisms, and pejorative terms.

Slang term	Origin
lab	laboratory
prepped	prepared
cathed	catheterized
intracathed	introduced an intravenous catheter
diabetic leg	leg of a diabetic patient
crock	"a crock of shit"
gomer	"get out of my emergency room"

Some of the less offensive terms of this kind occasionally turn up in formal papers, usually in those from inexperienced authors. They must be replaced by equivalents from the vocabulary acceptable in formal prose.

Less obtrusive than slang terms but worth eliminating are the worn-out phrases (clichés).

These *clinical pearls* have *stood the test of time.*
Parathyroid hormone assay is *the gold standard.* [reference standard]
One must have a *high clinical index of suspicion* for brucellosis.

MODIFIERS: STACKED AND AMBIGUOUS

17.15 Two frequent kinds of defective modifiers are stacked modifiers and those ambiguous in reference, usually because of faulty position.

The increasing complexity of science has been leading to increasing difficulties in coining concise terms for new equipment and procedures. Occasionally a felicitous coinage that condenses a long term becomes quickly and well established: *laser* for "light amplification by stimulated emission of radiation". More likely is a coinage that piles up adjectives and nouns serving as adjectives in front of the modified noun; the greater the number of modifiers, the greater is the probability that readers will not know what modifies what.

> . . . and the human spermatozoa-zona-free hamster in-vitro penetration test is a suitable assay for these sperm functions. [A close reading of the context revealed that the modifiers were built from "human spermatozoa", "penetration of hamster eggs that are zona-free", and "in vitro test", but readers should not be burdened with untangling such complex constructions.]

Sometimes such constructions can be broken up into linked phrases with clearer sense.

> ORIGINAL   the sperm-cervical mucus interaction
> REVISED FORM   the interaction of sperm with cervical mucus

A general rule can be helpful in deciding which of such constructions to revise: No noun should have more than 2 modifiers preceding it. This rule may have to be broken at times but it helps in spotting modifiers that do need revising.

17.16 Careless placement of modifiers can produce unintended meaning.

> NOT   . . . the precise molecular defect in ataxia-telangiectasia is not known. [the defect is not "precise"]
> BUT   . . . the molecular defect in ataxia-telangiectasia is not precisely known.
> OR   The specific molecular defect . . . is not known

> normal dog hearts ["hearts of normal dogs" or "normal hearts from dogs"]

In general, modifiers (adjectives, adverbs) should be kept close to the element they modify.

> Recently a few cases of neurologic toxicity from acyclovir therapy have been reported.
> BETTER   A few cases of neurologic toxicity from acyclovir therapy have been reported recently.

The fault called "dangling participle" tends to occur when the participle is used at a distance from the noun it modifies (see section 17.22).

SEX REFERENCES

17.17 Accurate writers take pains not to use terms or pronouns of solely mas-
culine or feminine reference where both sexes are in fact being referred
to. The solutions, in general, are changing the explicit reference to both
sexes or revising to substitute a plural form.

> . . . is a problem for today's physician. He must respond by . . .
> BETTER   . . . for today's physician. He or she must respond by . . .
> . . . for today's physicians. They must respond by . . .

A closely related question is when to abandon needed terms based on
a stem with sex reference, for example, such words as "chairman" and
"housewife". Some solutions do violence to reasonable and euphonious
idiom. Great care should be taken not to choose solutions that are as
destructive of euphony for readers who prefer unobstrusive idiom as the
uncorrected problem is irritating to readers with agendas in sexual po-
litics. The best compromise may be the choice of a functional synonym.

> . . . was elected chairman of the committee.
> ONE SOLUTION   . . . was elected chair of the committee. [This popular so-
> lution burdens *chair* with a new meaning.]
> A BETTER SOLUTION   . . . was elected convenor [or *leader*, or *moderator*]
> of the . . .

Several thorough discussions of problems with sex references are available (5,8,9). One of these (9) points out that "in parliamentary usage,
chairman is the official term and should not be changed".

SPELLING ERRORS

17.18 Most spelling errors in medical writing arise from relying on a judgment
based on the sound of a word and ignoring its etymologic origin or failing
to check the spelling of an unfamiliar word. The first basis accounts for
many frequent misspellings.

> "concensus" for *consensus*
> "erythematosis" for *erythematosus*
> "flourescent" for *fluorescent*
> "gentamycin" for *gentamicin*
> "principle" for *principal* [and the reverse error]
> "prevelent" or "prevalant" for *prevalent*
> "mucous" for *mucus*
> "discreet" for *discrete* [and the reverse error]
> "supercede" for *supersede*

Unfamiliar words and names should have their spelling verified in a medical or general dictionary.

> guaiac   liaison   meiotic   Papanicolaou   trachelismus

A journal should build and maintain a list of words frequently misspelled by its authors and undetected as misspelled by its manuscript editors.

VOGUE WORDS AND PHRASES

17.19   Some words and phrases come into vogue and become widely used without regard to the lack of need for them or the imprecision of their use: "employ" and "utilize" for *use*; "parameter" for *variable, index*; "cost-effective" for *beneficial, efficient*; coinages with the suffix "-wise" as in "therapywise". Many of these misuses and pompous substitutes are discussed in section 17.4.

But some apparently voguish words have precise and well-established meanings; manuscript editors must take care not to substitute erroneously for an apparent "vogue word", a hazard particularly with some technical terms like *parameter* and *cost effective* (10).

As for frequently misspelled words (section 17.18), a journal should build and maintain a list of vogue words and phrases that turn up frequently.

GRAMMATICAL RULES AND SYNTAX

AGREEMENT IN NUMBER: SUBJECT AND PREDICATE

17.20   The grammatical rule that the number of subject and of predicate must agree tends to get violated when the number of the subject is misunderstood or obscured by a modifying phrase with plural elements.

> NOT   Data is accumulating which suggests that . . .
> BUT   Accumulating data suggest that . . .
> [The author forgot that *data* is a plural form of *datum*, or did he mean "The accumulation of data suggests that . . . ?]
>
> NOT   The simultaneous occurrence of thyrotoxicosis and renal failure have rarely been reported.
> BUT   The simultaneous occurrence of thyrotoxicosis and renal failure has rarely been reported.
> [The author forgot that "occurrence" is the subject of "has rarely been reported", not "thyrotoxicosis and renal failure".]

AGREEMENT IN NUMBER: PRONOUN AND ANTECEDENT;
AMBIGUOUS ANTECEDENT

17.21   An author may obscure the antecedent of a pronoun when the two are separated by too great a distance.

> . . . are great problems for the deans of medical schools. But in view of the massive financial problems facing entire universities, they must . . .

[The author intended "they" to refer to "deans" and overlooked "universities" as a probable antecedent, for most readers, of "they".]

MODIFIERS; DANGLING AND MISPLACED

17.22 One of the most frequent faults in medical prose is the dangling participle, a present or past participle opening a phrase but with the noun to which the phrase refers remaining unstated, unclear, or inappropriate. This fault tends to occur most frequently when the phrase is at the beginning of the sentence.

> Based on our experience using four different venous access ports we would like to make some suggestions for optimal use.
> [What is "based"? An opening phrase of this kind is usually expected to be modifying the immediately following subject of the sentence. But here the subject "we" is not "based"; "suggestions" is "based". Also note that it was not "experience" that was "using" anything; "we used access ports".]
>
> POSSIBLE CORRECT VERSIONS   We used four different venous-access ports and from this experience wish to make some suggestions for optimal use. *Or:* On the basis of our having used four different venous-access ports, we wish to make some suggestions for their optimal use. [which could be properly rearranged as "We, having used . . . , wish to make . . ."]

The same error can occur when the participle lies deep in the sentence.

> Patients receiving methotrexate showed greater improvement, based on degree of joint swelling and tenderness, duration of morning stiffness, and subjective assessments of clinical condition, than those receiving placebo. ["improvement" was not "based" on criteria for improvement; "improvement" was "judged" by criteria]
> REVISED: . . . showed greater improvement, judged by degree of . . . than those receiving placebo.
>
> We recently observed bronchospastic reactions in an asthmatic patient after ingesting this drug. ["We, after ingesting this drug, observed . . ."?]
> REVISED: We recently observed . . . reactions in a patient after his ingesting the drug. *Or:* . . . after he ingested the drug.

A frequently misplaced modifier is the adverb and preposition *above*, often placed before a noun as an adjective. Do not use *above* as an adjective; use it only as an adverb and in the correct position.

> NOT   The above criteria . . .
> BUT   The criteria mentioned above . . . [Here *above* serves properly as an adverb modifying the past-participial adjective *mentioned*.]
> OR   The criteria above are . . . ["mentioned" or "described" implied]

VERB TENSES

17.23 Be sure that verb tenses accurately reflect the sequence of events. The past perfect tense indicates an event in the past of a past event.

NOT When he arrived at the emergency room, he was comatose for 2 hours.
BUT When he arrived at the emergency room, he had been comatose for
2 hours.

Errors in choice of tense frequently occur in statements about studies and published papers. The past tense is appropriate for events completed in the past and now only of historical importance.

For 2 years Smith and Jones studied the prevalence of hypercalcemia in sarcoidosis.
[The study was completed and is not ongoing.]

In 1973 Smith and Jones (45) reported their study of hypercalcemia.
[Their report is now chiefly of historical interest.]

The present perfect tense expresses actions begun in the past and continuing, or completed but still relevant to a current issue.

For 2 years Smith and Jones have studied the hypercalcemia of sarcoidosis.
[They began their study 2 years ago and it is still going on.]

Smith and Jones (45) have reported that hypercalcemia has a high prevalence in sarcoidosis.
[They published their findings 2 years ago but the prevalence of hypercalcemia in sarcoidosis is still an issue and their "report" (paper) still exists as relevant to this issue.]

If a date or adverb sets an event in the past, use the past tense.

Recently Smith and Jones (45) confirmed that . . .
[The "confirmation" was in the study; the paper reported the confirmation. When as in the preceding example the report is not set in the past by a date or an adverb, the "confirmation" can be regarded as being in the paper and of ongoing relevance: "Smith and Jones (45) have confirmed that . . .".]

An action going on at present that is characteristic of its agent and will go on indefinitely into the future is expressed by the present tense.

Competent physicians take detailed histories and examine patients carefully.

But present actions that will come to an end are expressed by the present progressive tense.

Smith and Jones are studying the prevalence of hypercalcemia in sarcoidosis.
[The action is going on but will come to an end.]

The same principle applies to continuing actions that were going on at a past time or will be going on at a future specified time.

Smith and Jones were studying sarcoidosis when they discovered the vitamin D derivative.

When Smith and Jones get a renewal of their grant next year, they will be studying new derivatives of vitamin D.

A notably thorough but clear and concise summary of verb tenses can be found in Quirk and Greenbaum's *A Concise Grammar of Contemporary English* (11).

REFERENCES

1. Morris W. The American heritage dictionary of the English language. Boston: Houghton Mifflin; 1981.
2. Room A. The Penguin dictionary of confusibles. New York: Penguin Books; 1980.
3. Read H. English prose style. New York: Pantheon Books; 1952:15–22.
4. Freedman BJ. Caucasian. Br Med J. 1984;288:696–8.
5. McGraw-Hill Book Company. Guidelines for bias-free publishing. New York: McGraw-Hill; [undated].
6. Kirkpatrick EM, ed. Chambers 20th century dictionary. Cambridge: Cambridge University Press; 1983.
7. Cowie AP, Mackin R. Oxford dictionary of current idiomatic English; Volume 1: Verbs with prepositions & particles. London: Oxford University Press; 1975.
8. Miller C, Swift K. The handbook of nonsexist writing. New York: Barnes & Noble; 1981.
9. American Psychological Association. Publication manual of the American Psychological Association. 3rd ed. Washington: American Psychological Association; 1983:43–9.
10. Doubilet P, Weinstein MC, McNeil BJ. Use and misuse of the term "cost-effective" in medicine. N Engl J Med. 1986;314:253–5.
11. Quirk R, Greenbaum S. A concise grammar of contemporary English. New York: Harcourt Brace Jovanovich; 1973:40–58.

Appendix A

Implementation of SI Units for Clinical Laboratory Data

Style Specifications and Conversion Tables

by Donald S Young, MB, PhD

INTRODUCTION

SI units are now used in many countries to report clinical laboratory data. Through 1987 and 1988 these units will be introduced to replace the various units that have been used until now to report laboratory information in the United States. This action, which has been initiated by the Medical and Health Coordinating Group of the American National Metric Council and endorsed by many professional societies including the American Medical Association, will lead to the reporting of clinical laboratory data in molar terms with the liter as the reference volume.

WHAT ARE SI UNITS?

"SI units" is the abbreviation for *le Système international d'Unités*. These units are the result of over a century of international cooperation to develop a universally acceptable system of units of measurement. The SI is an outgrowth

This document has been prepared by the Medical and Health Coordinating Group of the American National Metric Council and is recommended for adoption and use by health-care journals as part of a phased shift to the use of SI units. It is published here with the permission of the American National Metric Council, a private, nonprofit focal point for metric information, planning, coordinating, and government liaison activities.

Dr Young is Chairman, Laboratory Medicine Sector Committee, American National Metric Council, and Director, William Pepper Laboratory, Department of Pathology and Laboratory Medicine, Hospital of the University of Pennsylvania (3400 Spruce Street/2 Gibson, Philadelphia, PA 19104, USA).

For additional recommendations on SI units and their usage, see sections 13.12 to 13.18. Chapter 16 covers SI units in several specific fields: pharmacology, section 16.58; pulmonary medicine and respiratory physiology, section 16.61 and Table 16.20; and radiology, section 16.62 and Table 16.21. These recommendations in the chapters of this manual do not carry the endorsement of the American National Metric Council but are consistent with the recommendations in this appendix.

of the metric system that has been widely used throughout most of the world but which has had little impact outside scientific fields in the United States, even though Congress passed the Metric Conversion Act in 1975 which endorsed the SI.

The SI is a uniform system of reporting numerical values permitting interchangeability of information between nations and between disciplines. The SI not only provides a coherent system of units, but also ensures that units are uniform in concept and style. A coherent system is one in which interconversions between the units for different properties require the factor 1 only. With the SI, quantities can be more easily compared by means of the reduction in the number of multiples and submultiples in common use.

The SI has seven base units from which other units are derived. These seven cornerstones from which the other units have been developed are listed in Table A.1, together with the property or physical quantity to which they refer and their official symbol. Appropriate combinations of these base units can be made to express any property although, for simplicity, special names are given to some of the derived units. Representative examples are illustrated in Table A.2.

If only base units were used to report clinical laboratory data, some test values would be either unmanageably large or small. The SI uses a series of prefixes to the base unit to form decimal multiples and submultiples. The preferred multiples and submultiples change the quantity by increments of 10^3 or 10^{-3} as illustrated in Table A.3, but some increments or decrements of less than these factors are occasionally used. These exceptions are included in the box outlined in the

Table A.1: Base units of SI

Physical quantity	Base unit	SI symbol
length	meter	m
mass	kilogram	kg
time	second	s
amount of substance	mole	mol
thermodynamic temperature	kelvin	K
electric current	ampere	A
luminous intensity	candela	cd

Table A.2: Representative derived units

Derived unit	Name and symbol	Derivation from base units	
area	square meter	m^2	
volume	cubic meter	m^3	
force	newton (N)	$kg \cdot m \cdot s^{-2}$	
pressure	pascal (Pa)	$kg \cdot m^{-1} \cdot s^{-2}$	(N/m^2)
work, energy	joule (J)	$kg \cdot m^2 \cdot s^{-2}$	$(N \cdot m)$
mass density	kilogram per cubic meter	kg/m^3	
frequency	hertz (Hz)	s^{-1}	

Table A.3: Prefixes and symbols for decimal multiples and submultiples

Factor	Prefix	Symbol
10^{18}	exa	E
10^{15}	peta	P
10^{12}	tera	T
10^{9}	giga	G
10^{6}	mega	M
10^{3}	kilo	k
10^{2}	hecto	h
10^{1}	deka	da
10^{-1}	deci	d
10^{-2}	centi	c
10^{-3}	milli	m
10^{-6}	micro	μ
10^{-9}	nano	n
10^{-12}	pico	p
10^{-15}	femto	f
10^{-18}	atto	a

NOTE: Factors included in the rectangle do not conform to the preferred incremental changes of 10^{3} and 10^{-3} but are still used outside medicine.

table. The symbol for the prefix must be written as in the table and associated without a space with the unit: thus, kilopascal or kPa. For historical reasons the base unit for mass is the kilogram (kg). No prefixes may be combined with this base unit. One thousand kilograms is thus spoken of as 1 megagram (Mg) rather than as 1 kilokilogram. Although the correct symbol for micro is μ, it is proposed that u be accepted for use with automatic data processing systems at present.

The SI dictates certain matters of style. Thus symbols are printed in lowercase roman letters except when the name of a unit is derived from a proper name. When a unit derived from a proper name is written in full, not even the first letter is capitalized. The unit for pressure is accordingly pascal but is abbreviated to Pa. L, however, is now an accepted symbol for liter although it is not a proper name. This deviation from normal practice has been done to prevent confusion between the lowercase letter "l" and the numeral "1" which are the same or closely similar in certain type fonts. SI symbols are never followed by a period, except at the end of a sentence, and never pluralized. A name should not be combined with a symbol. When two or more names or symbols are used together, they should either be spelled out in full or in abbreviated form, but when measured values are printed it is preferable to use symbols for units rather than their complete names. A space must be left between a numeral and symbol, e.g., 50 mL and 37 °C. The product of two or more units is indicated by a dot above the line to distinguish it from a decimal point placed on the line. A zero should be placed

Table A.4: SI style specifications

Specifications	Example	Incorrect style	Correct style
Use lower case for symbols or abbreviations	kilogram	Kg	kg
Exceptions:	kelvin	k	K
	ampere	a	A
	liter	l	L
Symbols are not followed by period Exception: end of sentence	meter mole	m. mol.	m mol
Do not pluralize symbols	kilograms meters	kgs ms	kg m
Names and symbols are not to be combined	force	kilogram·meter·s⁻²	kg·m·s⁻² kg·m/s²
When numbers are printed symbols are preferred		100 meters 2 moles	100 m 2 mol
Space between number and symbol		50ml	50 mL
The product of units is indicated by a dot above the line		kg × m/s²	kg·m·s⁻² kg·m/s²
Only one solidus (/) per expression		mmol/L/s	mmol/(L·s)
Place zero before decimal		.01	0.01
Decimal numbers are preferable to fractions		3/4 75%	0.75 0.75
Spaces are used to separate long numbers		1,500,000	1 500 000
Exception: optional with four digit number		1,000	1000 or 1 000

before a decimal point in a numerical value and decimal numbers should be used in preference to fractions. Spaces should be used to separate long numbers into segments of 3 in both directions from the decimal point; a space is optional with 4-digit numbers. Commas should not be used so as to avoid possible confusion with the decimal point, which may be indicated by a comma in some European countries. These style requirements are summarized in Table A.4.

SI UNITS IN MEDICINE

The immediate rationale for reporting laboratory test data in SI units is that this is common practice in much of the world where such units are used on a daily basis in patient-care and in publications from research and other studies.

Nevertheless, the underlying reason for a change to SI units is that biological components react in vivo on a molar basis. When all data are expressed in uniform units relating to the actual amount of reactants in moles, a better understanding of the relative amounts of constituents of body fluids and of biological processes and of the interrelationships between different metabolic cycles is possible. When analytes are expressed in mass concentration units, for example, mg, regardless of the denominator or concentration unit, the relative amounts of the substances are obscured. There is seemingly 200 times as much albumin as bilirubin in the icteric neonate who has a serum bilirubin concentration of 20.0 mg/dL and an albumin concentration of 4.0 g/dL. Yet, there is only 1.7 times as much when these same concentrations are stated in molar terms, 340 μmol/L for bilirubin and 580 μmol/L for albumin. The influence of albumin concentration on the binding of bilirubin and other compounds, and the displacement of one compound by another, becomes more apparent.

With the use of SI it is possible to relate the amounts of reactants in different metabolic cycles involving, for example, amino acids, carbohydrates, and fats to each other. It is also possible to see the association of related compounds or metabolites in different tissues, for example, hemoglobin in erythrocytes and plasma, bilirubin and iron in plasma, together with urobilinogen in urine and feces.

IMPACT OF SI UNITS ON CURRENT MEDICAL PRACTICE

Although the SI allows the reporting of laboratory data in terms of mass concentration, use of mass units such as mg/L does not indicate the physiologically important amount of an analyte. To do this, units related to the amount of a substance must be used. These are expressed in terms of moles per liter. Although, by derivation, the cubic meter (m^3) should be the reference unit of volume, the liter (symbol L), a special name for cubic decimeter (dm^3), has now been accepted as the reference volume. The major changes affecting the reporting of clinical laboratory data are therefore referencing all values to the liter instead of units such as microliter (μL) or deciliter (dL) or 100 mL, and the concept of amount of substance which implies that a measured component will be described in moles or its subunits rather than in mass terms, for example, grams or milligrams. When the molecular mass of a compound is unknown, its concentration will continue to be reported in mass terms. See Table A.7.

The SI uses pascal (Pa) as the unit of pressure, but at present this unit is not recommended to report blood pressure. Nevertheless, it is accepted as the unit for partial pressures of gases instead of mmHg. The second (s) is the reference unit of time as this is the SI base unit, rather than the often used minute. Although not an SI unit, day (d) is still accepted for long periods of time rather than multiples of the second. The unit katal, abbreviated kat, corresponding to mol/s has been proposed as a special name to report catalytic activity. The Medical and Health Co-ordinating Group of the American National Metric Council recommends the use of kat/L to report enzyme activity because of the complexity of the official unit $mol \cdot s^{-1} \cdot L^{-1}$ or $mol/(s \cdot L)$ which is difficult both to write and for a computer to print. The new kat/L will replace international units per liter (U/L) as well as the plethora of units based on individuals' names. For those substances whose activity has been reported in terms of standardized biological units, for example, hormones, the same units should contiue to be used but with the liter as reference volume.

Thus, the immediate impact on the practice of medicine that implementation of reporting test values in SI units will have is the production of numbers that will initially be unfamiliar to the clinician. When mass concentrations are used, the values will generally be 10 times those with which physicians were familiar.

Implementation of SI units in many other countries has not been associated with problems for patients. Likewise, it should not be a problem in the United States provided all numerical data are *unequivocally* associated with their units. Additionally, it is recommended that numerical values on patient specimens be presented with the appropriate reference range or interval (normal values), at least until physicians have generally become accustomed to SI units.

SPECIAL SITUATIONS

HEMATOLOGY

With the reference volume becoming the liter, cell count values will increase by 10^6 from those obtained with μL or mm^3 as reference volume. However, the numerical values will remain the same if the multiplication factor is included as part of the unit, e.g., $\times 10^6/L$. Although much debate has centered on the reporting of hemoglobin concentrations with mass concentration (g/L) as well as substance concentration with both the monomer, Hb(Fe), and tetramer, Hb(4Fe), being advocated at different times, the International Committee for Standardization in Hematology (ICSH) indicates greater support for expressing hemoglobin as substance concentration in terms of the monomer. At least for the time being, MHCG recommends continued use of mass measurement of hemoglobin concentrations so the reporting unit is g/L.

With the SI, the concept of number fraction replaces percentage. Thus for mass fraction, volume fraction, and relative quantitites the unit 1 is used to replace former units. A hematocrit of 45% is reported as 0.45. When electrophoresis of hemoglobin or other blood constituents is done, each component should be reported as a mass fraction, e.g., 0.20 rather than 20%. Likewise, the number of cells in a peripheral smear or bone-marrow differential should be expressed as a number fraction of the total number of cells counted.

MICROBIOLOGY

Measurements of antibiotics both in serum and as inhibitory concentrations for growth of organisms in the clinical laboratory should be reported in molar units as for other drugs measured in the clinical laboratory. Colony counts should be referenced to the liter as unit of volume; the numerical value will remain unchanged. Bacteria counts on solid media should be referenced to the gram as denominator unit.

CLINICAL CHEMISTRY

Although drugs may continue to be administered in mass units, their concentrations in body fluids should be reported in molar terms so that these may be understood in relation to the concentration of other analytes. In the long term it is anticipated that drugs will also be administered in molar quantities. A difference in units for administered and measured drugs is not likely to lead to problems as the amount of drug absorbed and active in vivo is substantially different from the amount ingested when given orally. There is a greater rationale for using the same molar units when drugs are given intramuscularly or intravenously.

Although not an SI unit, the osmole should continue to be used for measurements of osmotic pressure rather than a recorded freezing point depression so that clinical understanding is not lessened; results should be expressed in terms of mol/kg. Hormone concentrations should be reported in terms of substance concentration, where possible, but if reported in terms of biological activity, international units (IU) should be used as before but with the liter as reference volume. Where the molecular mass of hormones or proteins is known then the concentrations of these constituents should be reported in moles in preference to grams or their submultiples.

STANDARDIZED REPORTING

Although the SI is only concerned with units of measurement, a major change in reporting practice provides the opportunity to standardize other practices. Certain abbreviations for tissues have been accepted to describe the material on which measurements have been made in many of the countries in which SI units have been adopted. It is proposed that the same abbreviations be implemented in the United States simultaneously with the introduction of SI units. These are illustrated in Table A.5. However, MHCG recommends that instead of describing a test as, e.g., S-glucose or U-calcium, the tests should be stated as glucose (S) and calcium (U), with a single space between the test name and the first parenthesis mark. This practice highlights the analyte that is measured, rather than the fluid, and recognizes current reporting practices where most results are grouped by fluid analyzed. It also facilitates computerized retrieval and display of data.

Various prefixes to provide complete definition of a material have also been accepted. These are also included in Table A.5. They are used without a space with the abbreviation for a "system" or tissue, e.g., aB for arterial blood.

It is recognized that several units are likely to continue in daily use even

Table A.5: Recommended abbreviations for tissues and descriptive prefixes

Amf	amniotic fluid	S	serum
B	blood	Semf	seminal fluid
Df	duodenal fluid	Sf	spinal fluid
Erc	erythrocyte (Ercs = plural)	Synf	synovial fluid
F	feces	T	tissue
Gf	gastric fluid	U	urine
H	hair	a	arterial
Lkc	leukocyte (Lkcs = plural)	c	capillary
P	plasma	d	day (24 h)
Perf	peritoneal fluid	f	fasting
Plf	pleural fluid	v	venous
Pt	patient		

NOTE: Several of these abbreviations were first used in Canada and have not been used in other countries.

though they do not conform to the SI and their use in medical practice is discouraged. Standardized symbols have been developed for various units of time. These are listed in Table A.6.

CONVERSION FACTORS

Tables A.7 [clinical chemistry] and A.8 [clinical hematology] list test names and the fluid in which measurements are made together with a typical normal range or reference interval in traditional units. The multiplication factor to convert from current metric to SI units is listed, as is the same reference interval in SI units with the correct symbols for SI units. To convert from SI to conventional units the numerical value in SI units is divided by the conversion factor. Tables A.7 and A.8 also list the appropriate number of significant digits and suggested minimal reporting increments to use so that no greater precision than pertains currently is implied in the data reported in SI units. The reporting intervals and suggested increments are related to the current level of imprecision in the relevant analytical procedures and are not necessarily clinically relevant. The test names listed are preferred over those sometimes used to describe the same ana-

Table A.6: Correct abbreviations of non-SI units of time

min	minute
h	hour
d	day
wk	week
mo	month
y	year

lyte as they reflect the state of the analyte under physiological conditions, for example, lactate dehydrogenase rather than lactic dehydrogenase, and pyruvate rather than pyruvic acid.

Note that the reference intervals cited in Tables A.7 and A.8, particularly those related to enzyme measurements, may be method dependent and should not be applied uncritically to the data obtained in any laboratory without verification that they are appropriate.

ACKNOWLEDGMENTS

Much of the material included here has been based on *The SI Manual in Health Care*, second edition, prepared by the Subcommittee of Metric Commission Canada, Sector 9.10 Health and Welfare, under the chairmanship of Mrs Genevieve Wilson. This publication includes a comprehensive section on SI units in hematology and clinical chemistry prepared by Dr M J McQueen.

Table A.7: SI units for clinical chemistry

Component	Present reference intervals (examples)	Present unit	Conversion factor	SI reference intervals	SI unit symbol	Significant digits	Suggested minimum increment
acetaminophen (P) – toxic	>5.0	mg/dL	66.16	>330	µmol/L	XX0	10 µmol/L
acetoacetate (S)	0.3–3.0	mg/dL	97.95	30–300	µmol/L	XX0	10 µmol/L
acetone (B,S)	0	mg/dL	172.2	0	µmol/L	XX0	10 µmol/L
acid phosphatase (S)	0–5.5	U/L	16.67	0–90	nkat/L	XX	2 nkat/L
adrenocorticotropin [ACTH] (P)	20–100	pg/mL	0.2202	4–22	pmol/L	XX	1 pmol/L
alanine aminotransferase [ALT] (S)	0–35	U/L	0.01667	0–0.58	µkat/L	X.XX	0.02 µkat/L
albumin (S)	4.0–6.0	g/dL	10.0	40–60	g/L	XX	1 g/L
aldolase (S)	0–6	U/L	16.67	0–100	nkat/L	XX0	20 nkat/L
aldosterone (S)							
normal salt diet	8.1–15.5	ng/dL	27.74	220–430	pmol/L	XX0	10 pmol/L
restricted salt diet	20.8–44.4	ng/dL	27.74	580–1240	pmol/L	XX0	10 pmol/L
aldosterone (U)– sodium excretion							
= 25 mmol/d	18–85	µg/24 h	2.774	50–235	nmol/d	XXX	5 nmol/d
= 75–125 mmol/d	5–26	µg/24 h	2.774	15–70	nmol/d	XXX	5 nmol/d
= 200 mmol/d	1.5–12.5	µg/24 h	2.774	5–35	nmol/d	XXX	5 nmol/d
alkaline phosphatase (S)	30–120	U/L	0.01667	0.5–2.0	µkat/L	X.X	0.1 µkat/L
alpha$_1$-antitrypsin (S)	150–350	mg/dL	0.01	1.5–3.5	g/L	X.X	0.1 g/L
alpha-fetoprotein (S)	0–20	ng/mL	1.00	0–20	µg/L	XX	1 µg/L
alpha-fetoprotein (Amf)	Depends on gestation	mg/dL	10	Depends on gestation	mg/L	XX	1 mg/L
alpha$_2$-macroglobulin (S)	145–410	mg/dL	0.01	1.5–4.1	g/L	X.X	0.1 g/L
aluminum (S)	0–15	µg/L	37.06	0–560	nmol/L	XX0	10 nmol/L

Table A.7: (continued)

Component	Present reference intervals (examples)	Present unit	Conversion factor	SI reference intervals	SI unit symbol	Significant digits	Suggested minimum increment
amino acid fractionation (P)							
alanine	2.2–4.5	mg/dL	112.2	245–500	μmol/L	XXX	5 μmol/L
alpha-aminobutyric acid	0.1–0.2	mg/dL	96.97	10–20	μmol/L	XXX	5 μmol/L
arginine	0.5–2.5	mg/dL	57.40	30–145	μmol/L	XXX	5 μmol/L
asparagine	0.5–0.6	mg/dL	75.69	35–45	μmol/L	XXX	5 μmol/L
aspartic acid	0.0–0.3	mg/dL	75.13	0–20	μmol/L	XXX	5 μmol/L
citrulline	0.2–1.0	mg/dL	57.08	15–55	μmol/L	XXX	5 μmol/L
cystine	0.2–2.2	mg/dL	41.61	10–90	μmol/L	XXX	5 μmol/L
glutamic acid	0.2–2.8	mg/dL	67.97	15–190	μmol/L	XXX	5 μmol/L
glutamine	6.1–10.2	mg/dL	68.42	420–700	μmol/L	XXX	5 μmol/L
glycine	0.9–4.2	mg/dL	133.2	120–560	μmol/L	XXX	5 μmol/L
histidine	0.5–1.7	mg/dL	64.45	30–110	μmol/L	XXX	5 μmol/L
hydroxyproline	0–trace	mg/dL	76.26	0–trace	μmol/L	XXX	5 μmol/L
isoleucine	0.5–1.3	mg/dL	76.24	40–100	μmol/L	XXX	5 μmol/L
leucine	1.0–2.3	mg/dL	76.24	75–175	μmol/L	XXX	5 μmol/L
lysine	1.2–3.5	mg/dL	68.40	80–240	μmol/L	XXX	5 μmol/L
methionine	0.1–0.6	mg/dL	67.02	5–40	μmol/L	XXX	5 μmol/L
ornithine	0.4–1.4	mg/dL	75.67	30–400	μmol/L	XXX	5 μmol/L
phenylalanine	0.6–1.5	mg/dL	60.54	35–90	μmol/L	XXX	5 μmol/L
proline	1.2–3.9	mg/dL	86.86	105–340	μmol/L	XXX	5 μmol/L
serine	0.8–1.8	mg/dL	95.16	75–170	μmol/L	XXX	5 μmol/L
taurine	0.3–2.1	mg/dL	79.91	25–170	μmol/L	XXX	5 μmol/L
threonine	0.9–2.5	mg/dL	83.95	75–210	μmol/L	XXX	5 μmol/L
tryptophan	0.5–2.5	mg/dL	48.97	25–125	μmol/L	XXX	5 μmol/L
tyrosine	0.4–1.6	mg/dL	55.19	20–90	μmol/L	XXX	5 μmol/L
valine	1.7–3.7	mg/dL	85.36	145–315	μmol/L	XXX	5 μmol/L

Component	Conventional Reference Interval	Conventional Unit	Factor	SI Reference Interval	SI Unit	Significant Digits	SI Increment
amino acid nitrogen (P)	4.0-6.0	mg/dL	0.7139	2.9-4.3	mmol/L	X.X	0.1 mmol/L
amino acid nitrogen (U)	50-200	mg/24 h	0.07139	3.6-14.3	mmol/d	X.X	0.1 mmol/d
delta-aminolevulinate [as levulinic acid] (U)	1.0-7.0	mg/24 h	7.626	8-53	μmol/d	XX	1 μmol/d
amitriptyline (P,S)—therapeutic	50-200	ng/mL	3.605	180-720	nmol/L	XX0	10 nmol/L
ammonia (vP)							
as ammonia [NH_3]	10-80	μg/dL	0.5872	5-50	μmol/L	XXX	5 μmol/L
as ammonium ion [NH_4^+]	10-85	μg/dL	0.5543	5-50	μmol/L	XXX	5 μmol/L
as nitrogen [N]	10-65	μg/dL	0.7139	5-50	μmol/L	XXX	5 μmol/L
amylase (S)	0-130	U/L	0.01667	0-2.17	μkat/L	XXX	0.01 μkat/L
androstenedione (S)							
male >18 years	0.2-3.0	μg/L	3.492	0.5-10.5	nmol/L	XX.X	0.5 nmol/L
female >18 years	0.8-3.0	μg/L	3.492	3.0-10.5	nmol/L	XX.X	0.5 nmol/L
angiotensin converting enzyme (S)	<40	nmol/mL/min	16.67	<670	nkat/L	XX0	10 nkat/L
arsenic (H) [as As]	<1	μg/g (ppm)	13.35	<13	nmol/g	XX.X	0.5 nmol/g
arsenic (U) [as As] [as As_2O_3]	0-5	μg/24 h	13.35	0-67	nmol/d	XX	1 nmol/d
	<25	μg/dL	0.05055	<1.3	μmol/L	XX.X	0.1 μmol/L
ascorbate (P) [as ascorbic acid]	0.6-2.0	mg/dL	56.78	30-110	μmol/L	X0	10 μmol/L
aspartate aminotransferase [AST] (S)	0-35	U/L	0.01667	0-0.58	μkat/L	0.XX	0.01 μkat/L
barbiturate (S)—overdose total expressed as:	Depends on composition of mixture. Usually not known.						
phenobarbital		mg/dL	43.06		μmol/L	XX	5 μmol/L
sodium phenobarbital		mg/dL	39.34		μmol/L	XX	5 μmol/L
barbitone		mg/dL	54.29		μmol/L	XX	5 μmol/L
barbiturate (S)—therapeutic							
see phenobarbital							
see pentobarbital							
see thiopental							

Table A.7: *(continued)*

Component	Present reference intervals (examples)	Present unit	Conversion factor	SI reference intervals	SI unit symbol	Significant digits	Suggested minimum increment
bile acids, total (S) [as chenodeoxycholic acid]	Trace–3.3	μg/mL	2.547	Trace–8.4	μmol/L	X.X	0.2 μmol/L
cholic acid	Trace–1.0	μg/mL	2.448	Trace–2.4	μmol/L	X.X	0.2 μmol/L
chenodeoxycholic acid	Trace–1.3	μg/mL	2.547	Trace–3.4	μmol/L	X.X	0.2 μmol/L
deoxycholic acid	Trace–1.0	μg/mL	2.547	Trace–2.6	μmol/L	X.X	0.2 μmol/L
lithocholic acid	Trace	μg/mL	2.656	Trace	μmol/L	X.X	0.2 μmol/L
bile acids (Df) [after cholecystokinin stimulation]	14.0–58.0	mg/mL	2.547	35.0–148.0	mmol/L	XX.X	0.2 mmol/L
total as chenodeoxy-cholic acid	2.4–33.0	mg/mL	2.448	6.8–81.0	mmol/L	XX.X	0.2 mmol/L
cholic acid	4.0–24.0	mg/mL	2.547	10.0–61.4	mmol/L	XX.X	0.2 mmol/L
chenodeoxycholic acid	0.8–6.9	mg/mL	2.547	2.0–18.0	mmol/L	XX.X	0.2 mmol/L
deoxycholic acid	0.3–0.8	mg/mL	2.656	0.8–2.0	mmol/L	XX.X	0.2 mmol/L
lithocholic acid	0.1–1.0	mg/dL	17.10	2–18	μmol/L	XX	2 μmol/L
bilirubin, total (S)	0–0.2	mg/dL	17.10	0–4	μmol/L	XX	2 μmol/L
bilirubin, conjugated (S)	>120	mg/dL	0.1252	>15	mmol/L	XX	1 mmol/L
bromide (S), toxic	>150	mg/dL	0.09719	>15	mmol/L	XX	1 mmol/L
as bromide ion	>15	mEq/L	1.00	>15	mmol/L	XX	1 mmol/L
as sodium bromide	<3	μg/dL	0.08897	<0.3	μmol/L	X.X	0.1 μmol/L
cadmium (S)	<100	pg/mL	1.00	<100	ng/L	XXX	10 ng/L
calcitonin (S)	8.8–10.3	mg/dL	0.2495	2.20–2.58	mmol/L	X.XX	0.02 mmol/L
calcium (S)	8.8–10.0	mg/dL	0.2495	2.20–2.50	mmol/L	X.XX	0.02 mmol/L
male	8.8–10.2	mg/dL	0.2495	2.20–2.56	mmol/L	X.XX	0.02 mmol/L
female <50 y	4.4–5.1	mEq/L	0.500	2.20–2.56	mmol/L	X.XX	0.02 mmol/L
female >50 y	2.00–2.30	mEq/L	0.500	1.00–1.15	mmol/L	X.XX	0.01 mmol/L
calcium ion (S)	4.00–4.60	mg/dL	0.2495	1.00–1.15	mmol/L	X.XX	0.01 mmol/L

Component	Present reference intervals	Present unit	Factor	SI reference intervals	SI unit	Significant digits	Suggested minimum increment
calcium (U), normal diet	<250	mg/24 h	0.02495	<6.2	mmol/d	X.X	0.1 mmol/d
carbamazepine (P) – therapeutic	4.0–10.0	mg/L	4.233	17–42	µmol/L	XX	1 µmol/L
carbon dioxide content (B,P,S) [bicarbonate + CO_2]	22–28	mEq/L	1.00	22–28	mmol/L	XX	1 mmol/L
carbon monoxide (B) [proportion of Hb which is COHb]	<15	%	0.01	<0.15	1	0.XX	0.01
beta-carotenes (S)	50–250	µg/dL	0.01863	0.9–4.6	µmol/L	X.X	0.1 µmol/L
catecholamines, total (U) [as norepinephrine]	<120	µg/24 h	5.911	<675	nmol/d	XX0	10 mg/d
ceruloplasmin (S)	20–35	mg/dL	10.0	200–350	mg/L	XX0	10 mg/L
chlordiazepoxide (P) therapeutic	0.5–5.0	mg/L	3.336	2–17	µmol/L	XX	1 µmol/L
toxic	>10.0	mg/L	3.336	>33	µmol/L	XX	1 µmol/L
chloride (S)	95–105	mEq/L	1.00	95–105	mmol/L	XXX	1 mmol/L
chlorimipramine (P) [includes desmethyl metabolite]	50–400	ng/mL	3.176	150–1270	nmol/L	XX0	10 nmol/L
chlorpromazine (P)	50–300	ng/mL	3.136	150–950	nmol/L	XX0	10 nmol/L
chlorpropamide (P) – therapeutic	75–250	mg/L	3.613	270–900	µmol/L	XX0	10 µmol/L
cholestanol (P) – [as a fraction of total cholesterol]	1–3	%	0.01	0.01–0.03	1	0.XX	0.01
cholesterol (P) <29 years	<200	mg/dL	0.02586	<5.20	mmol/L	X.XX	0.05 mmol/L
30–39 years	<225	mg/dL	0.02586	<5.85	mmol/L	X.XX	0.05 mmol/L
40–49 years	<245	mg/dL	0.02586	<6.35	mmol/L	X.XX	0.05 mmol/L
>50 years	<265	mg/dL	0.02586	<6.85	mmol/L	X.XX	0.05 mmol/L
cholesterol esters (P) [as a fraction of total cholesterol]	60–75	%	0.01	0.60–0.75	1	0.XX	0.01
cholinesterase (S)	620–1370	U/L	0.01667	10.3–22.8	µkat/L	XX.X	0.1 µkat/L

Table A.7: *(continued)*

Component	Present reference intervals (examples)	Present unit	Conversion factor	SI reference intervals	SI unit symbol	Significant digits	Suggested minimum increment
chorionic gonadotrophin (P) [beta-HCG]	0 if not pregnant	mIU/mL	1.00	0 if not pregnant	IU/L	XX	1 IU/L
citrate (B) [as citric acid]	1.2–3.0	mg/dL	52.05	60–160	µmol/L	XXX	5 µmol/L
complement, C3 (S)	70–160	mg/dL	0.01	0.7–1.6	g/L	X.X	0.1 g/L
complement, C4 (S)	20–40	mg/dL	0.01	0.2–0.4	g/L	X.X	0.1 g/L
copper (S)	70–140	µg/dL	0.1574	11.0–22.0	µmol/L	XX.X	0.2 µmol/L
copper (U)	<40	µg/24 h	0.01574	<0.6	µmol/d	X.X	0.2 µmol/d
coproporphyrins (U)	<200	µg/24 h	1.527	<300	nmol/d	XX0	10 nmol/d
cortisol (S)							
0800 h	4–19	µg/dL	27.59	110–520	nmol/L	XX0	10 nmol/L
1600 h	2–15	µg/dL	27.59	50–410	nmol/L	XX0	10 nmol/L
2400 h	5	µg/dL	27.59	140	nmol/L	XX0	10 nmol/L
cortisol, free (U)	10–110	µg/24 h	2.759	30–300	nmol/d	XX0	10 nmol/d
creatine (S)							
male	0.17–0.50	mg/dL	76.25	10–40	µmol/L	X0	10 µmol/L
female	0.35–0.93	mg/dL	76.25	30–70	µmol/L	X0	10 µmol/L
creatine (U)							
male	0–40	mg/24 h	7.625	0–300	µmol/d	XX0	10 µmol/d
female	0–80	mg/24 h	7.625	0–600	µmol/d	XX0	10 µmol/d
creatine kinase [CK] (S)	0–130	U/L	0.01667	0–2.16	µkat/L	X.XX	0.01 µkat/L
creatine kinase isoenzymes (S)– MB fraction	>5 in myocardial infarction	%	0.01	>0.05	1	0.XX	0.01
creatinine (S)	0.6–1.2	mg/dL	88.40	50–110	µmol/L	XX0	10 µmol/L
creatinine (U)	Variable	g/24 h	8.840	Variable	mmol/d	XX.X	0.1 mmol/d
creatinine clearance (S,U)	75–125	mL/min	0.01667	1.24–2.08	mL/s	X.XX	0.02 mL/s

$$\text{creatinine clearance corrected for body surface area} = \frac{\mu mol/L \ (\text{urine creatinine})}{\mu mol/L \ (\text{serum creatinine})} \times mL/s \times \frac{1.73}{A}$$

[where A is the body surface area in square metres (m²)]

cyanide (B) – lethal	>0.10	mg/dL	384.3	>40	µmol/L	XXX	5 µmol/L
cyanocobalamin (S) [vitamin B$_{12}$]	200–1000	pg/mL	0.7378	150–750	pmol/L	XX0	10 pmol/L
cyclic AMP (S)	2.6–6.6	µg/L	3.038	8–20	nmol/L	XXX	1 nmol/L
cyclic AMP (U)							
total urinary	2.9–5.6	µmol/g creat.	113.1	330–630	nmol/mmol creat.	XX0	10 nmol/mmol creatinine
renal tubular	<2.5	µmol/g creat.	113.1	<280	nmol/mmol creat.	XX0	10 nmol/mmol creatinine
cyclic GMP (S)	0.6–3.5	µg/L	2.897	1.7–10.1	nmol/L	XX.X	0.1 nmol/L
cyclic GMP (U)	0.3–1.8	µmol/g creat.	113.1	30–200	nmol/mmol creat.	XX0	10 nmol/mmol creatinine
cystine (U)	10–100	mg/24 h	4.161	40–420	µmol/d	XX0	10 µmol/d
dehydroepiandrosterone (P,S) [DHEA]							
1–4 years	0.2–0.4	µg/L	3.467	0.6–1.4	nmol/L	XX.X	0.2 nmol/L
4–8 years	0.1–1.9	µg/L	3.467	0.4–6.6	nmol/L	XX.X	0.2 nmol/L
8–10 years	0.2–2.9	µg/L	3.467	0.6–10.0	nmol/L	XX.X	0.2 nmol/L
10–12 years	0.5–9.2	µg/L	3.467	1.8–31.8	nmol/L	XX.X	0.2 nmol/L
12–14 years	0.9–20.0	µg/L	3.467	3.2–69.4	nmol/L	XX.X	0.2 nmol/L
14–16 years	2.5–20.0	µg/L	3.467	8.6–69.4	nmol/L	XX.X	0.2 nmol/L
premenopausal female	2.0–15.0	µg/L	3.467	7.0–52.0	nmol/L	XX.X	0.2 nmol/L
male	0.8–10.0	µg/L	3.467	2.8–34.6	nmol/L	XX.X	0.2 nmol/L
dehydroepiandrosterone (U)	*see* Steroids	Fractionation					
dehydroepiandrosterone sulphate [DHEA-S] (P,S)							
newborn	1670–3640	ng/mL	0.002714	4.5–9.9	µmol/L	XX.X	0.1 µmol/L
pre-pubertal children	100–600	ng/mL	0.002714	0.3–1.6	µmol/L	XX.X	0.1 µmol/L
male	2000–3350	ng/mL	0.002714	5.4–9.1	µmol/L	XX.X	0.1 µmol/L

Table A.7: (continued)

Component	Present reference intervals (examples)	Present unit	Conversion factor	SI reference intervals	SI unit symbol	Significant digits	Suggested minimum increment
female [premeno-pausal]	820–3380	ng/mL	0.002714	2.2–9.2	μmol/L	XX.X	0.1 μmol/L
female [post-menopausal]	110–610	ng/mL	0.002714	0.3–1.7	μmol/L	XX.X	0.1 μmol/L
pregnancy [term]	230–1170	ng/mL	0.002714	0.6–3.2	μmol/L	XX.X	0.1 μmol/L
11-deoxycortisol (S)	0–2	μg/dL	28.86	0–60	nmol/L	XX0	10 nmol/L
desipramine (P) – therapeutic	50–200	ng/mL	3.754	170–700	nmol/L	XX0	10 nmol/L
diazepam (P)							
therapeutic	0.10–0.25	mg/L	3512	350–900	nmol/L	XX0	10 nmol/L
toxic	>1.0	mg/L	3512	>3510	nmol/L	XX0	10 nmol/L
dicoumarol (P) – therapeutic	8–30	mg/L	2.974	25–90	μmol/L	XX	5 μmol/L
digoxin (P)							
therapeutic	0.5–2.2	ng/mL	1.281	0.6–2.8	nmol/L	X.X	0.1 nmol/L
	0.5–2.2	μg/L	1.281	0.6–2.8	nmol/L	X.X	0.1 nmol/L
toxic	>2.5	ng/mL	1.281	>3.2	nmol/L	X.X	0.1 nmol/L
dimethadione (P) – therapeutic	<1.00	g/L	7.745	<7.7	mmol/L	X.X	0.1 mmol/L
disopyramide (P) – therapeutic	2.0–6.0	mg/L	2.946	6–18	μmol/L	XX	1 μmol/L
doxepin (P) – therapeutic	50–200	ng/mL	3.579	180–720	nmol/L	XX0	10 nmol/L
electrophoresis, protein (S)							
albumin	60–65	%	0.01	0.60–0.65	1	0.XX	0.01
alpha₁-globulin	1.7–5.0	%	0.01	0.02–0.05	1	0.XX	0.01
alpha₂-globulin	6.7–12.5	%	0.01	0.07–0.13	1	0.XX	0.01
beta-globulin	8.3–16.3	%	0.01	0.08–0.16	1	0.XX	0.01
gamma-globulin	10.7–20.0	%	0.01	0.11–0.20	1	0.XX	0.01
albumin	3.6–5.2	g/dL	10.0	36–52	g/L	XX	1 g/L
alpha₁-globulin	0.1–0.4	g/dL	10.0	1–4	g/L	XX	1 g/L

beta-globulin	0.5-1.2	g/dL	10.0	5-12	g/L	XX	1 g/L
gamma-globulin	0.6-1.6	g/dL	10.0	6-16	g/L	XX	1 g/L
epinephrine (P)	31-95 (at rest for 15 min)	pg/mL	5.458	170-520	pmol/L	XX0	10 pmol/L
epinephrine (U)	<10	μg/24 h	5.458	<55	nmol/d	XX	5 nmol/d
estradiol (S) —male >18 years	15-40	pg/mL	3.671	55-150	pmol/L	XXX	1 pmol/L
estriol (U) [non-pregnant]							
onset of menstruation	4-25	μg/24 h	3.468	15-85	nmol/d	XXX	5 nmol/d
ovulation peak	28-99	μg/24 h	3.468	95-345	nmol/d	XXX	5 nmol/d
luteal peak	22-105	μg/24 h	3.468	75-365	nmol/d	XXX	5 nmol/d
menopausal women	1.4-19.6	μg/24 h	3.468	5-70	nmol/d	XXX	5 nmol/d
male	5-18	μg/24 h	3.468	15-60	nmol/d	XXX	5 nmol/d
estrogens (S) [as estradiol]							
female	20-300	pg/mL	3.671	70-1100	pmol/L	XXX0	10 pmol/L
peak production	200-800	pg/mL	3.671	750-2900	pmol/L	XXX0	10 pmol/L
male	<50	pg/mL	3.671	<180	pmol/L	XX0	10 pmol/L
estrogens, placental (U) [as estriol]	Depends on period of gestation	mg/24 h	3.468	Depends on period of gestation	μmol/d	XXX	1 μmol/d
estrogen receptors (T)							
negative	0-3	fmol estradiol bound/mg cytosol protein	1.00	0-3	fmol estradiol/ mg cytosol protein	XXX	1 fmol/mg protein
doubtful	4-10	fmol estradiol bound/mg cytosol protein	1.00	4-10	fmol estradiol/ mg cytosol protein	XXX	1 fmol/mg protein
positive	>10	fmol estradiol bound/mg cytosol protein	1.00	>10	fmol estradiol/ mg cytosol protein	XXX	1 fmol/mg protein

Table A.7: *(continued)*

Component	Present reference intervals (examples)	Present unit	Conversion factor	SI reference intervals	SI unit symbol	Significant digits	Suggested minimum increment
estrone (P,S)							
female 1–10 days of cycle	43–180	pg/mL	3.699	160–665	pmol/L	XXX	5 pmol/L
female 11–20 days of cycle	75–196	pg/mL	3.699	275–725	pmol/L	XXX	5 pmol/L
female 20–39 days of cycle	131–201	pg/mL	3.699	485–745	pmol/L	XXX	5 pmol/L
male	29–75	pg/mL	3.699	105–275	pmol/L	XXX	5 pmol/L
estrone (U)—female	2–25	μg/24 h	3.699	5–90	nmol/d	XXX	5 nmol/d
ethanol (P)							
legal limit [driving]	<80	mg/dL	0.2171	<17	mmol/L	XX	1 mmol/L
toxic	>100	mg/dL	0.2171	>22	mmol/L	XX	1 mmol/L
ethchlorvynol (P)—toxic	>40	mg/L	6.915	>280	μmol/L	XX0	10 μmol/L
ethosuximide (P)—therapeutic	40–110	mg/L	7.084	280–780	μmol/L	XX0	10 μmol/L
ethylene glycol (P)—toxic	>30	mg/dL	0.1611	>5	mmol/L	XX	1 mmol/L
fat (F) [as stearic acid]	2.0–6.0	g/24 h	3.515	7–21	mmol/d	XX	1 mmol/d
fatty acids, non-esterified (P)	8–20	mg/dL	10.00	80–200	mg/L	XX0	10 mg/L
ferritin (S)	18–300	ng/mL	1.00	18–300	μg/L	XX0	10 μg/L
fibrinogen (P)	200–400	mg/dL	0.01	2.0–4.0	g/L	X.X	0.1 g/L
fluoride (U)	<1.0	mg/24 h	52.63	<50	μmol/d	XX0	10 μmol/d
folate (S) [as pteroylglutamic acid]	2–10	ng/mL	2.266	4–22	nmol/L	XX	2 nmol/L
		μg/dL	22.66		nmol/L		2 nmol/L
folate (Erc)	140–960	ng/mL	2.266	550–2200	nmol/L	XX0	10 nmol/L

	Conventional Range	Conventional Unit	Factor	SI Range		SI Unit	Increment
follicle stimulating hormone [FSH] (P)							
female	2.0–15.0	mIU/mL	1.00	2–15	XX	IU/L	1 IU/L
peak production	20–50	mIU/mL	1.00	20–50	XX	IU/L	1 IU/L
male	1.0–10.0	mIU/mL	1.00	1–10	XX	IU/L	1 IU/L
follicle stimulating hormone [FSH] (U)							
follicular phase	2–15	IU/24 h	1.00	2–15	XXX	IU/d	1 IU/d
midcycle	8–40	IU/24 h	1.00	8–40	XXX	IU/d	1 IU/d
luteal phase	2–10	IU/24 h	1.00	2–10	XXX	IU/d	1 IU/d
menopausal women	35–100	IU/24 h	1.00	35–100	XXX	IU/d	1 IU/d
male	2–15	IU/24 h	1.00	2–15	XXX	IU/d	1 IU/d
fructose (P)	<10	mg/dL	0.05551	<0.6	X.XX	mmol/L	0.1 mmol/L
galactose (P) [children]	<20	mg/dL	0.05551	<1.1	X.XX	mmol/L	0.1 mmol/L
gases (aB)							
pO_2	75–105	mmHg (= Torr)	0.1333	10.0–14.0	XX.X	kPa	0.1 kPA
pCO_2	33–44	mmHg (= Torr)	0.1333	4.4–5.9	X.X	kPa	0.1 kPa
gamma-glutamyltransferase [GGT] (S)	0–30	U/L	0.01667	0–0.50	X.XX	μkat/L	0.01 μkat/L
gastrin (S)	0–180	pg/mL	1	0–180	XX0	ng/L	10 ng/L
globulins (S) [see immunoglobulins]							
glucagon (S)	50–100	pg/mL	1	50–100	XX0	ng/L	10 ng/L
glucose (P) – fasting	70–110	mg/dL	0.05551	3.9–6.1	XX.X	mmol/L	0.1 mmol/L
glucose (Sf)	50–80	mg/dL	0.05551	2.8–4.4	XX.X	mmol/L	0.1 mmol/L
glutethimide (P)							
therapeutic	<10	mg/L	4.603	<46	XX	μmol/L	1 μmol/L
toxic	>20	mg/L	4.603	>92	XX	μmol/L	1 μmol/L
glycerol, free (S)	<1.5	mg/dL	0.1086	<0.16	X.XX	mmol/L	0.01 mmol/L
gold (S) – therapeutic	300–800	μg/dL	0.05077	15.0–40.0	XX.X	μmol/L	0.1 μmol/L
gold (U)	<500	μg/24 h	0.005077	<2.5	X.X	μmol/d	0.1 μmol/d

Table A.7: *(continued)*

Component	Present reference intervals (examples)	Present unit	Conversion factor	SI reference intervals	SI unit symbol	Significant digits	Suggested minimum increment
growth hormone (P,S)							
male [fasting]	0.0–5.0	ng/mL	1.00	0.0–5.0	µg/L	XX.X	0.5 µg/L
female [fasting]	0.0–10.0	ng/mL	1.00	0.0–10.0	µg/L	XX.X	0.5 µg/L
haptoglobin (S)	50–220	mg/dL	0.01	0.50–2.20	g/L	X.XX	0.01 g/L
hemoglobin (B) [*see* Table A.8]							
male	14.0–18.0	g/dL	10.0	140–180	g/L	XXX	1 g/L
female	11.5–15.5	g/dL	10.0	115–155	g/L	XXX	1 g/L
homogentisate (U) [as homogentisic acid]	0	mg/24 h	5.947	0	µmol/d	XX	5 µmol/d
homovanillate (U) [as homovanillic acid]	<8	mg/24 h	5.489	<45	µmol/d	XX	5 µmol/d
beta-hydroxybutyrate (S) [as beta-hydroxybutyric acid]	<1.0	mg/dL	96.05	<100	µmol/L	XX0	10 µmol/L
5-hydroxyindoleacetate (U) [as 5-hydroxyindole acetic acid; 5 HIAA]	2–8	mg/24 h	5.230	10–40	µmol/d	XXX	5 µmol/d
17-alpha-hydroxy-progesterone (S,P)							
children	0.2–1.4	µg/L	3.026	0.5–4.5	nmol/L	XX.X	0.5 nmol/L
male	0.5–2.5	µg/L	3.026	1.5–7.5	nmol/L	XX.X	0.5 nmol/L
female	0.3–4.2	µg/L	3.026	1.0–13.0	nmol/L	XX.X	0.5 nmol/L
female, post-menopausal	0.3–1.7	µg/L	3.026	1.0–5.0	nmol/L	XX.X	0.5 nmol/L
hydroxyproline (U) 1 wk–1 y	55–220	mg/24 h/m²	7.626	420–1680	µmol/(d·m²)	XX0	10 µmol/(d·m²)

1–13 y	25–80	mg/24 h/m²	7.626	190–610	µmol/(d·m²)	XX0	10 µmol/(d·m²)
22–65 y	6–22	mg/24 h/m²	7.626	40–170	µmol/(d·m²)	XX0	10 µmol/(d·m²)
>65 y	5–17	mg/24 h/m²	7.626	40–130	µmol/(d·m²)	XX0	10 µmol/(d·m²)
immunoglobulins (S)							
IgG	500–1200	mg/dL	0.01	5.00–12.00	g/L	XX.XX	0.01 g/L
IgA	50–350	mg/dL	0.01	0.50–3.50	g/L	XX.XX	0.01 g/L
IgM	30–230	mg/dL	0.01	0.30–2.30	g/L	XX.XX	0.01 g/L
IgD	<6	mg/dL	10	<60	mg/L	XX0	10 mg/L
IgE							
0–3 years	0.5–10	IU/mL	2.4	1–24	µg/L	XX	1 µg/L
3–80 years	5–100	IU/mL	2.4	12–240	µg/L	XX	1 µg/L
imipramine (P)— therapeutic	50–200	ng/mL	3.566	180–710	nmol/L	XX0	10 nmol/L
insulin (P,S)	5–20	µU/mL	7.175	35–145	pmol/L	XXX	5 pmol/L
	5–20	mU/L	7.175	35–145	pmol/L	XXX	5 pmol/L
	0.20–0.84	µg/mL	172.2	35–145	pmol/L	XXX	5 pmol/L
iron (S)							
male	80–180	µg/dL	0.1791	14–32	µmol/L	XX	1 µmol/L
female	60–160	µg/dL	0.1791	11–29	µmol/L	XX	1 µmol/L
iron binding capacity (S)	250–460	µg/dL	0.1791	45–82	µmol/L	XX	1 µmol/L
isoniazid (P)							
therapeutic	<2.0	mg/L	7.291	<15	µmol/L	XX	1 µmol/L
toxic	>3.0	mg/L	7.291	>22	µmol/L	XX	1 µmol/L
isopropanol (P)	0	mg/dL	0.1664	0	mmol/L	XX	1 mmol/L
lactate (P) [as lactic acid]	0.5–2.0	mEq/L	1.00	0.5–2.0	mmol/L	X.X	0.1 mmol/L
	5–20	mg/dL	0.1110	0.5–2.0	mmol/L	X.X	0.1 mmol/L
lactate dehydrogenase (S)	50–150	U/L	0.01667	0.82–2.66	µkat/L	X.XX	0.02 µkat/L
lactate dehydrogenase isoenzymes (S)							
LD1	15–40	%	0.01	0.15–0.40	1	0.XX	0.01

Table A.7: (continued)

Component	Present reference intervals (examples)	Present unit	Conversion factor	SI reference intervals	SI unit symbol	Significant digits	Suggested minimum increment
LD2	20–45	%	0.01	0.20–0.45	1	0.XX	0.01
LD3	15–30	%	0.01	0.15–0.30	1	0.XX	0.01
LD4	5–20	%	0.01	0.05–0.20	1	0.XX	0.01
LD5	5–20	%	0.01	0.05–0.20	1	0.XX	0.01
LD1	10–60	U/L	0.01667	0.16–1.00	μkat/L	X.XX	0.02 μkat/L
LD2	20–70	U/L	0.01667	0.32–1.16	μkat/L	X.XX	0.02 μkat/L
LD3	10–45	U/L	0.01667	0.22–0.76	μkat/L	X.XX	0.02 μkat/L
LD4	5–30	U/L	0.01667	0.08–0.50	μkat/L	X.XX	0.02 μkat/L
LD5	5–30	U/L	0.01667	0.02–0.50	μkat/L	X.XX	0.02 μkat/L
lead (B)—toxic	>60	μg/dL	0.04826	>2.90	μmol/L	X.XX	0.05 μmol/L
		mg/dL	48.26		μmol/L	X.XX	0.05 μmol/L
lead (U)—toxic	>80	μg/24 h	0.004826	>0.40	μmol/d	X.XX	0.05 μmol/d
lidocaine (P) [Xylocaine]	1.0–5.0	mg/L	4.267	4.5–21.5	μmol/L	X.X	0.5 μmol/L
lipase (S)	0–160	U/L	0.01667	0–2.66	μkat/L	X.XX	0.02 μkat/L
lipids, total (P)	400–850	mg/dL	0.01	4.0–8.5	g/L	X.X	0.1 g/L
lipoproteins (P)							
low density [LDL]— as cholesterol	50–190	mg/dL	0.02586	1.30–4.90	mmol/L	X.XX	0.05 mmol/L
high density [HDL]— as cholesterol							
male	30–70	mg/dL	0.02586	0.80–1.80	mmol/L	X.XX	0.05 mmol/L
female	30–90	mg/dL	0.02586	0.80–2.35	mmol/L	X.XX	0.05 mmol/L
lithium ion (S)— therapeutic	0.50–1.50	mEq/L	1.00	0.50–1.50	mmol/L	X.XX	0.05 mmol/L
		μg/dL	0.001441		mmol/L	X.XX	0.05 mmol/L
		mg/dL	1.441		mmol/L		0.05 mmol/L
luteinizing hormone (S)							
male	3–25	mIU/mL	1.00	3–25	IU/L	XXX	1 IU/L
female	2–20	mIU/mL	1.00	2–20	IU/L	XXX	1 IU/L

Analyte	Present Reference Intervals	Present Unit	Conversion Factor	SI Reference Intervals	SI Unit Symbol	Significant Digits	Suggested Minimum Increment
peak production	30–140	mIU/mL	1.00	30–140	IU/L	XXX	1 IU/L
lysozyme (S) [muramidase]	1–15	µg/mL	1.00	1–15	mg/L	XXX	1 mg/L
lysozyme (U) [muramidase]	<2	µg/mL	1.00	<2	mg/L	XX	1 mg/L
magnesium (S)	1.8–3.0	mg/dL	0.4114	0.80–1.20	mmol/L	X.XX	0.02 mmol/L
	1.6–2.4	mEq/L	0.500	0.80–1.20	mmol/L	X.XX	0.02 mmol/L
	50–200	ng/mL	3.605	180–720	nmol/L	XX0	10 nmol/L
maprotiline (P) – therapeutic							
meprobamate (P) therapeutic	<20	mg/L	4.582	<90	µmol/L	XX0	10 µmol/L
toxic	>40	mg/L	4.582	>180	µmol/L	XX0	10 µmol/L
mercury (B) normal	<1.0	µg/dL	49.85	<50	nmol/L	XX0	10 nmol/L
chronic exposure	>20	µg/dL	0.04985	>1.00	µmol/L	X.XX	0.01 µmol/L
mercury (U) normal	<30	µg/24 h	4.985	<150	nmol/d	XX0	10 nmol/d
exposure – organic	>45	µg/24 h	4.985	>220	nmol/d	XX0	10 nmol/d
exposure – inorganic	>450	µg/24 h	0.004985	>2.20	µmol/d	XX.X	0.01 µmol/d
metanephrines (U) [as normetanephrine]	0–2.0	mg/24 h	5.458	0–11.0	µmol/d	XX.X	0.5 µmol/d
methanol (P)	0	mg/dL	0.3121	0	mmol/L	XX	1 mmol/L
methaqualone (P) therapeutic	<10	mg/L	3.995	<40	µmol/L	XX0	10 µmol/L
toxic	>30	mg/L	3.995	>120	µmol/L	XX0	10 µmol/L
methotrexate (S) – toxic	>2.3	mg/L	2.200	>5.0	µmol/L	X.X	0.1 µmol/L
methsuximide (P) (as desmethylsuximide) – therapeutic	10–40	mg/L	5.285	50–210	µmol/L	XX0	10 µmol/L
methyprylon (P) therapeutic	<10	mg/L	5.457	<50	µmol/L	XX0	10 µmol/L
toxic	>40	mg/L	5.457	>220	µmol/L	XX0	10 µmol/L
beta₂-microglobulin (S) – <50 y	0.80–2.40	mg/L	84.75	68–204	nmol/L	XXX	2 nmol/L

Table A.7: (*continued*)

Component	Present reference intervals (examples)	Present unit	Conversion factor	SI reference intervals	SI unit symbol	Significant digits	Suggested minimum increment
beta₂-microglobulin (U)—<50 y	<140	μg/24 h	0.08475	<12	nmol/d	XXX	2 nmol/L
nitrogen, total (U)	Diet dependent	g/24 h	71.38	Diet dependent	mmol/d	XX0	10 mmol/d
norepinephrine (P)	215–475 (at rest for 15 min)	pg/mL	0.005911	1.27–2.81	nmol/L	X.XX	0.01 nmol/L
norepinephrine (U)	<100	μg/24 h	5.911	<590	nmol/d	XX0	10 nmol/d
nortriptyline (P)—therapeutic	25–200	ng/mL	3.797	90–760	nmol/L	XX0	10 nmol/L
osmolality (P)	280–300	mOsm/kg	1.00	280–300	mmol/kg	XXX	1 mmol/kg
osmolality (U)	50–1200	mOsm/kg	1.00	50–1200	mmol/kg	XXX	1 mmol/kg
oxalate (U) [as anhydrous oxalic acid]	10–40	mg/24 h	11.11	110–440	μmol/d	XX0	10 μmol/d
palmitic acid (Amf)	Depends on gestation	mmol/L	1000	Depends on gestation	μmol/L	XXX	5 μmol/L
pentobarbital (P)	20–40	mg/L	4.419	90–170	μmol/L	XX	5 μmol/L
phenobarbital (P)—therapeutic	2–5	mg/dL	43.06	85–215	μmol/L	XXX	5 μmol/L
phensuximide (P)	4–8	mg/L	5.285	20–40	μmol/L	XX	5 μmol/L
phenylbutazone (P)—therapeutic	<100	mg/L	3.243	<320	μmol/L	XX0	10 μmol/L
phenytoin (P) therapeutic	10–20	mg/L	3.964	40–80	μmol/L	XX	5 μmol/L
toxic	>30	mg/L	3.964	>120	μmol/L	XX	5 μmol/L
phosphate (S) [as phosphorus, inorganic]	2.5–5.0	mg/dL	0.3229	0.80–1.60	mmol/L	X.XX	0.05 mmol/L
phosphate (U) [as phosphorus, inorganic]	Diet dependent	g/24 h	32.29	Diet dependent	mmol/d	XX.X	1 mmol/d

Component	Present Reference Intervals	Present Unit	Factor	SI Reference Intervals	SI Unit	Significant Digits	Suggested Minimum Increment
phospholipid phosphorus, total (P)	5–12	mg/dL	0.3229	1.60–3.90	mmol/L	X.XX	0.05 mmol/L
phospholipid phosphorus, total (Erc)	1.2–12	mg/dL	0.3229	0.40–3.90	mmol/L	X.XX	0.05 mmol/L
phospholipids (P)— substance fraction of total phospholipid							
phosphatidyl choline	65–70	% of total	0.01	0.65–0.70	1	0.XX	0.01
phosphatidyl ethanolamine	4–5	% of total	0.01	0.04–0.05	1	0.XX	0.01
sphingomyelin	15–20	% of total	0.01	0.15–0.20	1	0.XX	0.01
lysophosphatidyl choline	3–5	% of total	0.01	0.03–0.05	1	0.XX	0.01
phospholipids (Erc)— substance fraction of total phospholipid							
phosphatidyl choline	28–33	% of total	0.01	0.28–0.33	1	0.XX	0.01
phosphatidyl ethanolamine	24–31	% of total	0.01	0.24–0.31	1	0.XX	0.01
sphingomyelin	22–29	% of total	0.01	0.22–0.29	1	0.XX	0.01
phosphatidyl serine + phosphatidyl inositol	12–20	% of total	0.01	0.12–0.20	1	0.XX	0.01
lysophosphatidyl choline	1–2	% of total	0.01	0.01–0.02	1	0.XX	0.01
phytanic acid (P)	Trace–0.3	mg/dL	32.00	<10	μmol/L	XX	5 μmol/L
[human] placental lactogen (S) [HPL]	>4.0 (after 30 wk gestation)	μg/mL	46.30	>180	nmol/L	XX0	10 nmol/L
porphobilinogen (U)	0.0–2.0	mg/24 h	4.420	0–9.0	μmol/d	X.X	0.5 μmol/d
porphyrins							
coproporphyrin (U)	45–180	μg/24 h	1.527	68–276	nmol/d	XXX	2 nmol/d
protoporphyrin (Erc)	15–50	μg/dL	0.0177	0.28–0.90	μmol/L	X.XX	0.02 μmol/L
uroporphyrin (U)	5–20	μg/24 h	1.204	6–24	nmol/d	XX	2 nmol/d
uroporphyrinogen synthetase (Erc)	22–42	mmol/mL/h	0.2778	6.0–11.8	mmol/(L·s)	X.X	0.2 mmol/(L·s)

Table A.7: (*continued*)

Component	Present reference intervals (examples)	Present unit	Conversion factor	SI reference intervals	SI unit symbol	Significant digits	Suggested minimum increment
potassium ion (S)	3.5–5.0	mEq/L	1.00	3.5–5.0	mmol/L	X.X	0.1 mmol/L
		mg/dL	0.2558		mmol/L	X.X	0.1 mmol/L
potassium ion (U) [diet dependent]	25–100	mEq/24 h	1.00	25–100	mmol/d	XX	1 mmol/d
pregnanediol (U) normal	1.0–6.0	mg/24 h	3.120	3.0–18.5	µmol/d	XX.X	0.5 µmol/d
pregnancy	Depends on gestation						
pregnanetriol (U)	0.5–2.0	mg/24 h	2.972	1.5–6.0	µmol/d	XX.X	0.5 µmol/d
primidone (P) therapeutic	6.0–10.0	mg/L	4.582	25–46	µmol/L	XX	1 µmol/L
toxic	>10.0	mg/L	4.582	>46	µmol/L	XX	1 µmol/L
procainamide (P) therapeutic	4.0–8.0	mg/L	4.249	17–34	µmol/L	XX	1 µmol/L
toxic	>12.0	mg/L	4.249	>50	µmol/L	XX	1 µmol/L
N-acetylprocainamide (P)—therapeutic	4.0–8.0	mg/L	3.606	14–29	µmol/L	XX	1 µmol/L
progesterone (P) follicular phase	<2	ng/mL	3.180	<6	nmol/L	XX	2 nmol/L
luteal phase	2–20	ng/mL	3.180	6–64	nmol/L	XX	2 nmol/L
progesterone receptors (T) negative	0–3	fmol progesterone bound/mg cytosol protein	1.00	0–3	fmol progesterone bound/mg protein	XX	1 fmol/mg protein
doubtful	4–10	fmol progesterone bound/mg	1.00	4–10	fmol progesterone bound/mg	XX	1 fmol/mg protein

Analyte	Present Reference Intervals	Present Unit	Conversion Factor	SI Reference Intervals	SI Unit	Significant Digits	Suggested Minimum Increment
positive	>10	fmol progesterone bound/mg cytosol protein	1.00	>10	fmol progesterone bound/mg cytosol protein	XX	1 fmol/mg protein
prolactin (P)	<20	ng/mL	1.00	<20	µg/L	XX	1 µg/L
propoxyphene (P) – toxic	>2.0	mg/L	2.946	>5.9	µmol/L	X.X	0.1 µmol/L
propranolol (P) [Inderal] – therapeutic	50–200	ng/mL	3.856	190–770	nmol/L	XX0	10 nmol/L
protein, total (S)	6.0–8.0	g/dL	10.0	60–80	g/L	XX	1 g/L
protein, total (Sf)	<40	mg/dL	0.01	<0.40	g/L	X.XX	0.01 g/L
protein, total (U)	<150	mg/24 h	0.001	<0.15	g/d	X.XX	0.01 g/d
protriptyline (P)	100–300	ng/mL	3.797	380–1140	nmol/L	XX0	10 nmol/L
pyruvate (B) [as pyruvic acid]	0.30–0.90	mg/dL	113.6	35–100	µmol/L	XXX	1 µmol/L
quinidine (P) therapeutic	1.5–3.0	mg/L	3.082	4.6–9.2	µmol/L	X.X	0.1 µmol/L
toxic	>6.0	mg/L	3.082	>18.5	µmol/L	X.X	0.1 µmol/L
renin (P) normal sodium diet	1.1–4.1	ng/mL/h	0.2778	0.30–1.14	ng/(L·s)	X.XX	0.02 ng/(L·s)
restricted sodium diet	6.2–12.4	ng/mL/h	0.2778	1.72–3.44	ng/(L·s)	X.XX	0.02 ng/(L·s)
salicylate (S) [salicylic acid] – toxic	>20	mg/dL	0.07240	>1.45	mmol/L	X.XX	0.05 mmol/L
serotonin (B) [5-hydroxytryptamine]	8–21	µg/dL	0.05675	0.45–1.20	µmol/L	X.XX	0.05 µmol/L
sodium ion (S)	135–147	mEq/L	1.00	135–147	mmol/L	XXX	1 mmol/L
sodium ion (U)	Diet dependent	mEq/24 h	1.00	Diet dependent	mmol/d	XXX	1 mmol/d
Steroids							
17-hydroxycorticosteroids (U) [as cortisol] female	2.0–8.0	mg/24 h	2.759	5–25	µmol/d	XX	1 µmol/d
male	3.0–10.0	mg/24 h	2.759	10–30	µmol/d	XX	1 µmol/d

Table A.7: (*continued*)

Component	Present reference intervals (examples)	Present unit	Conversion factor	SI reference intervals	SI unit symbol	Significant digits	Suggested minimum increment
17-ketogenic steroids (U) [as dehydroepiandrosterone]							
female	7.0–12.0	mg/24 h	3.467	25–40	µmol/d	XX	1 µmol/d
male	9.0–17.0	mg/24 h	3.467	30–60	µmol/d	XX	1 µmol/d
17-ketosteroids (U) [as dehydroepiandrosterone]							
female	6.0–17.0	mg/24 h	3.467	20–60	µmol/d	XX	1 µmol/d
male	6.0–20.0	mg/24 h	3.467	20–70	µmol/d	XX	1 µmol/d
ketosteroid fractions (U)							
androsterone							
female	0.5–3.0	mg/24 h	3.443	1–10	µmol/d	XX	1 µmol/d
male	2.0–5.0	mg/24 h	3.443	7–17	µmol/d	XX	1 µmol/d
dehydroepiandrosterone							
female	0.2–1.8	mg/24 h	3.467	1–6	µmol/d	XX	1 µmol/d
male	0.2–2.0	mg/24 h	3.467	1–7	µmol/d	XX	1 µmol/d
etiocholanolone							
female	0.8–4.0	mg/24 h	3.443	2–14	µmol/d	XX	1 µmol/d
male	1.4–5.0	mg/24 h	3.443	4–17	µmol/d	XX	1 µmol/d
sulfonamides (B) [as sulfanilamide]– therapeutic	10.0–15.0	mg/dL	58.07	580–870	µmol/L	XX0	10 µmol/L
testosterone (P)							
female	0.6	ng/mL	3.467	2.0	nmol/L	XX.X	0.5 nmol/L
male	4.6–8.0	ng/mL	3.467	14.0–28.0	nmol/L	XX.X	0.5 nmol/L
theophylline (P)– therapeutic	10.0–20.0	mg/L	5.550	55–110	µmol/L	XX	1 µmol/L

	Present Reference Intervals	Present Unit	Factor	SI Reference Intervals	SI Unit	Significant Digits	Suggested Minimum Increment
thiocyanate (P) – (nitroprusside toxicity)	10.0	mg/dL	0.1722	1.7	mmol/L	X.XX	0.1 mmol/L
thiopental (P)	individual	mg/L	4.126	individual	µmol/L	XX	5 µmol/L
Thyroid tests							
thyroid stimulating hormone [TSH] (S)	2–11	µU/mL	1.00	2–11	mU/L	XX	1 mU/L
thyroxine [T₄] (S)	4.0–11.0	µg/dL	12.87	51–142	nmol/L	XXX	1 nmol/L
thyroxine binding globulin [TBG] (S) – [as thyroxine]	12.0–28.0	µg/dL	12.87	150–360	nmol/L	XX0	1 nmol/L
thyroxine, free (S)	0.8–2.8	ng/dL	12.87	10–36	pmol/L	XX	1 pmol/L
triiodothyronine [T₃] (S)	75–220	ng/dL	0.01536	1.2–3.4	nmol/L	X.X	0.1 nmol/L
T₃ uptake (S)	25–35	%	0.01	0.25–0.35	1	0.XX	0.01
tolbutamide (P) – therapeutic	50–120	mg/L	3.699	180–450	µmol/L	XX0	10 µmol/L
transferrin (S)	170–370	mg/dL	0.01	1.70–3.70	g/L	X.XX	0.01 g/L
triglycerides (P) [as triolein]	<160	mg/dL	0.01129	<1.80	mmol/L	X.XX	0.02 mmol/L
trimethadione (P) – therapeutic	<50	mg/L	6.986	<350	µmol/L	XX0	10 µmol/L
trimipramine (P) – therapeutic	50–200	ng/mL	3.397	170–680	nmol/L	XX0	10 nmol/L
urate (S) [as uric acid]	2.0–7.0	mg/dL	59.48	120–420	µmol/L	XX0	10 µmol/L
urate (U) [as uric acid]	Diet dependent	g/24 h	5.948	Diet dependent	mmol/d	XX	1 mmol/d
urea nitrogen (S)	8–18	mg/dL	0.3570	3.0–6.5	mmol/L urea	X.X	0.5 mmol/L
urea nitrogen (U)	12.0–20.0 diet dependent	g/24 h	35.700	450–700	mmol/d urea	XX0	10 mol/d
urobilinogen (U)	0.0–4.0	mg/24 h	1.693	0.0–6.8	µmol/d	X.X	0.1 µmol/d
valproic acid (P) – therapeutic	50–100	mg/L	6.934	350–700	µmol/L	XX0	10 µmol/L

Table A.7: *(continued)*

Component	Present reference intervals (examples)	Present unit	Conversion factor	SI reference intervals	SI unit symbol	Significant digits	Suggested minimum increment
vanillylmandelic acid [VMA] (U)*	<6.8	mg/24 h	5.046	<35	µmol/d	XX	1 µmol/d
vitamin A [retinol] (P,S)	10–50	µg/dL	0.03491	0.35–1.75	µmol/L	X.XX	0.05 µmol/L
vitamin B₁ [thiamine hydrochloride] (U)	60–500	µg/24 h	0.002965	0.18–1.48	µmol/d	X.XX	0.01 µmol/d
vitamin B₂ [riboflavin] (S)	2.6–3.7	µg/dL	26.57	70–100	nmol/L	XXX	5 nmol/L
vitamin B₆ [pyridoxal] (B)	20–90	ng/mL	5.982	120–540	nmol/L	XXXX	5 nmol/L
vitamin B₁₂ [cyanocobalamin] (P,S)	200–1000	pg/mL ng/dL	0.7378 7.378	150–750	pmol/L pmol/L	XX0	10 pmol/L
vitamin C [see ascorbate] (B,P,S)							
vitamin D₃ [cholecalciferol] (P)	24–40	µg/mL	2.599	60–105	nmol/L	XXX	5 nmol/L
25 OH-cholecalciferol	18–36	ng/mL	2.496	45–90	nmol/L	XXX	5 mmol/L
vitamin E [alpha-tocopherol] (P,S)	0.78–1.25	mg/dL	23.22	18–29	µmol/L	XX	1 µmol/L
warfarin (P)—therapeutic	1.0–3.0	mg/L	3.243	3.3–9.8	µmol/L	XX.X	0.1 µmol/L
xanthine (U)—hypoxanthine	5–30	mg/24 h mg/24 h	6.574 7.347	30–200	µmol/d µmol/d	XX0 XX0	10 µmol/d 10 µmol/d
D-xylose (B) [25 g dose]	30–40 (30–60 min)	mg/dL	0.06661	2.0–2.7 (30–60 min)	mmol/L	X.X	0.1 mmol/L
D-xylose excretion (U) [25 g dose]	21–31 (excreted in 5 h)	%	0.01	0.21–0.31 (excreted in 5 h)	1	0.XX	0.01
zinc (S)	75–120	µg/dL	0.1530	11.5–18.5	µmol/L	XX.X	0.1 µmol/L
zinc (U)	150–1200	µg/24 h	0.01530	2.3–18.3	µmol/d	XX.X	0.1 µmol/d

* This is a misnomer, but because of its popularity the name VMA has been retained in this publication. In many publications it is being referred to as 4-hydroxy-3-methoxy mandelic acid.

Table A.8: SI units for clinical hematology

Component	Present reference intervals (examples)	Present unit	Conversion factor	SI reference intervals	SI unit symbol	Significant digits	Suggested minimum increment
erythrocyte count (B)							
female	3.5–5.0	$10^6/mm^3$	1	3.5–5.0	$10^{12}/L$	X.X	$0.1\ 10^{12}/L$
male	4.3–5.9	$10^6/mm^3$	1	4.3–5.9	$10^{12}/L$	X.X	$0.1\ 10^{12}/L$
erythrocyte count (Sf)	0	mm^{-3}	1	0	$10^6/L$	XX	$1\ 10^6/L$
erythrocyte sedimentation rate [ESR] (BErc)							
female	0–30	mm/h	1	0–30	mm/h	XX	1 mm/h
male	0–20	mm/h	1	0–20	mm/h	XX	1 mm/h
hematocrit (BErcs) vol. fraction							
female	33–43	%	0.01	0.33–0.43	1	0.XX	0.01
male	39–49	%	0.01	0.39–0.49	1	0.XX	0.01
hemoglobin (B) mass concentration							
female	12.0–15.0	g/dL	10	120–150	g/L	XXX	1 g/L
male	13.6–17.2	g/dL	10	136–172	g/L	XXX	1 g/L
substance conc. Hb [Fe]							
female	12.0–15.0	g/dL	0.6206	7.45–9.30	mmol/L	XX.XX	0.05 mmol/L
male	13.6–17.2	g/dL	0.6206	8.45–10.65	mmol/L	XX.XX	0.05 mmol/L
leukocyte count (B) number fraction ["differential"]	3200–9800	mm^{-3}	0.001	3.2–9.8	$10^9/L$	XX.X	$0.1\ 10^9/L$
		%	0.01		1	0.XX	0.01
leukocyte count (Sf)	0–5	mm^{-3}	1	0–5	$10^6/L$	XX	$1\ 10^6/L$
mean corpuscular hemoglobin [MCH] (BErc)							
mass	27–33	pg	1	27–33	pg	XX	1 pg
amount of substance Hb [Fe]	27–33	pg	0.06206	1.70–2.05	fmol	X.XX	0.05 fmol

Table A.8: (continued)

Component	Present reference intervals (examples)	Present unit	Conversion factor	SI reference intervals	SI unit symbol	Significant digits	Suggested minimum increment
mean corpuscular hemoglobin concentration [MCHC] (BErc)							
mass concentration	33–37	g/dL	10	330–370	g/L	XX0	10 g/L
substance conc. Hb [Fe]	33–37	g/dL	0.6206	20–23	mmol/L	XX	1 mmol/L
mean corpuscular volume [MCV] (BErc) —erythrocyte volume	76–100	μm^3	1	76–100	fL	XXX	1 fL
platelet count (B)	130–400	$10^3/mm^3$	1	130–400	$10^9/L$	XXX	5 $10^9/L$
reticulocyte count (B)–	10,000–75,000	mm^{-3}	0.001	10–75	$10^9/L$	XX	1 $10^9/L$
adults number fraction	1–24	0/00 (number per 1000 erythrocytes)	0.001	0.001–0.024	1	0.XXXX	0.001
	0.1–2.4	%	0.001	0.001–0.024	1	0.XXX	0.001

Appendix B

Abbreviations and Unabbreviated Terms for Journal Titles in Bibliographic References

This appendix lists the abbreviated and unabbreviated terms to be used for journal titles in bibliographic references (see section 15.18). The terms have been derived from the abbreviation listing published annually in the National Library of Medicine's *List of Journals Indexed in Index Medicus* (1).

PROCEDURE FOR FORMING ABBREVIATED TITLES

In combining abbreviations to form the abbreviated versions of titles, prefatory articles and connectives are omitted (such as "the" and "of" in *The New England Journal of Medicine* and *Journal of the Tennessee Medical Association*; additional examples are *and, della, et, in*). Each abbreviated element is capitalized (also see section 15.18). A period is placed at the end of the abbreviated title to mark the close of the collective-title group of bibliographic elements (see sections 15.17 and 15.24 and Tables 15.1 and 15.2); periods are not used after each element of the abbreviated title.

The New England Journal of Medicine	N Engl J Med
Journal of the Tennessee Medical Association	J Tenn Med Assoc
Advances in Lipid Research	Adv Lipid Res
Archives des Maladies du Coeur et des Vaisseaux	Arch Mal Coeur

Single-word journal titles and some words within longer titles are not abbreviated: the journal titles *Blood, Circulation*, and *Gut*, for example, retain their full form; "Lipid" in the title *Advances in Lipid Research* illustrated above is not abbreviated but remains "Lipid".

Gut	Gut
Circulation	Circulation
BUT: Circulation Research	Circ Res

Note that the Abbreviation or Term columns in this appendix include some unabbreviated terms that represent the complete titles of some journals or unabbreviated terms to be used in abbreviated titles.

For a small number of titles some terminal elements may be dropped when no ambiguity would result (as for "Arch Mal Coeur" in the first group of examples above); check long titles in the *Index Medicus* list (1) for such omissions. The abbreviations of journal titles that are already abbreviations drop the unabbreviated part of the original title.

Advances in Nephrology from the Necker Hospital	Adv Nephrol
AJNR. American Journal of Roentgenology	AJNR
IMJ. Illinois Medical Journal	IMJ

Hyphenated terms are either combined or separated; see examples in the list. Slant lines are omitted. Diacritical marks (see Table 9.1) are omitted.

The list in this appendix is selective and omits some abbreviations, notably those for transliterations of words in Chinese and Japanese titles. Emphasis in the selection of terms has been put on those in the titles of journals adhering to the Vancouver agreement (see section 15.4) and other journals in the free world. The correct forms of abbreviated titles can be verified for a large number of journals in reference 1, but the list below and the principles set forth above can be used to construct abbreviated titles for journals not covered by *Index Medicus*.

The Library's abbreviations are based on the *International Standard ISO-4-1972: Documentation-International Code for the Abbreviation of Titles of Periodicals* (2).

Word	Abbreviation or Term	Word	Abbreviation or Term
Abnormal	Abnorm	Aeronautica	Aeronaut
Abuse	Abuse	Aesthetic	Aesthetic
Academia	Acad	Affairs	Aff
Academiae	Acad	Affective	Affective
Academie	Acad	African	Afr
Academy	Acad	Age	Age
Acoustical	Acoust	Ageing	Ageing
Acta	Acta	Agents	Agents
Actas	Actas	Aging	Aging
Actions	Actions	Agressologie	Agressologie
Activitas	Act	Air	Air
Acupuncture	Acupunct	AJNR	AJNR
Acute	Acute	AJR	AJR
Addiction	Addict	Akademie	Akad
Addictions	Addict	Aktuelle	Aktuel
Addictive	Addict	Alabama	Ala
Additives	Addit	Alaska	Alaska
Adolescence	Adolescence	Alcohol	Alcohol
Adolescent	Adolesc	Alcoholism	Alcohol
Advanced	Adv	Alergia	Alergia
Advancement	Adv	Allergie	Allerg
Advances	Adv	Allergologia	Allergol
Adverse	Adverse	Allergy	Allergy

Word	Abbreviation or Term	Word	Abbreviation or Term
Allied	Allied	AORN	AORN
AMB	AMB	Aparato	Apar
America	Am	Apheresis	Apheresis
American	Am	Appetite	Appetite
Anaesthesia	Anaesth	Applied	Appl
Anaesthesie	Anaesth	Arbeiten	Arb
Anaesthesiologica	Anaesthesiol	Archiv	Arch
Anaesthetist	Anaesthetist	Archive	Arch
Anaesthetists	Anaesth	Archives	Arch
Anais	An	Archivio	Arch
Anales	An	Archivos	Arch
Analgesia	Analg	Archivum	Arch
Analyst	Analyst	Archiwum	Arch
Analytical	Anal	Argentina	Argent
Anasthesie	Anasth	Arizona	Ariz
Anatomia	Anat	Arkansas	Arkansas
Anatomica	Anat	Army	Army
Anatomical	Anat	Arquivos	Arq
Anatomie	Anat	Arteriosclerosis	Arteriosclerosis
Anatomischer	Anat	Artery	Artery
Anatomistes	Anat	Arthritis	Arthritis
Anatomy	Anat	Artificial	Artif
Andrologia	Andrologia	Arzneimittel-	Arzneimittelforschung
Andrology	Androl	forschung	
Anestesiologica	Anestesiol	Arztliche	Artzl
Anaestesiologia	Anestesiol	ASDC	ASDC
Anesthesia	Anesth	ASHA	ASHA
Anesthesie	Anesth	Asian	Asian
Anesthesiologie	Anesthesiol	Asia-Oceania	Asia Oceania
Anesthesiology	Anesthesiology	Asociacion	Asoc
Angeiologie	Angeiol	Assessment	Assess
Angewandte	Angew	Association	Assoc
Angiologia	Angiologia	Asthma	Asthma
Angiology	Angiology	Ateneo	Ateneo
Angle	Angle	Atherosclerosis	Atherosclerosis
Animal	Anim	Audiology	Audiology
Ankle	Ankle	Audiovisual	Audiov
Annales	Ann	Auditory	Aud
Annali	Ann	Auris	Auris
Annals	Ann	Australia	Aust
Annee	Annee	Australian	Aust
Annual	Annu	Austriaca	Austriaca
ANS	ANS	Autism	Autism
Anthropogenetica	Anthropogenet	Autonomic	Auton
Anthropologischer	Anthropol	Avian	Avian
Anthropology	Anthropol	Aviation	Aviat
Antibiotics	Antibiot	Bangladesh	Bangladesh
Anticancer	Anticancer	Basel	Basel
Antigens	Antigens	Basic	Basic
Antimicrobial	Antimicrob	Bacteriology	Bacteriol
Antiviral	Antiviral	Batteriologia	Batteriol
Anzeiger	Anz	Behavior	Behav

Word	Abbreviation or Term
Behavioral	Behav
Behaviors	Behav
Behavioural	Behav
Beitrage	Beitr
Belge	Belg
Belges	Belg
Belgica	Belg
Belgiques	Belg
Berliner	Berl
Beruf	Beruf
Bibliotheca	Bibl
Biken	Biken
Bilddiagnostik	Bilddiagn
Bilten	Bilten
Biochemical	Biochem
Biochemistry	Biochem
Biochimica	Biochim
Biochimie	Biochim
Biocommunications	Biocommun
Bioelectromagnetics	Bioelectromagnetics
Bioenergetics	Bioenerg
Biofeedback	Biofeedback
Biologia	Biol
Biologica	Biol
Biological	Biol
Biologicos	Biol
Biologie	Biol
Biologique	Biol
Biology	Biol
Biomaterials	Biomater
Biomechanical	Biomech
Biomechanics	Biomech
Biomedica	Biomed
Bio-Medica	Biomed
Biomedical	Biomed
Bio-medical	Biomed
Biomedicine	Biomed
Biomedizinische	Biomed
Biomembranes	Biomembr
Biometeorology	Biometeorol
Biometrics	Biometrics
Biopharmaceutics	Biopharm
Biophysica	Biophys
Biophysical	Biophys
Biophysics	Biophys
Biopolymers	Biopolymers
Biorheology	Biorheology
Bioscience	Biosci
Biosocial	Biosoc
Biosystems	Biosystems
Biotechnological	Biotechnol
Biotechnology	Biotechnol

Word	Abbreviation or Term
Biotheoretica	Biotheor
Birth	Birth
Blood	Blood
Blut	Blut
Blutalkohol	Blutalkahol
Bluttransfusion	Bluttransfus
Boden-	Boden
Boletin	Bol
Bollettino	Boll
Bone	Bone
Brain	Brain
Brasileira	Bras
Brasileiros	Bras
Brazilian	Braz
Breast	Breast
British	Br
Bruxelles	Brux
Buccale	Buccale
Bulgarica	Bulg
Bulletin	Bull
Burns	Burns
CA	CA
Cahiers	Cah
Calcified	Calcif
Calcium	Calcium
Canadian	Can
Canadienne	Can
Cancer	Cancer
Carbohydrate	Carbohydr
Carcinogenesis	Carcinog
Carcinogenic	Carcinog
Cardioangiologica	Cardioangiol
Cajal	Cajal
Cardiography	Cardiogr
Cardiologia	Cardiol
Cardiologica	Cardiol
Cardiologie	Cardiol
Cardiology	Cardiol
Cardiovascular	Cardiovasc
Care	Care
Caries	Caries
Carolinae	Carol
Catheterization	Cathet
Cell	Cell
Cells	Cells
Cellular	Cell
Central	Cent
Cephalagia	Cephalagia
Cerebral	Cereb
Cervico-faciale	Cervicofac
Ceylon	Ceylon
Chemica	Chem

Word	Abbreviation or Term	Word	Abbreviation or Term
Chemical	Chem	Communication	Commun
Chemicals	Chem	Communications	Commun
Chemico-biological	Chem Biol	Community	Community
Chemie	Chem	Comparative	Comp
Chemioterapia	Chemiotherapia	Comparee	Comp
Chemistry	Chem	Complement	Complement
Chemists	Chem	Comprehensive	Compr
Chemotherapy	Chemother	Comptes	C
Chest	Chest	Computerized	Comput
Child	Child	Computers	Comput
Childs	Childs	Connecticut	Conn
Childhood	Child	Connective	Connect
Children	Child	Consulting	Consult
Chilena	Chil	Contact	Contact
Chileno	Chil	Contaminants	Contam
Chimico	Chim	Contamination	Contam
Chinese	Chin	Contemporary	Contemp
Chirurgica	Chir	Contributions	Contrib
Chirurgia	Chir	Control	Control
Chirurgiae	Chir	Controlled	Controlled
Chirurgie	Chir	Copenhagen	Copenh
Chronic	Chronic	Cornea	Cornea
Chromatographic	Chromatogr	Cornell	Cornell
Chromatography	Chromatogr	Corps	Corps
Chromosoma	Chromosoma	Cortex	Cortex
Chronicle	Chron	Council	Counc
Chronobiologia	Chronobiologia	Craniofacial	Craniofac
Ciba	Ciba	CRC	CRC
Ciencias	Cienc	Critical	Crit
Cientifica	Cient	Cryobiology	Cryobiology
Circulation	Circulation	Culture	Cult
Circulation	Circ	Current	Curr
Circulatory	Circ	Currents	Curr
Cirurgia	Cir	Cutanea	Cutan
CLAO	CLAO	Cutaneous	Cutan
Cleft	Cleft	Cutis	Cutis
Cleveland	Cleve	Cybernetics	Cybern
Clinic	Clin	Cyclic	Cyclic
Clinics	Clin	Cytobios	Cytobios
Clinica	Clin	Cytogenetics	Cytogenet
Clinical	Clin	Cytologica	Cytol
Clinicas	Clin	Cytologie	Cytol
Clinique	Clin	Cytology	Cytol
Clio	Clio	Cytometry	Cytometry
Coeur	Coeur	Dairy	Dairy
Cognition	Cogn	Dakar	Dakar
Cold Spring Harbor	Cold Spring Harbor	Danish	Dan
Collagen	Coll	Darm	Darm
College	Coll	Deaf	Deaf
Colon	Colon	Decision	Decis
Colorado	Colo	Defects	Defects
Communicable	Commun	Deficiency	Defic

Word	Abbreviation or Term	Word	Abbreviation or Term
Delivery	Deliv	DNA	DNA
Demographie	Demogr	Documenta	Doc
Demography	Demography	Doencas	Doencas
Dental	Dent	Drug	Drug
Dentistry	Dent	Drug-Nutrient	Drug Nutr
Dependencies	Depend	Drugs	Drugs
Dermatitis	Dermatitis	DTW	DTW
Dermatologia	Dermatol	Duodecim	Duodecim
Dermatologica	Dermatologica	Ear	Ear
Dermatological	Dermatol	Early	Early
Dermatologie	Dermatol	East African	East Afr
Dermatologische	Dermatol	Economic	Econ
Dermatology	Dermatol	Ecotoxicology	Ecotoxicol
Dermatopathology	Derrmatopathol	Educacion	Educ
Dermatosen	Derm	Educational	Educ
Dermato-Venereolog-ica	Derm Venereol	EEG/EMG	EEG EMG
		Egyptian	Egypt
Detection	Detect	Electrocardiology	Electrocardiol
Deutsche	Dtsch	Electroencephalo-graphy	Electroencephalogr
Deutschen	Dtsch		
De Vecchi	De Vecchi	Electromyography	Electromyogr
Development	Dev	Electron	Electron
Developpement	Dev	Electro-therapeutics	Electrother
Devices	Devices	Elevage	Elev
Diabete	Diabete	EMBO	EMBO
Diabetes	Diabetes	Embriologia	Embriol
Diabetologia	Diabetologia	Embryo	Embryo
Diabetologica	Diabetol	Embryologia	Embryol
Diabetologie	Diabetol	Embryologie	Embryol
Diagnosis	Diagn	Embryology	Embryol
Diagnostic	Diagn	Endeavour	Endeavour
Diagnostica	Diagn	Emergency	Emerg
Dialysis	Dial	Encephale	Encephale
Diarrhoeal	Diarrhoeal	Endocrine	Endocr
Diergeneeskunde	Diergeneeskd	Endocrinologia	Endocr
Dieta	Dieta	Endocrinologica	Endocrinol
Dietetic	Diet	Endocrinological	Endocrinol
Dietologica	Dietol	Endocrinologie	Endocrinol
Differentiation	Differ	Endocrinology	Endocrinology
Digestion	Digestion	Endoscopy	Endosc
Digestive	Dig	Endoscopy	Endoscopy
Digestivo	Dig	Enfermadades	Enferm
Digitale	Digitale	Engineering	Eng
Dimensions	Dimens	Enteral	Enteral
Directions	Dir	Entomology	Entomol
Directors	Dir	Environmental	Environ
Discussions	Discuss	Enzyme	Enzyme
Disease	Disease	Enzymologica	Enzymol
Diseases	Dis	Enzymology	Enzymol
Disorders	Disord	Epidemiologie	Epidemiol
Disposition	Dispos	Epidemiologic	Epidemiol
DM	DM	Epidemiology	Epidemiol

Word	Abbreviation or Term	Word	Abbreviation or Term
Epilepsia	Epilepsia	Florida	Fla
Erganzungsband	Erganzungsband	Folia	Folia
Ergebnisse	Ergeb	Food	Food
Ergology	Ergol	Foot	Foot
Ergonomics	Ergonomics	Forensic	Forensic
Ernahrung	Ernahr	Fortschritte	Fortschr
Ernahrungsforschung	Ernahrungsforsch	Foundation	Found
Ernahrungswissen-schaft	Ernahrungswiss	Francais	Fr
		Francaises	Fr
Espanola	Esp	Frauenheilkunde	Frauenheilkd
Espanolas	Esp	Function	Funct
Espanoles	Esp	Fundamental	Fundam
Essays	Essays	Gaceta	Gac
Esthetique	Esthet	Gastroenterologia	Gastroenterol
Estomatologia	Estomatol	Gastroenterologica	Gastroenterol
Ethics	Ethics	Gastroenterologie	Gastroenterol
Ethnopharmacology	Ethnopharmacol	Gastroenterology	Gastroenterol
Eugenics	Eugen	Gastroenterology	Gastroenterology
Europaea	Eur	Gastrointestinal	Gastrointest
European	Eur	Gebiete	Geb
Evaluation	Eval	Geburtshilfe	Geburtshilfe
Exotique	Exot	Gemellologiae	Gemellol
Experimental	Exp	GEN	GEN
Experimentale	Exp	Gene	Gene
Experimentales	Exp	Geneeskunde	Geneeskd
Exceptional	Except	General	Gen
Exercise	Exerc	Genetic	Genet
Experientia	Experientia	Genetica	Genet
Experimentalis	Exp	Geneticae	Genet
Experimentelle	Exp	Genetical	Genet
Eye	Eye	Genetics	Genetics
Factors	Factors	Genetics	Genet
Faculdade	Fac	Genetika	Genet
Facultad	Fac	Genetique	Genet
Facultatis	Fac	Geneve	Geneve
Family	Fam	Genitourinary	Genitourin
FAO	FAO	Geographical	Geogr
Faraday	Faraday	Georgia	Ga
Farmaceutico	Farm	Geriatric	Geriatr
Farmacie	Farm	Geriatrics	Geriatr
Farmaco	Farmaco	Geriatrie	Geriatr
Farmacologia	Farmacol	Gerichtlichen	Gerichtl
FDA	FDA	Gerontologie	Gerontol
FEBS	FEBS	Gerontologist	Gerontologist
Federation	Fed	Gerontology	Gerontol
Fennicae	Fenn	Gesamte	Gesamte
Fertilitatas	Fertil	Gesamtgebiete	Gesamtgeb
Fertility	Fertil	Geschwulstforschung	Geschwulstforsch
Filiales	Filiales	Gesellschaft	Ges
Finnish	Finn	Gesichts-chirurgie	Gesichtschir
Fisiologia	Fisiol	Gesundheitswesen	Gesundheitswes
Fitness	Fitness	Ginecologia	Ginecol

Word	Abbreviation or Term	Word	Abbreviation or Term
Ginecologica	Ginecol	Hiroshima	Hiroshima
Giornale	G	Histochemica	Histochem
Grenzgebiete	Grenzgeb	Histochemical	Histochem
Group	Group	Histochemistry	Histochem
Groupement	Group	Histochemistry	Histochemistry
Groups	Groups	Histologicum	Histol
Growth	Growth	Histologie	Histol
Gut	Gut	Histology	Histol
Gynaecologiae	Gynaecol	Histopathology	Histopathology
Gynaecological	Gynaecol	History	Hist
Gynaecology	Gynaecol	HNO	HNO
Gynakologe	Gynakologe	Homosexuality	Homosex
Gynakologische	Gynakol	Hoppe-Seyler	Hoppe Seyler
Gynecologic	Gynecol	Horizons	Horiz
Gynecologica	Gynecol	Hormone	Horm
Gynecology	Gynecol	Hormones	Horm
Haematologia	Haematol	Hospital	Hosp
Haematologica	Haematol	Hospitals	Hospitals
Haematology	Haematol	Humaine	Hum
Haemostasis	Haemostasis	Human	Hum
Hamatolgie	Hamatol	Humans	Hum
Handchirurgie	Handchir	Hungarica	Hung
Hansenologia	Hansenol	Hungaricae	Hung
Harefuah	Harefuah	Hybridoma	Hybridoma
Harvey	Harvey	Hygie	Hygie
Hastings Center	Hastings Cent	Hygiene	Hyg
Hautarzt	Hautarzt	Hypertension	Hypertens
Hautkrankheiten	Hautkr	Hypertension	Hypertension
Hawaii	Hawaii	Hypnosis	Hypn
Head	Head	Hypotheses	Hypotheses
Headache	Headache	IARC	IARC
Health	Health	Iberoamericanos	Ibero Am
Hearing	Hear	Ibero-latino-ameri- cana	Ibero Lat Am
Heart	Heart		
Helminthology	Helminthol	ICRP	ICRP
Helvetiae	Helv	IEEE	IEEE
Helvetica	Helv	Igiene	Ig
Hematological	Hematol	Imaging	Imaging
Hematology	Hematol	IMJ	IMJ
Hemoglobin	Hemoglobin	Immunitat	Immun
Hemostasis	Hemost	Immunity	Immun
Hepato-gastroentero- logy	Hepatogastroentero- logy	Immunoassay	Immunoassay
		Immunobiology	Immunobiol
Hepatology	Hepatology	Immunogenetics	Immunogenetics
Hereditas	Hereditas	Immuno-hemato- logie	Immunohematol
Heredity	Heredity		
Herz	Herz	Immunologia	Immunol
Herz-	Herz	Immunologiae	Immunol
Higiene	Hig	Immunologica	Immunol
Hindustan	Hindustan	Immunological	Immunol
Hip	Hip	Immunologie	Immunol
Hirnforschung	Hirnforsch	Immunology	Immunol

Word	Abbreviation or Term	Word	Abbreviation or Term
Immunopathologia	Immunopathol	Investigative	Invest
Immunopharmacol-ogy	Immunopharmacol-ogy	Iowa	Iowa
		Irish	Ir
Immunotherapy	Immunother	ISA	ISA
Implant	Implant	Isis	Isis
In	In	Isotopes	Isot
Including	Incl	Isozymes	Isozymes
India	India	Israel	Isr
Indian	Indian	Issues	Issues
Indiana	Indiana	Istanbul	Istanbul
Indonesiana	Indones	Istituto	Ist
Industria	Ind	Italiana	Ital
Industrial	Ind	Italiani	Ital
Infantil	Infant	Italiano	Ital
Infection	Infect	Italiennes	Ital
Infectious	Infect	Iugoslavica	Iugosl
Infektion	Infekt	Jahrbuch	Jahrb
Inflammation	Inflamm	JAMA	JAMA
Informatics	Inf	Japanese	Jpn
Infusionstherapie	Infusionther	Japonica	Jpn
Inherited	Inherited	Japonicum	Jpn
Injury	Inj	JCU	JCU
Injury	Injury	Joint	Jt
Inneren	Inn	Journal	J
Inorganic	Inorg	JPEN	JPEN
Inquiry	Inquiry	JPMA	JPMA
Institu	Inst	Jungenkunde	Jungendkd
Institut	Inst	Kansas	Kans
Institutes	Inst	Kardiologie	Kardiol
Instituto	Inst	Keio	Keio
Instrumentation	Instrum	Kekkaku	Kekkaku
Insurance	Insur	Kentucky	Ky
Intelligence	Intell	Kidney	Kidney
Intensive	Intensive	Kiefer-	Kiefer
Intensivtherapie	Intensivther	Kieferorthopadie	Kieferorthop
Interactions	Interact	Kinderchirurgie	Kinderchir
Interferon	Interferon	Kindergeneeskunde	Kindergeneeskd
Internal	Intern	Kinderheilkunde	Kinderheilkd
International	Int	Kinderpsychiatrie	Kinderpsychiatr
Internationales	Int	Kinderpsychologie	Kinderpsychol
Internationalis	Int	Kinetics	Kinet
Interne	Interne	Klinische	Klin
Internist	Internist	Kobe	Kobe
Interventional	Intervent	Koninklijke	K
Intervirology	Intervirology	Kreislaufforschung	Kreislaufforsch
Intra-ocular	Intraocul	Kriminologie	Kriminol
Invasion	Invasion	Kunstliche	Kunstliche
Invertebrate	Invertebr	Kurume	Kurume
Investigacion	Invest	Laboratorio	Lab
Investigation	Invest	Laboratoriumsdiag-nostik	Lab Diagn
Investigational	Invest		
Investigations	Invest	Laboratory	Lab

Word	Abbreviation or Term	Word	Abbreviation or Term
Laegeforening	Laegeforen	Malaysian	Malays
Laeger	Laeger	Management	Manage
Lancet	Lancet	Manipulative	Manipulative
Landwirtschaft	Landwirtsch	Maria	Maria
Language	Lang	Mariae	Mariae
Laryngologie	Laryngol	Marital	Marital
Laryngology	Laryngol	Maritime	Marit
Laryngoscope	Laryngoscope	Maroc	Maroc
Larynx	Larynx	Maryland	Md
Lasers	Lasers	Mass	Mass
Latina	Lat	Masui	Masui
Latinoamericana	Latinoam	Mathematical	Math
Latinoamericanos	Latinoam	Maturitas	Maturitas
Lavoro	Lav	Mayo	Mayo
Law	Law	Maxillofacial	Maxillofac
Lebensmittel-unter-	Lebensm Unters	Maxillofacialis	Maxillofac
suchung		Maxilofacial	Maxilofac
Leber	Leber	Measurement	Meas
Lectures	Lect	Mechanisms	Mech
Legal	Leg	Medecine	Med
Legalis	Leg	Media	Media
Leidensia	L	Medica	Med
Leiden	Leiden	Medicae	Med
Leprologica	Leprol	Medical	Med
Leprosy	Lepr	Medicale	Med
Letters	Lett	Medicales	Med
Leucocyte	Leucocyte	Mediche	Med
Leukotriene	Leukotriene	Medicina	Med
Leukotrienes	Leukotrienes	Medicinae	Med
Library	Libr	Medicinal	Med
Liege	Liege	Medicine	Med
Life	Life	Medico	Med
Life-threatening	Life Threat	Medico-chirurgica	Med Chir
Lipid	Lipid	Medico-Psychologi-	Med Psychol
Lipids	Lipids	ques	
Literature	Lit	Medizinische	Med
Louisiana	La	Medizinischen	Med
Lufthygiene	Lufthyg	Membrane	Membr
Lung	Lung	Memoires	Mem
Luso-Espanolas	Luso Esp	Menninger	Menninger
Lymphokine	Lymphokine	Mental	Ment
Lymphologie	Lymphol	Mentale	Ment
Lymphology	Lymphology	Metabolic	Metab
Madagascar	Madagascar	Metabolism	Metab
Magen	Magen	Metabolisme	Metab
Magnesium	Magnesium	Metastasis	Metastasis
Magnetic	Magn	Methods	Methods
Main	Main	Mexico	Mex
Making	Making	Michigan	Mich
Maladies	Mal	Microbial	Microb
Malariologia	Malariol	Microbiologia	Microbiol
Malaysia	Malaysia	Microbiologica	Microbiol

Word	Abbreviation or Term	Word	Abbreviation or Term
Microbiological	Microbiol	Neck	Neck
Microbiologie	Microbiol	Nederlands	Ned
Microbiology	Microbiol	Neerlando-Scand-	Neerl Scand
Microbios	Microbios	inavica	
Microcirculation	Microcirc	Nefrologica	Nefrol
Microscopique	Microsc	Neglect	Negl
Microvascular	Microvasc	Neonate	Neonate
Microwave	Microwave	Nephrology	Nephrol
Mikrochirurgie	Mikrochir	Nephron	Nephron
Military	Milit	Nervenarzt	Nervenarzt
Mineral	Miner	Nervosa	Nerv
Minerva	Minerva	Nervous	Nerv
Minnesota	Minn	Netherlands	Neth
Mississippi	Miss	Neural	Neural
Missouri	Mo	Neurobehavioral	Neurobehav
Mitteilungen	Mitt	Neurobiologia	Neurobiol
MMWR	MMWR	Neurobiologiae	Neurobiol
Modification	Modif	Neurobiology	Neurobiol
Molecular	Mol	Neurochemistry	Neurochem
Monatsschrift	Monatsschr	Neurochirurgia	Neurochirurgia
Monographia	Monogr	Neurochirurgica	Neurochir
Monographien	Monogr	Neuro-chirurgie	Neurochirurgie
Monographs	Monogr	Neurocytology	Neurocytol
Morphologica	Morphol	Neuroendocrinology	Neuroendocrinology
Morphologie	Morphol	Neurogenetics	Neurogenet
Morphologisches	Morphol	Neuroimmunology	Neuroimmunol
Motility	Motil	Neurologia	Neurol
Movimento	Mov	Neurologic	Neurol
Mount Sinai	Mt Sinai	Neurologica	Neurol
Munchener	Munch	Neurological	Neurol
Muscle	Muscle	Neurologie	Neurol
Mutagenesis	Mutagen	Neurologique	Neurol
Mutation	Mutat	Neurology	Neurol
Mycobacterial	Mycobact	Neuro-oncology	Neurooncol
Mycopathologia	Mycopathologia	Neuro-ophthalmology	Neuro Ophthalmol
Mykosen	Mykosen	Neuropathologica	Neuropathol
Nacional	Nac	Neuropathology	Neuropathol
Nagoya	Nagoya	Neuropediatrics	Neuropediatrics
Nahrung	Nahrung	Neuropeptides	Neuropeptides
Narcotics	Narc	Neuropharmacology	Neuropharmacology
Nasus	Nasus	Neurophysiology	Neurophysiol
National	Natl	Neuropsychobiology	Neuropsychobiology
Nationale	Natl	Neuropsychologia	Neuropsychologia
Natural	Nat	Neuro-psychopharm-	Neuropsychopharm-
Nature	Nature	acology	acol
Naturstoffe	Naturst	Neuro-psiquiatria	Neuropsiquiatr
Naturwissenschaften	Naturwissenschaften	Neuropsychology	Neuropsychol
Naunyn-Schmiede-	Naunyn Schmiede-	Neuroradiology	Neuroradiol
bergs	bergs	Neuroradiology	Neuroradiology
Naval	Nav	Neuroscience	Neurosci
Navarra	Navarra	Neurosurgery	Neurosurg
Nebraska	Nebr	Neurosurgery	Neurosurgery

Word	Abbreviation or Term	Word	Abbreviation or Term
Neurosurgical	Neurosurg	Organi	Organi
Neurotoxicology	Neurotoxicology	Organischer	Org
New	New	Organization	Organ
New England	N Engl	Organs	Organs
New Jersey	NJ	ORL	ORL
New Orleans	New Orleans	Orthodontics	Orthod
New York	NY	Orthodontist	Orthod
New Zealand	NZ	Orthopade	Orthopade
NIPH	NIPH	Orthopadie	Orthop
Nordisk	Nord	Orthopaedic	Orthop
Normale	Norm	Orthopaedica	Orthop
Norske	Nor	Orthopaedicae	Orthop
North America	North Am	Orthopsychiatry	Orthopsychiatry
North Carolina	NC	Orthotics	Orthot
Notfallmedizin	Notfallmed	Osaka	Osaka
Nose	Nose	Oslo	Oslo
Nouvelle	Nouv	Ospedale	Osp
Nuclear	Nucl	Osteo-articulaires	Osteoartic
Nucleotide	Nucleotide	Osteopathic	Osteopath
Nuklearmedizin	Nuklearmed	Ostetricia	Ostet
Nuovi	Nuovi	Oto-laryngologica	Otolaryngol
Nursing	Nurs	Oto-laryngologie	Otolaryngol
Nutricion	Nutr	Otolaryngology	Otolaryngol
Nutritio	Nutr	Otologie	Otol
Nutrition	Nutr	Otology	Otol
Nutritional	Nutr	Oto-rhino-laryngol-	Otorhinolaryngol
Obesity	Obes	ogica	
Obstetric	Obstet	Oto-rhino-laryngol-	Otorhinolaryngol
Obstetricia	Obstet	ogy	
Obstetrics	Obstet	Otorrinolaringolog-	Otorrinolaringol
Occupational	Occup	icos	
Oculaire	Ocul	Oxford	Oxford
Olomucensis	Olomuc	Pace	Pace
Odontologica	Odontol	Padagogische	Padagog
Odontologie	Odontol	Padiatrie	Padiatr
Offentliche	Off	Padologie	Padol
Official	Off	Paediatric	Paediatr
Oficina	Of	Paediatrica	Paediatr
Ohio	Ohio	Paediatrics	Paediatr
Oklahoma	Okla	Paedopsychiatrica	Paedopsychiatr
Oncologia	Oncol	Palate	Palate
Oncology	Oncol	Panama	Panama
Ophtalmologie	Ophtalmol	Pan American	Pan Am
Ophthalmologica	Ophthalmol	Panamericana	Panam
Ophthalmological	Ophthalmol	Panminerva	Panminerva
Ophthalmology	Ophthalmol	Paper	Pap
Optical	Opt	Papua New Guinea	Papua New Guinea
Optics	Opt	Paraplegia	Paraplegia
Optometric	Optom	Parasite	Parasite
Optometry	Optom	Parasitenkunde	Parasitenkd
Oral	Oral	Parasitologia	Parasitol
Organe	Organe	Parasitologica	Parasitol

Word	Abbreviation or Term	Word	Abbreviation or Term
Parasitologie	Parasitol	Phlebologie	Phlebologie
Parasitology	Parasitol	Phonetica	Phonetica
Parassitologia	Parassitologia	Phoniatrica	Phoniatr
Parenteral	Parenter	Phosphorylation	Phosphorylation
Pasteur	Pasteur	Photobiology	Photobiol
Pathologe	Pathologe	Photochemistry	Photochem
Pathologica	Pathol	Photo-dermatology	Photodermatol
Pathologie	Pathol	Photography	Photogr
Pathologiques	Pathol	Physica	Phys
Pathology	Pathol	Physical	Phys
Patologia	Patol	Physician	Physician
Patologica	Patol	Physicians	Physicians
Paulista	Paul	Physics	Phys
Pays	Pays	Physiologica	Physiol
Pediatria	Pediatr	Physiological	Physiol
Pediatrica	Pediatr	Physiologie	Physiol
Pediatrician	Pediatrician	Physiology	Physiol
Pediatrics	Pediatr	Physiopathologie	Physiopathol
Pediatrie	Pediatr	Placenta	Placenta
Pediatrique	Pediatr	Planning	Plann
Pennsylvania	Pa	Planta	Planta
Peptide	Pept	Plastic	Plast
Peptides	Pept	Plastica	Plast
Peptides	Peptides	Plasticae	Plast
Perception	Perception	Plastiche	Plast
Perceptual	Percept	Plastique	Plast
Perinatal	Perinat	Pneumologie	Pneumol
Perinatale	Perinat	Podiatric	Podiatr
Perinatology	Perinatol	Podiatry	Podiatry
Periodontal	Periodont	Poisoning	Poisoning
Periodontology	Periodontol	Policy	Policy
Personality	Pers	Politics	Polit
Perspectives	Perspect	Pollution	Pollut
Pflugers	Pflugers	Population	Popul
Pharmaceutica	Pharm	Portuguesa	Port
Pharmaceutical	Pharm	Postgraduate	Postgrad
Pharmaceutiques	Pharm	Poultry	Poult
Pharmaceutisch	Pharm	Practice	Pract
Pharmacobio-dy-namics	Pharmacobiodyn	Practitioners	Pract
		Praxis	Prax
Pharmacodynamie	Pharmacodyn	Pregnancy	Pregnancy
Pharmacokinetics	Pharmacokinet	Prenatal	Prenat
Pharmacologica	Pharmacol	Preparative	Prep
Pharmacology	Pharmacol	Presse	Presse
Pharmacopsychiatry	Pharmacopsychiatry	Prevention	Prev
Pharmacotherapy	Pharmacother	Preventive	Prev
Pharmacy	Pharm	Primary	Primary
Pharmatherapeutica	Pharmatherapeutica	Primatologica	Primatol
Pharmazeuten	Pharm	Primatology	Primatol
Pharmazie	Pharm	Probleme	Probl
Pharos	Pharos	Proceedings	Proc
Philosophical	Philos	Process	Process

Word	Abbreviation or Term	Word	Abbreviation or Term
Processes	Processes	Radiobiologia	Radiobiol
Products	Prod	Radiography	Radiogr
Programs	Programs	Radioisotopes	Radioisotopes
Progress	Prog	Radiologe	Radiologe
Progressi	Prog	Radiologia	Radiol
Prostaglandin	Prostaglandin	Radiologica	Radiol
Prostaglandins	Prostaglandins	Radiologie	Radiol
Prostate	Prostate	Radiologists	Radiol
Prosthetic	Prosthet	Radiology	Radiol
Prosthetics	Prosthet	Radiology	Radiology
Protein	Protein	Radiotherapia	Radiother
Protozoology	Protozool	Rational	Ration
Psichiatrica	Psichiatr	Reactions	React
Psicologica	Psicol	Real	R
Psiquiatrica	Psiquiatr	Reanimacion	Reanim
Psiquiatria	Psiquiatr	Reanimation	Reanim
Psyche	Psyche	Recenti	Recenti
Psychiatric	Psychiatr	Recherche	Rech
Psychiatrica	Psychiatr	Recherches	Rech
Psychiatrie	Psychiatr	Rechtsmedizin	Rechtsmed
Psychiatry	Psychiatry	Recombinant	Recomb
Psychoactive	Psychoactive	Reconstructive	Reconstr
Psychoanalysis	Psychoanal	Record	Rec
Psycho-analysis	Psychoanal	Rectum	Rectum
Psychoanalytic	Psychoanal	Regional	Reg
Psycholinguistic	Psycholinguist	Regulation	Regul
Psychologica	Psychol	Regulatory	Regul
Psychologie	Psychol	Rehabilitation	Rehabil
Psychologist	Psychol	Renal	Renal
Psychology	Psychol	Rendus	R
Psychoneuroendo-	Psychoneuroendo-	Report	Rep
crinology	crinology	Reports	Rep
Psychopathology	Psychopathology	Reproduction	Reprod
Psychopharmacology	Psychopharmacol	Reproductive	Reprod
Psychophysiology	Psychophysiology	Research	Res
Psychosocial	Psychosoc	Residue	Residue
Psychosomatic	Psychosom	Resonance	Reson
Psychosomatics	Psychosom	Respiration	Respir
Psychosomatik	Psychosom	Respiration	Respiration
Psychotherapie	Psychother	Respiratoire	Respir
Psychotherapy	Psychother	Respiratory	Respir
Pubblicazioni	Pubbl	Response	Response
Public	Public	Resuscitation	Resuscitation
Publica	Publica	Retardation	Retard
Publique	Publique	Retina	Retina
Puerto Rico	PR	Review	Rev
Putti	Putti	Reviews	Rev
QRB	QRB	Revista	Rev
Quantitative	Quant	Revue	Rev
Quarterly	Q	Rheumatic	Rheum
Rada	Rada	Rheumatism	Rheum
Radiation	Radiat	Rheumatologie	Rheumatol

Word	Abbreviation or Term	Word	Abbreviation or Term
Rheumatology	Rheumatol	Sleep	Sleep
Rhinologie	Rhinol	Social	Soc
Rhinology	Rhinol	Societe	Soc
Rhode Island	RI	Societes	Soc
Rhumatisme	Rhum	Societies	Soc
Ricerca	Ric	Society	Soc
Rivista	Riv	Sociological	Sociol
ROFO	ROFO	Sociologie	Sociol
Romande	Romande	Sociology	Sociol
Rontgen-blatter	Rontgenblatter	Somatic	Somatic
Rontgenpraxis	Rontgenpraxis	Somatosensory	Somatosens
Rontgenstrahlen	Rontgenstr	South African	S Afr
Roumaines	Roum	South Carolina	SC
Royale	R	South Dakota	SD
Sabouraudia	Sabouraudia	Southeast	Southeast
Safety	Safety	Southern	South
Salud	Salud	Sozial-	Soz
Sangre	Sangre	Sozialmedizin	Sozialmed
Sanguinis	Sang	Space	Space
Sanidad	Sanid	Spaziale	Spaz
Sanita	Sanita	Spectrometry	Spectrom
Sanitaria	Sanit	Speech	Speech
Saude	Saude	Sperimentale	Sper
Scandinavian	Scand	Spine	Spine
Scandinavica	Scand	Sportmedizin	Sportmed
Scanning	Scan	Sports	Sports
Schizophrenia	Schizophr	Springer	Springer
School	Sch	Stain	Stain
Schriftenreihe	Schriftr	Standardization	Stand
Schweizerische	Schweiz	Standards	Stand
Schweizerischen	Schweiz	Statistical	Stat
Science	Sci	Stazione	Stn
Sciences	Sci	Steroid	Steroid
Scientia	Sci	Steroids	Steroids
Scientiarum	Sci	Stetinepsis	Stetin
Scientific	Sci	Stockholm	Stockh
Scientifique	Sci	Stoffwechselkrank-	Stoffwechselk
Scienza	Sci	heiten	
Scottish	Scott	Stomatologica	Stomatol
Security	Secur	Stomatologie	Stomatol
Seminars	Semin	Strabismus	Strabismus
Series	Ser	Strahlenschutz	Strahlenschutz
Service	Serv	Strahlentherapie	Strahlentherapie
Sex	Sex	Stress	Stress
Sexual	Sex	Stroke	Stroke
Sexually	Sex	Structure	Struct
Sexualforschung	Sexualforsch	Studies	Stud
Shock	Shock	Sub-cellular	Subcell
Sieroterapico	Sieroter	Submicroscopic	Submicrosc
Singapore	Singapore	Substance	Subst
Sinica	Sin	Subtropicale	Subtrop
Skeletal	Skeletal	Sudhoffs	Sudhoffs

Word	Abbreviation or Term	Word	Abbreviation or Term
Suecica	Suec	Torino	Torino
Suicide	Suicide	Total	Total
Superior	Super	Toxicologia	Toxicol
Superiore	Super	Toxicologic	Toxicol
Supplementum	Suppl	Toxicologica	Toxicol
Support	Support	Toxicological	Toxicol
Surgeon	Surg	Toxicology	Toxicol
Surgeons	Surg	Toxikologie	Toxikol
Surgery	Surg	Trabajos	Trab
Surgical	Surg	Trachome	Trach
Swedish	Swed	Traditional	Tradit
Symposia	Symp	Transactions	Trans
Symposium	Symp	Transfer	Transfer
System	Syst	Transfusion	Transfusion
Systems	Syst	Transmission	Transm
Technical	Tech	Transmitted	Transm
Technik	Tech	Transplant	Transplant
Technology	Technol	Transplantation	Transplantation
Tennessee	Tenn	Traumatic	Trauma
Terapeutica	Ter	Traumatologiae	Traumatol
Teratogenesis	Teratogenesis	Traumatologie	Traumatol
Teratology	Teratol	Tropica	Trop
Thailand	Thai	Tropicais	Trop
Theoretical	Theor	Tropical	Trop
Therapeutics	Ther	Tropicale	Trop
Therapeutique	Ther	Tropicaux	Trop
Therapeutische	Ther	Tropischen	Trop
Therapiae	Ther	Tubercle	Tubercle
Therapie	Ther	Tuberculosis	Tuberc
Therapies	Ther	Tumori	Tumori
Therapy	Ther	Tumour	Tumour
Thermal	Therm	Tunis	Tunis
Thoracic	Thorac	Tunisie	Tunis
Thorax	Thorax	Turkish	Turk
Throat	Throat	Ugeskrift	Ugeskr
Thrombosis	Thromb	Ulster	Ulster
Thromboxane	Thromboxane	Ultramicroscopy	Ultramicroscopy
Thymus	Thymus	Ultraschall	Ultraschall
Tidsskrift	Tidsskr	Ultrasonic	Ultrason
Tierarztliche	Tierarztliche	Ultrasonics	Ultrasonics
Tierernahrung	Tierernahr	Ultrasound	Ultrasound
Tierheilkunde	Tierheilkd	Ultrastructural	Ultrastruct
Tijdschrift	Tijdschr	Ultrastructure	Ultrastruct
Tissue	Tissue	Umschau	Umsch
Today	Today	Umwelt	Umwelt
Tohoku	Tohoku	Undersea	Undersea
Tokai	Tokai	Unfallchirurg	Unfallchirurg
Tokushima	Tokushima	Unfallchirurgie	Unfallchirurgie
Tokyo	Tokyo	Union	Union
Tomography	Tomogr	Universitatis	Univ
Topics	Top	Upsala	Ups
Torace	Torace	Uremia	Uremia

Word	Abbreviation or Term	Word	Abbreviation or Term
Urologe	Urologe	Visual	Vis
Urologia	Urol	Vital	Vital
Urologic	Urol	Vitamin-	Vitam
Urologica	Urol	Vitaminologica	Vitaminol
Urologicas	Urol	Vitaminology	Vitaminol
Urologie	Urol	Vitamins	Vitam
Urology	Urol	Vitro	Vitro
Vaccine	Vaccine	Vittoria	Vittoria
Vasa	Vasa	Vox	Vox
Venereologia	Venereol	Wasser-	Wasser
Venereologie	Venereol	Weekblad	Weekbl
Venezolana	Venez	Welfare	Welfare
Verdauungs-	Verdau	Western	West
Vereins	Ver	West Indian	West Indian
Verhandelingen	Verh	West Virginia	W Va
Verhandlungen	Verh	Wiener	Wien
Veroffentlichungen	Veroff	Wildlife	Wildl
Vessels	Vessels	Wisconsin	Wis
Veterinaermedicin	Vet	Wissenschaften	Wiss
Veterinaires	Vet	Wochenschrift	Wochenschr
Veterinaria	Vet	World Health Or-	WHO
Veterinarian	Vet	ganization	
Veterinarmedizin	Veterinarmed	Womens	Wom
Veterinary	Vet	Xenobiotica	Xenobiotica
Virginia	Va	Yale	Yale
Virologia	Virol	Zahnmedizin	Zahnmed
Virologica	Virol	Zeitschrift	Z
Virological	Virol	Zoologica	Zool
Virology	Virol	Zoology	Zool
Virus	Virus	Zoonoses	Zoonoses

REFERENCES

1. National Library of Medicine. List of journals indexed in Index Medicus. Bethesda, Maryland: National Library of Medicine; [Annual]. This list is published each year in the January issue of Index Medicus and is also available as a separate publication from the Superintendent of Documents, US Government Printing Office, Washington, DC 20402.
2. International Organization for Standardization. International standard ISO-4-1972(E): Documentation-international code for the abbreviation of titles of periodicals. Geneva: International Organization for Standardization; 1972. Available from the American National Standards Institute, 1430 Broadway, New York, NY 10018.

Appendix C

Annotated Bibliography

The books briefly described here represent the core of a reference library for editorial offices of journals in the medical sciences. Other valuable reference books are cited in Chapters 10, 13, and 16.

STYLE MANUALS

Style Manuals of the English-speaking World: A Guide. JB Howell. Phoenix, Arizona: Oryx; 1983.

An exhaustive and annotated-in-detail bibliography of style manuals for English-language literature. Covers commercial, governmental, and university-press manuals: general manuals and those for specific disciplines.

GENERAL MANUALS

The Chicago Manual of Style. 13th ed. Chicago: University of Chicago Press; 1982.

The basic and detailed style manual for scholarly publishing. Strongest on style for general literature and the humanities; does not cover many aspects of scientific style.

Hart's Rules for Compositors and Readers at the University Press Oxford. 39th ed. Oxford: Oxford University Press; 1983.

A short, pocket manual. Useful on British preferences in style.

The McGraw-Hill Style Manual: A Concise Guide for Writers and Editors. M Longyear, ed. New York: McGraw-Hill; 1983.

Good detail on many aspects of scientific style, notably mathematics and physics.

The MLA Style Manual. WS Achtert, J Gibaldi. New York: Modern Language Association of America; 1985.

A standard manual for the humanities. Its chapter on bibliographic references is particularly helpful with regard to many types of documents infrequently cited in scientific literature, but its style for references is not, of course, the Vancouver style. Has a helpful appendix on scholarly abbreviations and publisher names.

United States Government Printing Office Style Manual: 1984. Washington: US Government Printing Office; 1984.

Has a wealth of detail, often in tabular form, not found in other manuals. Particularly valuable for details of style with reference to countries other than the United States: currency, languages, names.

Webster's Standard American Style Manual. Springfield, Massachusetts: Merriam-Webster; 1985.

A general manual. Well-organized with attention to types of particular style problems.

Words into Type. 3rd ed. Englewood Cliffs, New Jersey: Prentice-Hall; 1974.

An exhaustingly detailed manual but without much coverage of scientific style. A new edition may be available in 1987.

STYLE MANUALS IN THE SCIENCES

The ACS Style Guide: A Manual for Authors and Editors. JS Dodd, ed. Washington: American Chemical Society; 1986.

A basic and clear manual on style for all aspects of chemistry. Should be on the reference shelf in editorial offices of medical journals.

ASM Style Manual for Journals and Books. Washington: American Society for Microbiology; 1985.

An exhaustively detailed manual for style in bacteriology, mycology, and virology, including genetic aspects of these fields. Thorough coverage of style and format problems in tables and illustrations.

CBE Style Manual: A Guide for Authors, Editors, and Publishers in the Biological Sciences. 5th ed. CBE Style Manual Committee. Bethesda, Maryland: Council of Biology Editors; 1983.

A classic among scientific style manuals. Despite its title does cover many aspects of style in the medical sciences. Particularly helpful in fields not covered by style manuals in chemistry and medicine, notably botany, other plant sciences, and zoology. Has an authoritative compilation of abbreviations and a useful annotated bibliography.

Manual for Authors & Editors: Editorial Style and Manuscript Preparation. WR Barclay, M Therese Southgate, Robert W Mayo. Los Altos, California: Lange Medical Publications; 1981. Compiled for the American Medical Association.

The details of publication style specified for the journals published by the American Medical Association (AMA). Note that although the AMA journals are in the Vancouver agreement, not all of the details of style for bibliographic references are in accord with the Vancouver style. A new edition may be available in 1987.

Mathematics into Type: Copy Editing and Proofreading of Mathematics for Editorial Assistants and Authors. Rev ed. E Swanson. Providence, Rhode Island: American Mathematical Society; 1979.

A clear, detailed and basic manual for all aspects of style in mathematical text and equations.

Publication Manual of the American Psychological Association. 3rd ed. Washington: American Psychological Association; 1983.

Style specified for the journals published by the American Psychological Association. The style for bibliographic references is not that of the Vancouver style. Has a good short section on problems in prose style and helpful discussions of sex reference and ethics in scholarly publishing.

Style Manual for Guidance in the Preparation of Papers for Journals Published by the American Institute of Physics and Its Member Societies. 3rd ed. D Hathwell, AWK Metzner. New York: American Institute of Physics; 1978.

Style for the journals published by the American Institute of Physics. Its section on mathematical style is not as helpful as the manual published by the American Mathematical Society.

Suggestions to Authors of the Reports of the United States Geological Survey. 6th ed. Washington: US Geological Survey; 1978. Available from the Superintendent of Documents, US Government Printing Office, Washington, DC.

An authority on nomenclature and style for geologic eras, paleontology, and stratigraphy. A new edition may be available in 1987.

DICTIONARIES

GENERAL DICTIONARIES

The American Heritage Dictionary of the English Language. W Morris, ed. Boston: Houghton Mifflin; 1981.

Chambers 20th Century Dictionary. EM Kirkpatrick, ed. Cambridge: Cambridge University Press; 1983.

The Penguin Dictionary of Confusibles. A Room. New York: Penguin Books; 1980.

Oxford Dictionary of Current Idiomatic English.
Volume 1: Verbs with Prepositions & Particles. AP Cowie, R Mackin. London: Oxford University Press; 1975.
Volume 2: Phrase, Clause & Sentence Idioms. AP Cowie, R Mackin, IR McCaig. London: Oxford University Press; 1983.

Webster's II New Riverside University Dictionary. Boston: Riverside; 1984.

Webster's Ninth New Collegiate Dictionary. Springfield, Massachusetts: Merriam-Webster; 1983.

Among the general desk dictionaries, *The American Heritage Dictionary* is probably the most useful, for its usage notes. "Chambers" specifies both British and American spelling and usage. *Volume 1: Verbs with Prepositions & Particles* of the *Oxford Dictionary of Current Idiomatic English* should be helpful to authors and editors for whom English is not their original language; the misuse of prepositions is a frequent problem for such authors who otherwise write acceptably idiomatic English.

MEDICAL DICTIONARIES

Butterworths Medical Dictionary. 2nd ed. M Critchley, ed. London: Butterworths; 1978.

A comprehensive, authoritative medical dictionary oriented to British usage. Through its capitalizing of generic drug and chemical names and failing to observe the rules for italicization in taxonomic names used as entry terms, it may confuse some users on widely accepted conventions of style.

Dorland's Illustrated Medical Dictionary. 26th ed. Philadelphia: WB Saunders; 1985.

Like "Butterworths", fails to italicize taxonomic names used as entry terms that are names properly italicized in taxonomic conventions. Generic drug names are, however, lowercased as entry terms to distinguish them from brand names.

Illustrated Stedman's Medical Dictionary. 24th ed. Baltimore: Williams & Wilkins; 1982.

A standard dictionary in the same class as "Butterworths" and "Dorlands".

International Dictionary of Medicine and Biology. SI Landau, ed. New York: John Wiley; 1986.

A new 3-volume dictionary that owes its great length mainly to long definitions for anatomic terms and its coverage of biology. Unlike "Butterworths", "Dorland's", and "Stedman's", it does follow the conventions for italicization of taxonomic terms when they are entry terms. Generous coverage of taxonomic names in biology usually not given in medical dictionaries. Useful notes on older synonyms for many presently preferred terms. If the editorial office of a medical journal can afford only one scientific dictionary, this is the one it should have despite its price.

SCIENTIFIC DICTIONARIES

McGraw-Hill Concise Encyclopedia of Science and Technology. SP Parker, ed. New York: McGraw-Hill; 1984.

The Oxford Dictionary of Natural History. M Allaby, ed. New York: Oxford University Press; 1986.

Two comprehensive sources in which to verify spelling and usage for many scientific terms, including taxonomic terms, in fields such as botany, geology, and zoology not covered in detail in some style manuals.

USAGE AND PROSE STYLE

A Dictionary of Modern English Usage. 2nd ed. HW Fowler. New York: Oxford University Press; 1965.

The classic commentary on innumerable details of prose style in formal English. Some modern authors might consider some of Fowler's views to be antique, but Fowler always rationalized his views thoroughly and with care.

Guidelines for Bias-Free Publishing. New York: McGraw-Hill; [undated]. 38 p.

The Handbook of Nonsexist Writing: For Writers, Editors and Speakers. C Miller, K Swift. New York: Barnes & Noble; 1981.

Two thorough discussions of issues and styles with reference to sex discrimination and other biases.

American Usage and Style: The Consensus. RH Copperud. New York: Van Nostrand Reinhold; 1980.

Harper Dictionary of Contemporary Usage. W Morris, M Morris. New York: Harper & Row; 1975.

A number of commentaries on American usage are available; these may be the best, for their scope and clarity. Copperud's is notably attractive for his drawing in the views of other authorities.

The King's English. 3rd ed. HW Fowler, FG Fowler. Oxford: Oxford University Press; 1931.

The other "Fowler". A systematic discussion of vocabulary, syntax, "Airs and Graces" (rhetorical devices, good and bad), punctuation, and other details of prose style in English.

The Oxford Guide to English Usage. ESC Weiner. Oxford: Oxford University Press; 1983.

A handbook on word formation, pronunciation, vocabulary, and grammar. Useful as a supplement to an abridged general dictionary. Has a British orientation but pays ample attention to American usage.

Style: Ten Lessons in Clarity & Grace. 2nd ed. JM Williams. Glenview, Illinois: Scott Foresman; 1985.

A textbook but useful for its reasoned analyses of defects in prose style.

The Words Between: A Handbook for Scientists Needing English, with Examples Mainly from Biology and Medicine. 2nd ed. JM Perttunen. Helsinki: Kustannus oy Duodecim; 1986.

A thorough analysis of the traps in English prose style for authors reared in another language.

UNITS OF MEASUREMENT

The SI for the Health Professions. Geneva: World Health Organization; 1977.

SI Units in Medicine: An Introduction to the International System of Units with Conversion Tables and Normal Ranges. H Lippert, HP Lehmann. Baltimore: Urban & Schwarzenberg; 1978.

Extensive discussions of SI units and their use and style. Would be useful supplements to the basic document represented by Appendix A of this manual.

Units of Measurement: An Encyclopaedic Dictionary of Units Both Scientific and Popular and the Quantities They Measure. S Dresner. New York: Hastings House; 1972.

An excellent source on antique, exotic, and otherwise obscure units of measurement: symbols, definitions, equivalents, historical notes, and other details.

REFERENCES ON DRUGS AND CHEMICALS

Handbook of Nonprescription Drugs. 8th ed. Washington: American Pharmaceutical Association: 1986.

Despite its title, this compendium also covers products not accurately covered by the term *drugs*, such as skin lotions, depilatories, hard-lens products, needles, condoms. Its tables provide brand names, identify manufacturers, and specify active and inert ingredients by generic names.

Martindale: The Extra Pharmacopoeia. 28th ed. JEF Reynolds. London: Pharmaceutical Press; 1982.

An excellent reference work in which to verify the generic names official for many drugs in many countries.

The Merck Index: An Encyclopedia of Chemicals, Drugs, and Biologicals. 10th ed. M Windholz, ed. Rahway, New Jersey: Merck; 1983.

The best single reference work in which to verify the spelling and style for the names of a great number of chemicals and drugs.

Pharmacological and Chemical Synonyms. 7th ed. EEJ Marler. Amsterdam: Excerpta Medica; 1983.

A comprehensive international list of generic and brand names, with systematic chemical names.

USAN and the USP Dictionary of Drug Names. MC Griffiths, ed. Rockville, Maryland: United States Pharmacopeial Convention. Published annually.

The standard American reference work on official drug names and the chemical-name equivalents. Its annual revision makes it more useful for American journals than "Martindale" and the book by Marley.

NOMENCLATURE AND TAXONOMY

Synopsis and Classification of Living Organisms. SP Parker, ed. New York: McGraw-Hill; 1982.

A Synoptic Classification of Living Organisms. RSK Barnes, ed. Oxford: Blackwell; 1984. Available in the United States from Sinauer, Sunderland, Massachusetts.

Useful supplements to the medical dictionaries for taxonomic names.

OTHER REFERENCE WORKS

The Oxford Companion to Medicine. J Walton, PB Beeson, R Bodley Scott. Oxford: Oxford University Press; 1986.

A 2-volume mini-encyclopedia on historical and modern medicine. Although it has been prepared as a reference work for a wide audience, it can serve well as a compact source in which to check on details in the history and biography of medicine. It includes lengthy appendixes giving abbreviations for medical degrees and honors (qualifications) and other medical abbreviations, including those for organizations.

GUIDES TO INFORMATION SOURCES

Guide to Information Sources in the Botanical Sciences. E Davis. Littleton, Colorado: Libraries Unlimited; 1987.

Guide to the Literature of Pharmacy and the Pharmaceutical Sciences. T Andrews. Littleton, Colorado: Libraries Unlimited; 1986. 383 p.

Information Sources in the Medical Sciences. 3rd ed. LT Morton, S Godbolt, eds. London: Butterworths; 1984.

Introduction to Reference Sources in the Health Sciences. 2nd ed. FW Roper, JA Boorkman. Chicago: Medical Library Association; 1984.

These guides to reference works, databases, textbooks, government documents are valuable for editors wishing to build an adequate reference library for their editorial offices.

Index